Cardio-Obstetrics

The past: To my mother who instilled the pursuit of excellence in me and for her love and guidance.

The present: To all mothers with heart disease who embarked upon their journey to motherhood.

The future: To my husband and our triplet daughters who aspire to make this world a better place.

—ABH

Dedicated to my parents who nourished and enriched me,

to all women with heart disease who endured childbirth and to those who wish for motherhood,

and finally to my husband and daughter who enlighten me daily.

—DSW

Cardio-Obstetrics

A Practical Guide to Care
for Pregnant Cardiac Patients

Edited by

Afshan B. Hameed, MD, FACC, FACOG
Professor of Maternal-Fetal Medicine and Cardiology
University of California, Irvine

Diana S. Wolfe, MD, MPH, FACOG
Associate Professor of Maternal-Fetal Medicine
Einstein/Montefiore Medical Center, New York

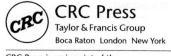

CRC Press
Taylor & Francis Group
Boca Raton London New York

CRC Press is an imprint of the
Taylor & Francis Group, an **informa** business

First edition published [2020]
by CRC Press
6000 Broken Sound Parkway NW, Suite 300, Boca Raton, FL 33487-2742

and by CRC Press
2 Park Square, Milton Park, Abingdon, Oxon, OX14 4RN

© 2020 Taylor & Francis Group, LLC

CRC Press is an imprint of Taylor & Francis Group, LLC

Library of Congress Cataloging-in-Publication Data

Names: Hameed, Afshan B., editor. | Wolfe, Diana, editor.
Title: Cardio-obstetrics : a practical guide to care for pregnant cardiac patients / edited by Afshan B. Hameed, Diana Wolfe.
Description: First edition. | Boca Raton : CRC Press, 2020. | Includes bibliographical references and index. |
Identifiers: LCCN 2020000259 (print) | LCCN 2020000260 (ebook) | ISBN 9781138317918 (paperback) | ISBN 9781138317963 (hardback) | ISBN 9780429454912 (ebook)
Subjects: MESH: Pregnancy Complications, Cardiovascular--diagnosis | Pregnancy Complications, Cardiovascular--therapy | Heart Diseases | Pregnancy, High Risk
Classification: LCC RG580.H4 (print) | LCC RG580.H4 (ebook) | NLM WQ 244 | DDC 618.3/61--dc23
LC record available at https://lccn.loc.gov/2020000259
LC ebook record available at https://lccn.loc.gov/2020000260

ISBN: 978-1-138-31796-3 (hbk)
ISBN: 978-1-138-31791-8 (pbk)
ISBN: 978-0-429-45491-2 (ebk)

Contents

Contributors

Katherine W. Arendt
Department of Anesthesiology and Perioperative
   Medicine
Mayo Clinic
Rochester, Minnesota

Dana Senderoff Berger
Department of Obstetrics & Gynecology
University of California, Irvine
Irvine, California

Anna E. Bortnick
Department of Medicine
Division of Cardiology
Einstein/Montefiore Medical Center
Bronx, New York

Thomas Boucher
Department of Medicine
Division of Cardiology
Einstein/Montefiore Medical Center
Bronx, New York

Joan Briller
Department of Medicine
Division of Cardiology
The University of Illinois
Chicago, Illinois

Mary M. Canobbio
Department of Nursing
Division of Pediatric Cardiology
University of California, Los Angeles
Los Angeles, California

Alice Chan
Department of Nursing
Icahn School of Medicine at Mount Sinai
New York, New York

Judith H. Chung
Department of Obstetrics & Gynecology
Division of Maternal Fetal Medicine
University of California, Irvine
Irvine, California

Melinda B. Davis
Department of Medicine
Division of Cardiovascular Medicine
University of Michigan
Ann Arbor, Michigan

Uri Elkayam
Department of Medicine
Division of Cardiology
Keck School of Medicine of the University of Southern California
Los Angeles, California

Nisha Garg
Department of Obstetrics and Gynecology
University of California, Irvine
Irvine, California

Dena Goffman
Department of Obstetrics and Gynecology
Division of Maternal Fetal Medicine
Columbia University Irving Medical Center
New York, New York

Tanush Gupta
Department of Medicine
Division of Cardiology
Einstein/Montefiore Medical Center
Bronx, New York

Afshan B. Hameed
Department of Obstetrics & Gynecology
Division of Maternal Fetal Medicine
University of California, Irvine
Irvine, California

Jennifer Haythe
Department of Medicine
Division of Cardiology
Columbia University Irving Medical Center
New York, New York

Ann K. Lal
Department of Obstetrics & Gynecology
Division of Maternal Fetal Medicine
Loyola University Medical Center
Maywood, Illinois

Jeannette P. Lin
Department of Medicine
Division of Cardiology
University of California, Los Angeles
Los Angeles, California

Kathryn Lindley
Department of Medicine
Division of Cardiology
Washington University School of Medicine in St Louis
St Louis, Missouri

Elliott Main
Department of Obstetrics & Gynecology
Stanford University
Palo Alto, California

Stephanie Martin
Clinical Concepts in Obstetrics
Maternal Fetal Medicine
Colorado Springs, Colorado

Ather Mehboob
Department of Medicine
Division of Hematology and Oncology
Adventist Health AIS Cancer Center
Bakersfield, California

Marie-Louise Meng
Department of Anesthesiology
Columbia University Irving Medical Center
New York, New York

Gassan Moady
Department of Medicine
Division of Cardiology
Keck School of Medicine of the University of Southern
    California
Los Angeles, California

Rachel A. Newman
Department of Obstetrics & Gynecology
University of California, Irvine
Irvine, California

Lee Brian Padove
Department of Medicine
Division of Cardiology
Atlanta, Georgia

Melissa Perez
Department of Obstetrics & Gynecology
University of California, Irvine
Irvine, California

Rachel Perry
Department of Obstetrics & Gynecology
University of California, Irvine
Irvine, California

Lauren A. Plante
Department of Obstetrics and Gynecology
Division of Maternal Fetal Medicine
Drexel University College of Medicine
Philadelphia, Pennsylvania

Pavan Reddy
Department of Medicine
Division of Cardiology
Keck School of Medicine of the University of Southern California
Los Angeles, California

Jessica Spiegelman
Department of Obstetrics and Gynecology
Division of Maternal Fetal Medicine
Columbia University Irving Medical Center
New York, New York

Edlira Tam
Department of Medicine
Division of Cardiology
Einstein/Montefiore Medical Center
Bronx, New York

Cynthia Taub
Department of Medicine
Division of Cardiology
Einstein/Montefiore Medical Center
Bronx, New York

Arthur J. Vaught
Department of Obstetrics and Gynecology
Division of Maternal Fetal Medicine
Johns Hopkins University Medical Center
Baltimore, Maryland

Thaddeus P. Waters
Department of Obstetrics and Gynecology
Division of Maternal Fetal Medicine
Loyola University Medical Center
Maywood, Illinois

Diana S. Wolfe
Department of Obstetrics & Gynecology and Women's Health
Division of Maternal Fetal Medicine
Einstein/Montefiore Medical Center
Bronx, New York

Ali N. Zaidi
Department of Medicine & Pediatrics
Division of Adult Congenital Heart Disease
Icahn School of Medicine at Mount Sinai
New York, New York

Blake Zwerling
Department of Obstetrics & Gynecology
University of California, Irvine
Irvine, California

1

Burden of Cardiovascular Disease

Diana S. Wolfe, Afshan B. Hameed, and Elliott Main

KEY POINTS

- The United States is one of eight countries in the world with a rising maternal mortality rate [1]
- Cardiovascular disease is the leading cause of indirect maternal deaths in the United States [2]
- Qualitative maternal mortality reviews are essential in addition to vital statistics to comprehend maternal mortality [3]

- Implementation of toolkits, quality improvement projects, and safety bundles have been proven to decrease maternal mortality rates in California [4]
- Perinatal quality collaboratives essentially bring stakeholders together to a common goal of improving maternal morbidity and mortality [5]

Introduction

There has been a global effort to establish reliable statistics on maternal mortality. This has been a challenge due to differences in reporting systems; however, the World Health Organization (WHO), United Nations International Children's Emergency Fund (UNICEF), United Nations Fund for Population Activities (UNFPA), World Bank Group, and the United National Population Division recently published an executive summary on mortality statistics between 1990–2015 [17]. Their goal was in part to establish accurate and internationally comparable measures of maternal mortality to help accomplish the United Nations new millennium goal to decrease maternal mortality by 2015. Their refined measuring system allowed for comparability and a measure of uncertainty around the country-specific estimates. Globally, the maternal mortality ratio has fallen by 44%; however, the burden remains high especially for low-resource countries which accounted for 99% of global maternal deaths in 2015. Region-specific distributions are displayed in Figure 1.1 [15]. Sub-Saharan Africa accounts for the majority load of maternal deaths at 66%.

A WHO systematic study on etiology of maternal mortality worldwide analyzed and combined data from the years 2003–2009 [1,6]; a total of 73% of cases were due to direct obstetric causes of death, including hemorrhage 27%, hypertensive disorders 14%, embolism 2%, sepsis 10%, abortion 9%, and other direct causes 24%, leaving approximately 27% accounted for indirect obstetric causes. Internationally, HIV/AIDS accounts for only a small proportion (1.6%) of maternal deaths.

Maternal mortality in the United States has gained recent attention because of the surprising increase in its rate, contrary to all other high-resource countries. Approximately 700 women die each year in the United States due to pregnancy or related complications [7]. There are also stark racial and ethnic disparities with black and Native American women having rates two to four times those of white or Asian women [8,2] (Figure 1.2). This disparity in maternal mortality is the largest disparity noted for any public health metric and has led to the mobilization of multiple organizations for important local and national efforts. Maternal mortality data is produced by two branches of the Centers for Disease Control and Prevention (CDC) [9]. The National Center for Health Statistics (NCHS) produces data to calculate the WHO definition of maternal mortality (death during or within 42 days after the termination of a pregnancy from a cause related to the pregnancy or its treatment). This determination is made by review of International Classification of Disease (ICD) codes from the death certificate alone. Death certificate causes of death are publicly available from the CDC, but there is serious concern over the quality of the data and the limitations of the 42-day boundary. For these reasons, NCHS has not released an official U.S. maternal mortality rate since 2007.

The Reproductive Health branch of the CDC established the Pregnancy Mortality Surveillance System (PMSS) in collaboration with the American College of Obstetricians and Gynecologists in 1986 to understand the causes of death and risk factors and thus provide a more comprehensive review of maternal deaths. Starting with all deaths from any cause during or within 12 months of a birth/loss (cohort of pregnancy-associated mortalities), case reviews of all data on the death certificate and more recently on linked birth certificates, is used to establish whether the death was causally related to the pregnancy or its care (pregnancy-related mortalities) [10,11]. (See Box 1.1.)

The most recent report on U.S. pregnancy-associated mortality rates, covering the years 2007–2016, identifies 16.7 deaths per

1

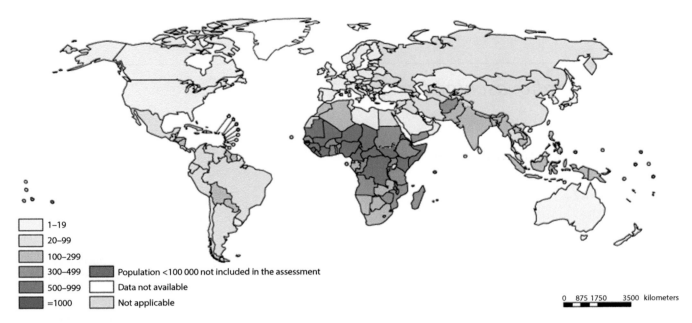

FIGURE 1.1 Worldwide map of rates of maternal mortality per 100 000 live births. (From WHO, UNICEF, UNFPA, World Bank Group, and the United Nations Population Division. *Trends in Maternal Mortality: 1990 to 2015.* Geneva: WHO; 2015. With permission.)

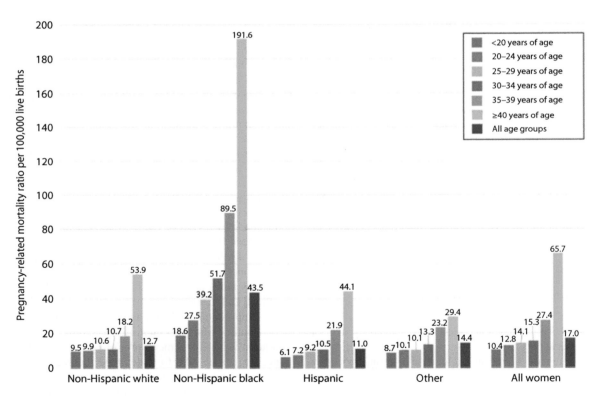

FIGURE 1.2 U.S. maternal mortality ratios by age, race-ethnicity, and overall for 2011–2013. (From Creanga AA et al. *Obstet Gynecol.* 2015;125(1):5–12. With permission.)

100,000 live births [7,8]. The top causes include cardiovascular diseases (26.5%) ranking first, combining cardiovascular conditions (15.5%) and cardiomyopathy (11.0%) (Figure 1.3). These were followed by other medical conditions reflecting preexisting illnesses (14.5%), infection (12.7%), hemorrhage (11.4%), and cardiomyopathy (11.0%) [7]. Relative to data covering the period 2006–2010, the contribution of hemorrhage, hypertensive disorders of pregnancy, and anesthesia complications have all declined. In contrast, cardiovascular and other medical conditions have significantly increased (Figure 1.3).

Pregnancy Mortality Reviews

The current focus is to reestablish state-based maternal mortality review committees (MMRCs) in all 50 U.S. states. New York City and Washington, DC have their own independent MMRC and are included. The aim is to review all maternal deaths in the country for causation, preventability, and improvement opportunities. Currently, MMRCs have been established in about two-thirds of states [3]. They consist of multidisciplinary committees to identify, review, and analyze maternal deaths using all available data sources (e.g., medical records, autopsy reports, and community information) rather than death certificates alone.

Impact on Women of Reproductive Age

Global indirect causes of maternal mortality that are of concern and focus include cardiovascular, respiratory, diabetes, and cancer. This burden of disease has identified an important challenge for health care providers to resolve. That is, to coordinate care among specialists to optimize outcomes for most cases. At the national level in the United States, studies have shown a rise in pregnant women with chronic diseases as well, including hypertension, diabetes, and chronic heart disease. A call to action from the professional community is in place to determine the underlying characteristics of U.S. women who die during childbirth. Black race, age over 35, and no prenatal care have been identified as major associated characteristics with maternal death in the United States [9].

MMRC compared to national vital statistics allows for investigation and ultimately action to prevent maternal mortality. The ability to turn reviews into action has focused on the development of state perinatal quality collaboratives, which represent state-level partnerships among public health agencies, professional organizations, hospital associations, and patient advocates. The National Partnership for Maternal Safety, established in 2014, has taken quality improvement lessons from MMRCs and developed national safety bundles for the most preventable causes of maternal mortality, including hemorrhage, hypertension, and venous thromboembolism. The California Maternal Quality Care Collaborative (see www.CMQCC.org) has led the nation for widespread adoption of safety bundles (see Box 1.2) and publication of key implementation toolkits. California has subsequently noted a major decline in their maternal mortality rates from 16.9 deaths per 100,000 live births in 2006 to 7.3 deaths per 100,000 live births in 2013 [4]. These publications were followed by the initiation of the cardiovascular disease in pregnancy toolkit, also initiated by CMQCC. (see also California Maternal Quality Care Collaborative, State of California, Department of Public Health, California Birth and Death Statistical Master Files, 1999–2013; www.cmqcc.org). Details of the cardiovascular disease toolkit are discussed in Chapter 6.

While many states have adopted perinatal quality collaboratives (PQCs), there are potential challenges involved when

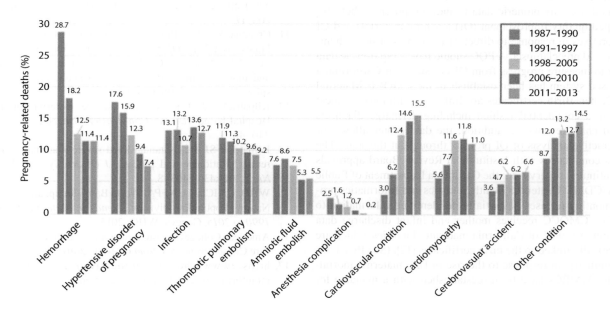

FIGURE 1.3   Causes of U.S. maternal mortality for five time periods. (From Creanga AA et al. *Obstet Gynecol.* 2015;125(1):5–12. With permission.)

**BOX 1.2 BASIC STEPS TO IMPLEMENT
A SAFETY BUNDLE: AN EXAMPLE**

**COUNSEL ON PATIENT SAFETY
IN WOMEN'S HEALTH CARE**

The team approach: Technical leader, clinical expertise, day-to-day leadership, project sponsor

Goal setting: What, who, by how much, by when will we improve it?

SMART (specific, measurable, attainable, relevant, time-bound) goals

Driver diagram

PDSA (plan, do, study, act) cycle

Measures

Models for change

Building sustainability and encouraging spread

**BOX 1.3 BASIC STEPS TO SUSTAIN QI
INITIATIVES AT YOUR HOSPITAL [16]**

Public health burden/population impact of issue

Clinician enthusiasm/existence of champions

Availability of funding

Alignment with state and national priorities

Established benchmarks for best practices

Evidence-based/evidence-supported interventions available

Documented variation in outcomes

Prior successes elsewhere

Feasibility: Implementation and measurement

multiple organizations and disciplines work together [5]. In California, the state Maternal Mortality Review Committee facilitated not only numeric data to indicate progress, but also developed quality improvement (QI) teaching materials and QI collaboratives in response to direct cases such as obstetric hemorrhage and preeclampsia. A PQC should have a rapid-cycle data system to measure progress from QI measures. In California, a web-based system has been established, the CMQCC Maternal Data Center. Birth certificates are linked to additional medical charts in a confidential fashion including discharge diagnosis file and chart reviews. In addition, the data center allows for an interactive analysis of QI projects throughout the state. The process commences with Institutional Review Board approvals and continuing supervision; the California Department of Public Health (CDPH) Center for Health Statistics and Informatics provides monthly releases of partially de-identified information to CMQCC. CMQCC receives mother and infant discharge data files from over 96% of California maternity facilities, which are automatically linked to the birth certificates [12]. (See Box 1.3.)

In summary, in response to the rise in U.S. maternal mortality state, MMRCs have been reestablished with a mandate for translating their findings into action using state perinatal quality collaboratives. While this model is still early in its development in many states, established states including California, Illinois, Michigan, and North Carolina are showing encouraging results.

REFERENCES

1. Say L et al. Global causes of maternal death: A WHO systematic analysis. *Lancet Glob Health.* 2014;2(6):e323–33.
2. Creanga AA et al. Pregnancy-related mortality in the United States, 2006-2010. *Obstet Gynecol.* 2015;125(1):5–12.
3. Creanga AA. Maternal mortality in the United States: A review of contemporary data and their limitations. *Clin Obstet Gynecol.* 2018;61(2):296–306.
4. Main EK. Reducing maternal mortality and severe maternal morbidity through state-based quality improvement initiatives. *Clin Obstet Gynecol.* 2018;61(2):319–31.
5. Henderson ZT et al. The National Network of State Perinatal Quality Collaboratives: A growing movement to improve maternal and infant health. *J Womens Health (Larchmt).* 2018; 27(3):221–26.
6. Waiswa P et al. Status of birth and pregnancy outcome capture in health demographic surveillance sites in 13 countries. *Int J Public Health.* 2019;64(6):909–20.
7. Petersen EE et al. Vital signs: Pregnancy-Related Deaths, United States, 2011–2015, and Strategies for Prevention, 13 States, 2013–2017. *MMWR Morb Mortal Wkly Rep.* 2019; 68(18):423–29.
8. Petersen EE et al. Racial/ethnic disparities in pregnancy-related deaths—United States, 2007-2016. *MMWR Morb Mortal Wkly Rep.* 2019;68(35):762–65.
9. MacDorman MF, Declercq E, Thoma ME. Trends in maternal mortality by sociodemographic characteristics and cause of death in 27 states and the District of Columbia. *Obstet Gynecol.* 2017;129(5):811–18.
10. Creanga AA. Maternal mortality in the developed world: A review of surveillance methods, levels and causes of maternal deaths during 2006-2010. *Minerva Ginecol.* 2017;69(6): 608–17.
11. Creanga AA et al. Pregnancy-related mortality in the United States, 2011-2013. *Obstet Gynecol.* 2017;130(2):366–73.
12. Main EK, Markow C, Gould J. Addressing maternal mortality and morbidity in California through public-private partnerships. *Health Aff.* 2018;37(9):1484–93.
13. Kilpatrick SJ. Understanding severe maternal morbidity: Hospital-based review. *Clin Obstet Gynecol.* 2018. 61(2): 340–46.
14. Kilpatrick SJ et al. Standardized severe maternal morbidity review: Rationale and process. *J Obstet Gynecol Neonatal Nurs.* 2014;43(4):403–8.
15. WHO, UNICEF, UNFPA, World Bank Group, and the United Nations Population Division. *Trends in Maternal Mortality: 1990 to 2015.* Geneva: WHO; 2015.
16. American College of Obstetricians and Gynecologists. Obstetric care Consensus no. 5. *Obstet Gynecol.* 2016;128:e54–e60.
17. https://www.who.int/reproductivehealth/publications/monitoring/maternal-mortality-2015/en/

2

The Cardio-Obstetric Team

Diana S. Wolfe

KEY POINTS

- Care of a pregnant woman with cardiac disease requires collaboration between various disciplines
- The multidisciplinary team bridges the gap in communication, promoting appropriate care of the pregnant cardiac patient
- Academic, administrative, and logistic support is needed to create a cardio-obstetric team at a given institution

- A "Triad" solution to improve maternal mortality due to cardiovascular disease includes patient education, universal cardiovascular disease screening, and a multidisciplinary team approach
- Advocacy for establishing a cardio-obstetric team should continue at local and national levels

Introduction

The concept of team effort to care for a patient is not novel, especially when there is a high risk of morbidity and mortality. The goal is to bring together skill sets from maternal-fetal medicine (MFM), cardiology, anesthesia, neonatology, and other subspecialties as needed to optimize patient care. Cardiovascular disease in pregnancy is the number one indirect obstetric cause of pregnancy-related mortality ratio in the United States [1]. The 2006–2010 pregnancy-related mortality ratio was 16.0 deaths per 100,000 live births, a total of 14.6% due to cardiovascular conditions and 11.8% due to cardiomyopathy [1]. Improved data collection of severe maternal morbidity and maternal near-miss (SMM/MNM) has illustrated that cardiac disease is a significant contributing indicator in the United States [2]. The definition of SMM/MNM has evolved from the initial WHO definition that attempted to establish a comparable description across facilities to encourage health quality improvement [13]. The 2011 SMM/MNM definition includes five disease-specific, four management, and seven organ dysfunction–based criteria including cardiovascular dysfunction. In the United States, the Centers for Disease Control and Prevention (CDC) uses a large all-payer hospital inpatient care database for SMM/MNM surveillance. These indicators are based on three guiding principles [3]:

1. State-level availability of data in most states, territories, and large metropolitan areas
2. Presence of an established evidence base in the literature
3. Quality of the indicator was sufficient for population level surveillance and the planning and evaluation of public health interventions

A validation study of the CDC SMM/MNM index was applied to 67,468 deliveries across 16 California hospitals and found a sensitivity of 0.99 and a positive predictive value of 0.44 [4]. The American College of Obstetricians and Gynecologists (ACOG) and the Alliance for Innovation on Maternal Health updated the 2009 set of 25 CDC SMM/MNM indicators [3]. Based on the revised 21 indicator index, rates for the majority of SMM/MNM indicators increased in the United States between 1993–2014 [4]. Acute myocardial infarction was among those indicators that increased. This information implies the need for public health surveillance and clinical audit to ultimately improve quality obstetric care. A team of experts is required to care for complex obstetric patients including the cardiac pregnant patient.

Multidisciplinary Team

The *cardio-obstetric team* comprises a multidisciplinary team of the patient, physicians, nurses, and administration that includes the following team members at the minimum: MFM, cardiology, anesthesia, neonatology, labor and delivery (L&D), and critical care staff. The approach mirrors the "heart team" model, traditionally known as a team of cardiologists and cardiothoracic surgeons who manage most at-risk cardiac surgical patients [5]. The pregnancy heart team is now employed internationally, and outlined in the most recent European Society of Cardiology Guidelines [6]. The mobilization of this framework came from the devastating findings of the U.S. maternal mortality rate in recent years whereby cardiac disease is the number one contributor in the United States [1]. Due to the complexity of the cardiac pregnant patient, an exchange of expertise and knowledge among experts including MFM and cardiology is strongly advisable to optimize maternal and fetal outcomes.

Our Experience

At Einstein/Montefiore in the Bronx, New York, we created an MFM–Cardiology outpatient joint program in February 2015 in response to the rising contribution of cardiovascular conditions to pregnancy-related morbidity and mortality [1]. The aim was to establish a multidisciplinary program to optimize the care of high-risk pregnant patients with known or suspected cardiac disease. In these instances, there is a real potential for communication barriers or gaps in care when specialists individually see patients at different times, locations, and/or health systems.

To create a cardio-obstetric team, an institution needs administrative and academic support from both departments, i.e., obstetrics and gynecology and cardiology. The office space where patients are seen is a key component because it has to be designed to accommodate both maternal and fetal testing. The logistics including billing are often a challenge because each specialty and its staff are most accustomed to their own needs for detailed physical exam and testing. However, a collaborative environment can be established with administrative support from both specialties. Trainee participation is key to modeling this multidisciplinary work and therefore academic support to build this into fellows' required rotations is recommended. In addition to the outpatient setting described, an inpatient team is essential for management of the pregnant cardiac patient.

At Einstein/Montefiore we have established an outpatient cardio-obstetric team that is composed of both MFM and cardiology attendings and fellows who see patients together in the same space at least 3 times per month. The cardiologists include subspecialists in interventional cardiology, noninvasive imaging, and congenital heart disease. The space where we see our patients has multiple expert areas within cardiology including pulmonary hypertension, heart failure, electrophysiology, and so on. Our office is able to provide a risk assessment through both maternal and fetal assessment. We have cardiac testing readily available including echocardiogram, EKG, pacemaker interrogation, and other vascular studies including lower extremity Doppler studies. We utilize sonograms and Doppler tones to assess fetal well-being as well as fetal echocardiography study within the same space. Our examination rooms consist of a gynecology table with the appropriate lighting and examination tools to provide for our pregnant patients and also to serve our postpartum and preconception patients. In this environment, as a team, together we have the ability to establish risk assessment each trimester (Table 2.1) and commence delivery planning. For our postpartum

TABLE 2.1

Sample Pregnancy Follow-Up Checklist

| | Frequency of Follow-Up | | |
	Cardiologist	Laboratory	Diagnostic Testing
First trimester	☐ Once ☐ Every 4 weeks ☐ Every 2 weeks ☐ Every week	☐ BNP ☐ CBC ☐ TSH ☐ INR ☐ Other	☐ EKG ☐ Echocardiogram ☐ Holter monitor ☐ Exercise stress test ☐ Other
☐ Pregnancy termination			
Second trimester	☐ Once ☐ Every 4 weeks ☐ Every 2 weeks ☐ Every week	☐ BNP ☐ CBC ☐ TSH ☐ INR ☐ Other	☐ EKG ☐ Echocardiogram ☐ Holter monitor ☐ Exercise stress test ☐ Other
☐ Anesthesia consultation ☐ Multidisciplinary meeting ☐ Delivery planning ☐ Contraception plan			
Third trimester	☐ Once ☐ Every 4 weeks ☐ Every 2 weeks ☐ Every week	☐ BNP ☐ CBC ☐ TSH ☐ INR ☐ Other	☐ EKG ☐ Echocardiogram ☐ Holter monitor ☐ Other
☐ Contraception ☐ Medication review ☐ Follow-up plan with cardiology			
Postpartum	☐ 1 week ☐ 2 weeks ☐ 4 weeks	☐ BNP ☐ CBC ☐ TSH ☐ INR ☐ Other	☐ EKG ☐ Echocardiogram ☐ Holter monitor ☐ Other

Abbreviations: BNP, B-type natriuretic peptide; CBC, complete blood count; TSH, thyroid stimulating hormone; INR, international normalized ratio; EKG, electrocardiogram.

and preconception patients, reproductive life planning and birth control counseling is emphasized. The team demonstrates their collaboration to the patient, delivering the same message, clarifying any confusion while they are counseled in person by both MFM and cardiology. In addition to our outpatient team, we have an inpatient cardio-obstetric team where the delivery plans are finalized. We meet monthly in the cardiac intensive care conference room. All members of the team are represented to review the major concerns and exchange an understanding of both cardiac and obstetric risks (Figure 2.1). We use a template (see Figure 2.2) to present the case and a review checklist as a reminder of all aspects of the intrapartum and peripartum time period.

The checklist begins with a description of the pathophysiology of the patient and a review of their cardiac history including surgeries and any comorbidities. Step 2 is to review of all imaging studies. This will raise any major concerns and culminate an exchange of thoughts from MFM, cardiology, anesthesia, and L&D staff to think through the possible scenarios during labor and delivery. This leads to the next steps, which involve choosing timing and location of delivery. At Einstein/Montefiore, most of our patients deliver by 39 weeks at our larger location, where we have a cardiac intensive care unit (CICU) and therefore cardiology consult available 24/7. Very few patients require delivery outside of L&D, that is, main operating room or CICU. Your institution should assess the safest place for these patients and consider where and when all equipment and experts are readily available. We deliver our patients at 39 weeks or earlier due to need for a scheduled delivery where the most skilled experts, including nursing, for the specific cardiac pathology are available. The L&D nurse at our institution is not telemetry trained and therefore we often have two nurses monitoring our patient—obstetrics and CICU nursing. Equipment is readily available on L&D to manage indwelling pacemakers and implantable defibrillators, as an example. For the rare case that may require delivery outside of the L&D unit, cesarean delivery and neonatal trays are housed adjacent to or inside the patient's room for any unforeseen emergency. Cardiac medications and those on L&D for various indications are reviewed with the team to assess their

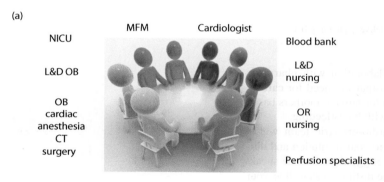

(a)

(b)

Team Member	Role
Maternal-fetal medicine	1. Present the patient 2. Present obstetric concerns 3. Determine safe management in labor and postpartum
Cardiologist	1. Present the cardiac pathophysiology 2. Review the cardiac studies with team 3. Determine safe management in labor and postpartum
Neonatology	Availability for receival of fetus at time of delivery
Blood bank	All blood products available
Labor and delivery OB staff	Availability to deliver patient
Labor and delivery OB Nursing	Coordinate 1:1 nursing at delivery and postpartum
Cardiac and obstetric Anesthesia	Tailor safe anesthesia plan, cardiac monitoring
OR nursing	Coordinate delivery and cardiac monitoring
Cardiothoracic surgery	Availability where risk of CT surgery warranted
Perfusion specialists	Availability where risk of heart failure elevated

FIGURE 2.1 Cardio-obstetric team: (a) Personnel; (b) roles.

Attendees: Services Represented				
☐ MFM	☐ Cardiology	☐ L&D Att	☐ L&D Director	☐ Patient Safety
☐ Anesthesia	☐ Pediatrics	☐ L&D Nursing	☐ Blood Bank	☐ Other _____

Patient Information

Name _____ MRN _____
Age _____ EDC _____ BMI _____ Parity _____
Health Care Proxy _____
Major Medical Co-Morbidities _____

Prior Cardiac Surgery _____
Prior Cardiac Disease _____
Birth Control Recommendation _____
Birth Control Plan _____
Desire future fertility?   ☐ Yes   ☐ No
BTL papers signed?   ☐ Yes   ☐ No

Cardiac Studies

Structural heart disease?   ☐ Yes   ☐ No
Arrhythmia?   ☐ Yes   ☐ No
Maternal Echocardiogram: _____
_____
_____
Holter: _____

Fetal Echo: _____

Date and Time of IOL or CD: (check one)   Place of Delivery:
   ☐ Date _____   ☐ Time _____   ☐ Weiler   ☐ Wakefield

Intrapartum Plan:	☐ Yes	☐ No	*If Yes:* Pulse Oximetry Other _____
CCU	☐ Yes	☐ No	If Yes ☐ Telemetry ☐ Cardiac
Lines	☐ Yes	☐ No	If Yes ☐ CVP ☐ A-line ☐ Other ___
Fluid Monitoring	☐ Yes	☐ No	If Yes ☐ Strict I/O ☐ Other ___

Postpartum Plan:	☐ Yes	☐ No	*If Yes:* Pulse Oximetry Other _____
CCU	☐ Yes	☐ No	If Yes ☐ Telemetry ☐ Cardiac
Lines	☐ Yes	☐ No	If Yes ☐ CVP ☐ A-line ☐ Other ___
Fluid Monitoring	☐ Yes	☐ No	If Yes ☐ Strict I/O ☐ Other ___

Summary of Delivery Plan

Overall Risk of Mortality: ☐ High   ☐ Moderate   ☐ Low
Mode of Delivery: ☐ Safe to Labor   ☐ Cesarean   ☐ Assisted Second Stage
Special Situation: Preeclampsia _____
                              Hemorrhage _____
                              Medication to Avoid _____
Anesthesia: ☐ Regional   ☐ General   ☐ Other _____

EMERGENCY PLAN

Back-Up
   ☐ Cardiologist _____
   ☐ Critical Care _____
   ☐ Anesthesia _____
   ☐ Other _____

Disclaimer: The above is intended to serve as guidelines and not intended to be a standard of care. Care should be based on the judgment of the physician based on the individual patient's condition.

FIGURE 2.2   Multidisciplinary labor and delivery planning list.

maternal and neonatal safety in collaboration with pharmacy specialists and the neonatal team. Postpartum need for cardiac medications should be individualized for nursing mothers based on the indications and compatibility with breastfeeding.

I recommend advocating for a cardio-obstetric team within your community to increase referrals to your institution and ultimately to establish safe motherhood. Suggestions include speaking at Grand Rounds within your home institution as well as your city and region. Creation of continuing medical education courses within your community can attract the attention of providers and lead to positive collaborations. An emphasis on patient education and why screening for cardiovascular disease should be universal for all pregnant and postpartum patients is beneficial. Patient education should include a review of the normal physiological changes and symptoms that occur in pregnancy, including its impact on the heart. Patients with cardiac disease need to be advised about warning signs that should prompt them to seek medical attention, because benign symptoms of pregnancy may mimic worsening cardiac disease. In addition, patients need to be counseled that a cesarean delivery is not an absolute requirement for all patients with cardiac disease, and that a normal spontaneous vaginal delivery and breastfeeding postpartum are optimal [7].

The Triad

A triad solution (Figure 2.3) including patient education, cardiovascular screening, and the multidisciplinary team has been proposed to address maternal mortality and morbidity associated with cardiovascular disease of pregnancy [7]. Preconception counseling for all women with known heart disease is recommended. Review of their reproductive goals and an understanding of their disease and potential physiologic cardiac changes in a future pregnancy is recommended [8,9]. A contraceptive plan is essential to optimize

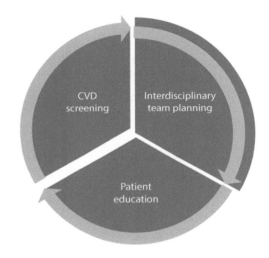

FIGURE 2.3   Triad algorithm: Patient education, screening, maternal cardiology team.

pregnancy planning and birth spacing [10]. This counseling can be done in a multidisciplinary setting whereby a cardiologist and MFM subspecialist can assess the patient's options together. The third aspect of the triad is a cardiovascular screening toolkit that has been proposed by the California Maternal Quality Care Collaborative based on a retrospective review of peripartum cardiomyopathy case deaths [11]. This screening tool is used to identify pregnant and postpartum patients at risk for cardiovascular disease who therefore need to be referred to the maternal cardiology team. It is well established that many symptoms of pregnancy overlap common symptoms of heart disease. The challenge of distinguishing between the two has been proposed in Table 6.1 of the Practice Bulletin on Pregnancy and Heart Disease, ACOG [12]; see Chapter 6 of this book.

Conclusion

High-risk cardiac patients contemplating pregnancy or who are currently pregnant should have expedited, streamlined evaluation by cardiology and MFM specialists. The team approach as supported by ACC/AHA guideline includes collaboration with cardiology, MFM/obstetricians, anesthesiologists, cardiothoracic surgery, and additional subspecialists as needed. The cardio-obstetric team (Figure 2.1) and the multidisciplinary planning list (Figure 2.2) provide key components needed to create a cardio-obstetric team and how to utilize available resources to achieve an appropriate level of care for the pregnant cardiac patient.

REFERENCES

1. Creanga AA et al. Pregnancy-related mortality in the United States, 2006–2010. *Obstet Gynecol.* 2015;125(1):5–12.
2. Kuklina EV, Goodman DA. Severe maternal or near miss morbidity: Implications for public health surveillance and clinical audit. *Clin Obstet Gynecol.* 2018;61(2):307–18.
3. Callaghan WM, Creanga AA, Kuklina EV. Severe maternal morbidity among delivery and postpartum hospitalizations in the United States. *Obstet Gynecol.* 2012;120(5):1029–36.
4. Main EK et al. Measuring severe maternal morbidity: Validation of potential measures. *Am J Obstet Gynecol.* 2016;214(5):643 e1–10.
5. European Society of Gynecology (ESG) et al. ESC guidelines on the management of cardiovascular diseases during pregnancy: The Task Force on the Management of Cardiovascular Diseases during Pregnancy of the European Society of Cardiology (ESC). *Eur Heart J.* 2011;32(24):3147–97.
6. Regitz-Zagrosek V et al. 2018 ESC Guidelines for the management of cardiovascular diseases during pregnancy. *Eur Heart J.* 2018;39(34):3165–241.
7. Wolfe DS et al. Addressing maternal mortality: The pregnant cardiac patient. *Am J Obstet Gynecol.* 2019;220(2):167 e1–8.
8. Ladouceur M et al. Educational needs of adolescents with congenital heart disease: Impact of a transition intervention programme. *Arch Cardiovasc Dis.* 2017;110(5):317–24.
9. Mittal P, Dandekar A, Hessler D. Use of a modified reproductive life plan to improve awareness of preconception health in women with chronic disease. *Perm J.* 2014;18(2):28–32.
10. Roos-Hesselink JW et al. Contraception and cardiovascular disease. *Eur Heart J.* 2015;36(27):1728–34, 1734a–b.
11. Hameed AB et al. Pregnancy-related cardiovascular deaths in California: Beyond peripartum cardiomyopathy. *Am J Obstet Gynecol.* 2015;213(3):379 e1–10.
12. ACOG Practice Bulletin No. 212: Pregnancy and Heart Disease. *Obstet Gynecol.* 2019;133(5):e320–56.
13. WHO, Department of Reproductive Health and Research. *Evaluating the Quality of Care for Severe Pregnancy Complications: The WHO Near-miss Approach for Maternal Health.* Geneva: WHO; 2011.

3

Cardiovascular Physiology of Pregnancy and Clinical Implications

Jessica Spiegelman, Marie-Louise Meng, Jennifer Haythe, and Dena Goffman

KEY POINTS

- Pregnancy can expose undiagnosed cardiac pathology, or it can cause cardiac pathology in otherwise healthy people
- Heart rate, blood volume, and cardiac output all increase, while systemic vascular resistance and blood pressure decrease
- Heart rate >100 beats per minute in pregnancy should be regarded as abnormal until proven otherwise

- Many of the symptoms of normal pregnancy are similar to the symptoms of cardiac disease
- A systematic approach is required to evaluate any pregnant or postpartum patient with suspected cardiovascular disease in order to differentiate physiologic change from a pathologic process

Introduction

Pregnancy is unique as the only non-pathologic state that causes dramatic alterations in physiology. The integral components of pregnancy physiology that promote fetal growth and development are cardiovascular adaptations [1]. The maternal heart undergoes significant structural and functional changes beginning soon after conception that evolve as the pregnancy progresses to serve the changing demands of the developing fetus and in anticipation of blood loss at delivery [2]. Disruptions in this physiologic system may lead to both maternal and fetal morbidity at all stages of pregnancy. In the intrapartum period, increased perfusion of the uterus, pain-related tachycardia, and fluid shifts lead to additional hemodynamic variation. Most of these cardiovascular adaptations of pregnancy return to baseline in the postpartum period; however, some may persist for up to 6 months after delivery, emphasizing the need for maternal care in the "fourth trimester."

Because many of the cardiovascular adaptations of pregnancy are marked departures from the nonpregnant physiology, pregnancy may unmask previously unrecognized cardiac disease such as rheumatic mitral stenosis that can lead to significant morbidity and mortality. Not surprisingly, cardiovascular disease remains the leading cause of maternal mortality in the United States [3]. Normal pregnancy symptoms may overlap with those of cardiovascular disease. An understanding of the maternal adaptations that may elicit or exacerbate cardiovascular disease is essential for any obstetric provider. Appropriate triage and follow-up is essential in women with cardiovascular disease during pregnancy and the postpartum period.

Cardiovascular Physiologic Adaptations

The hemodynamic parameters that adapt during pregnancy include heart rate (HR), systemic vascular resistance (SVR), blood volume, cardiac output (CO), and blood pressure (BP) (Box 3.1). Each parameter is reviewed and the interplay between them is demonstrated in Figure 3.1. *Most changes begin in the first trimester, peak in the late second or early third trimester, and then plateau for the remainder of pregnancy with a return to pre-pregnancy values during the postpartum period* [4].

Heart Rate

Maternal HR increases steadily throughout pregnancy and has been shown in some studies to be the first hemodynamic parameter to change after conception as early as 5 weeks of gestation [5,6]. Unlike most other hemodynamic parameters, which change at rapid rates until a plateau point in the second trimester, HR increases steadily throughout pregnancy [2]. Peak increase in HR is generally between 10–20 beats per minute (bpm), or 20%–25%, above pre-pregnancy values [7]. The upper limit of normal heart rate in pregnancy is generally no higher than 95 bpm, and therefore heart rates >100 bpm should be regarded as abnormal until proven otherwise [2]. Later in pregnancy, this increase in HR is the primary contributor to the rise in CO. Maternal position may cause variations in HR, with slightly lower rates noted in the left lateral position than in the supine position, most likely due to alterations in preload with position changes [8]. HR typically returns to pre-pregnancy values in the immediate postpartum period, that is, within 6 hours postpartum [9].

BOX 3.1 THE HEMODYNAMICS OF UNCOMPLICATED PREGNANCIES: ANTEPARTUM, INTRAPARTUM, AND POSTPARTUM CHANGES

	Heart Rate	Systemic Vascular Resistance	Plasma Volume	RBC Volume	Cardiac Output	Blood Pressure
1st trimester	Increase	Decrease	Increase	Increase	Sharp increase	Decrease
2nd trimester	Steady increase	Rapid decrease	Rapid increase	Steady increase	Slower increase	Continued decrease, nadir
3rd trimester	Steady increase	Slight increase after 32 weeks	Slower increase after 28 weeks	Steady increase	Plateau	Increase
Intrapartum	Continues to increase	No significant change	Decrease due to blood loss	Decrease due to blood loss	Increase	Increase
Postpartum	Return to pre-pregnancy within 6–48 hours	Return to pre-pregnancy values soon after delivery	Vaginal delivery: decrease over 10 days Cesarean delivery: no change	Vaginal delivery: decrease over 10 days Cesarean delivery: no change	Rapid decrease in first 2 weeks, slower decrease for up to 6 months	Return to pre-pregnancy, unknown time frame
Earliest change	5 weeks	5 weeks	6 weeks	8–10 weeks	Before 8 weeks	7 weeks
Peak/nadir above/ below pre-pregnancy values	+20%–25%	−30%	+45%	+20%–30% (with iron), +15%–20% (no iron)	+30%–50%	−5–10 mmHg (systolic); up to −15 mmHg (diastolic)
GA at peak/nadir	Intrapartum	32 weeks	32 weeks	Term	25–35 weeks	20–24 weeks

Systemic Vascular Resistance

The decrease in SVR occurs as early as 5 weeks of gestation and prior to full development of the placenta [4]. In the first trimester, SVR decreases by about 10%, primarily due to the vasodilatory effects of progesterone, estrogen, prostaglandins, and relaxin [10]. Increased nitric oxide production in pregnancy likely also plays a role in the decrease in SVR [11]. As the placenta develops, it further decreases the SVR by adding a high-flow, low-resistance component to the maternal circulation. Decreased SVR leads to a decrease in BP, more specifically diastolic BP, and a widening of pulse pressure [12].

Decreased SVR in the renal vasculature activates the renin-angiotensin-aldosterone (RAA) system. Increased angiotensin leads to salt and water retention at the level of the kidneys and thus to an increase in blood volume and maintenance of blood pressure

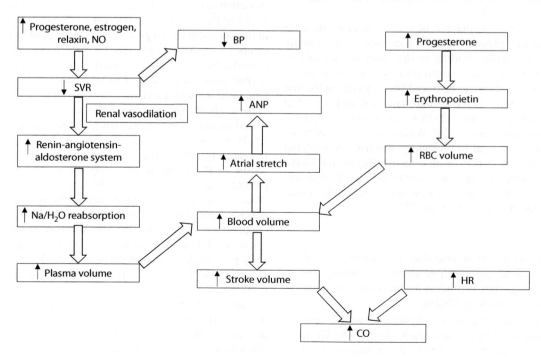

FIGURE 3.1 Relationship of parameters.

[13]. Decreased SVR is therefore at least partially responsible for an increase in blood volume and stroke volume. The combination of decreased SVR and increased HR leads to the increased cardiac output (Figure 3.1), with a larger contribution from HR in later pregnancy. SVR nadirs in the second trimester at about 30% lower than the baseline, and then plateaus until about 32 weeks, after which time it increases slightly [14]. At term, SVR remains up to 21% lower than pre-pregnancy values [15]. The pattern of SVR change during pregnancy is generally inverse to that of cardiac output, leading to a minimal change in the mean arterial pressure [14].

Blood Volume

Increased blood volume in pregnancy is evident from studies dating as far back as the 1930s [16]. Both plasma and red blood cell (RBC) expansion contribute to the total blood volume increase of pregnancy. Plasma volume expansion is primarily mediated by the upregulation of the RAA system, which begins as early as 6 weeks' gestation and continues to increase rapidly throughout pregnancy, with the steepest increase in the second trimester [17]. After 28 weeks, the rate of plasma volume increase slows; plasma volume reaches its peak at approximately 32 weeks' gestation [18]. To quantify plasma volume expansion in pregnancy, a 2017 meta-analysis of 30 studies found that plasma volume rose by 180 mL in the first trimester, by 570 mL in the second trimester, and by 1090 mL by 35 weeks. By 41 weeks' gestation, the total plasma volume expansion was 1130 mL above pre-pregnancy values [19].

RBC expansion is in part the result of a progesterone-driven increase in erythropoietin and helps support the increased oxygen demand of pregnancy [20,21]. RBC mass increases beginning at 8–10 weeks' gestation and steadily rises, reaching a 20%–30% increase by the end of pregnancy in women taking iron supplementation, or a 15%–20% increase in women not taking supplemental iron [22].

Although both plasma and red blood cell volume increase during pregnancy, plasma volume increases more rapidly than erythrocyte volume, leading to the dilutional anemia of pregnancy [23]. In one study, normal reference ranges for maternal hemoglobin were shown to be from 11.6–13.9 g/dL in the first trimester, 9.7–14.8 g/dL in the second trimester, and 9.5–15 g/dL in the third trimester; with 12–15.8 g/dL used as a reference range for nonpregnant females [24]. While some degree of "anemia" is considered normal in pregnancy, maternal hemoglobin levels below these values may result from insufficient iron intake to meet the demands of increased erythropoiesis. Pregnancy-related anemia responds well to iron supplementation. Other causes of anemia should be ruled out [25].

Clinical Implications

1. Anemia may lead to adverse obstetric outcomes including low birth weight, therefore attention to hemoglobin levels in pregnancy is prudent for prevention of maternal and fetal morbidity [18,26].
2. Conversely, the absence of physiologic anemia may be detrimental. Hemoglobin levels above 14.6 g/dL in early pregnancy are associated with an increased risk of intrauterine fetal demise [27].

Increasing blood volume traversing through the heart leads to an increased atrial natriuretic peptide (ANP), released in response to atrial stretch. ANP acts as a peripheral vasodilator and a diuretic, thus exerting a check on volume expansion and contributing to a further decrease in SVR in order to compensate for the increase in blood volume [28]. Increased total blood volume during pregnancy serves several purposes: (i) To meet the increased metabolic demands of the gravid uterus and its enlarged vasculature with up to 750 mL/min directed to the uterus at term gestation [29]. (ii) It prepares maternal blood volume for the blood loss experienced at delivery. (iii) Increased blood flow to the placenta provides the fetus with the oxygen and nutrients necessary for normal development.

Clinical Implications

1. The degree of blood volume expansion is proportional to birth weight in multiple studies, and diminished plasma volume increase has been associated with pre-eclampsia and growth restriction [30].
2. Fetal growth restriction has been shown to be preceded by inadequate volume expansion even as early as 8 weeks of pregnancy [31].

Cardiac Output

CO is the product of stroke volume and HR that reflects the capacity of the heart to respond to the perfusion requirement of the body. CO has been the focus of many studies assessing the hemodynamics of pregnancy that have universally shown a rise during pregnancy. Measurement of CO can be either invasive or noninvasive. Invasive methods using thermodilution technique remain the gold standard for calculating cardiac output. Many studies have understandably focused on identifying noninvasive techniques that can best replicate the measurements obtained invasively, such as 2D or Doppler echocardiography [32–34]. Due to differences in measurement techniques and feasibility of obtaining measurements, the precise degree of the CO increase and the mechanisms behind it have not been universally agreed upon [35]. Studies of normal maternal physiology in relation to these changes in CO remain an important area for future research.

Typically, the sharpest rise in CO occurs by 8 weeks, with continued increase into the second trimester and a peak between 25–35 weeks [36]. In some studies, CO has been shown to be increased by 50% during pregnancy; however, there is no consensus in the literature regarding the precise magnitude and pattern of change in CO. A 2016 meta-analysis looking at 39 studies assessing CO data in uncomplicated, singleton pregnancies showed that CO increased by 1.5 L/min, or 31%, above nonpregnant values [14]. This increase was steady, though nonlinear, until its peak at 31 weeks, with a subsequent plateau. In early pregnancy, stroke volume was the major contributor to the increase in CO, and in late pregnancy, HR became increasingly influential [14,35].

Maternal position affects CO, which has implications during obstetric procedures, imaging studies, and during labor and delivery. In the supine position, the gravid uterus compresses the inferior vena cava, decreasing venous return to the heart and causing a significant decrease in CO [8]. The magnitude of decrease correlates with the size of the uterus, as is evident from twin studies [37]. Evidence has shown that in twin gestations, CO is 20% higher than in singleton pregnancies, and that compression of the vena cava by the uterus is even more pronounced [38]. CO is directly related to weight and height, with an increase in CO noted as weight increases in women above 160 cm in height. CO is inversely related to age, with higher CO in women under the age of 25 [39].

The need to augment CO in pregnancy and delivery is a major contributing factor to the potential decompensation of women with cardiac disease if this augmentation is compromised due to the underlying cardiac structure and function.

Blood Pressure

Despite marked blood volume expansion, pregnant women usually remain normotensive throughout pregnancy, and have been traditionally thought to have an overall decrease in BP [40]. Data from longitudinal studies have demonstrated that, like SVR, arterial BP begins to decrease in the first trimester, as early as 7 weeks [41]. BP nadirs in the second trimester, but the majority of the decrease in BP occurs at 6–8 weeks. It is therefore important, if possible, to compare pregnancy BPs to true preconception BPs, as BPs in early pregnancy are likely already displaying the effects of pregnancy [2]. Systolic blood pressure, diastolic blood pressure, and mean arterial pressure all decrease, but diastolic blood pressure and mean arterial pressure decrease more than systolic blood pressure, leading to a widened pulse pressure [12]. In the third trimester, BP begins to increase, and it returns to pre-pregnancy values in the postpartum period, though the precise timeline of BP normalization is not clear.

Some recent studies have challenged the traditional thinking that BP is lower in pregnancy than in the nonpregnant state. A study of third trimester BP from 2016 showed significantly higher systolic and diastolic BPs in pregnant compared to nonpregnant women, by 18 and 12 mmHg, respectively [42]. In 2002, a retrospective study of 1599 women showed that women with a high initial BP had a fall in BP during pregnancy, while those with low initial BP had either a much smaller fall or a rise in BP as pregnancy progressed [43]. In addition, a 2011 study demonstrated a progressive increase in blood pressure throughout pregnancy [44]. The Generation R study, meanwhile, demonstrated that women with lower education levels did not experience a midpregnancy fall in diastolic blood pressure, and this difference was not explained by body mass index or weight change during pregnancy [45]. These factors should be taken into consideration when assessing maternal blood pressure.

Correct patient positioning, timing, and cuff size are all extremely important in the measurement of blood pressure.

- Blood pressure should be taken after the patient has rested, ideally for at least 10 minutes.
- The patient should be seated with her legs uncrossed and her back supported, and her arm should be positioned at the level of her heart.
- If blood pressure must be taken in a recumbent position, which is often the case in the intrapartum setting,

the patient should be placed in a left lateral decubitus position and the cuff should be at the level of the right atrium.

- An appropriately sized cuff has a length that is 1.5 times the upper arm circumference, or a bladder that encircles at least 80% of the arm and a width of at least 40% of the arm circumference [46].
- BPs are generally higher in the sitting position than in the recumbent position, because compression of the vena cava by the gravid uterus in the supine position leads to a decrease in venous return and therefore cardiac output. Normally, there is a compensatory increase in peripheral vascular resistance that helps maintain the maternal BP; however, occasionally supine position may lead to an increase in HR and decrease in BP which may result in significant dizziness, lightheadedness, nausea, or syncope [8]]. These hemodynamic changes in response to positioning must be kept in mind when evaluating a pregnant patient.

Cardiac Structure

Pregnancy and exercise are the two non-pathological states known to cause cardiac hypertrophy [48]. In pathologic cardiac hypertrophy, pressure and volume overload lead to either concentric or eccentric changes in ventricular geometry. Concentric hypertrophy is an increase in ventricular wall thickness with decrease in ventricular cavity size that may lead to diastolic heart dysfunction, and eccentric hypertrophy is a thinning of the ventricular wall leading to a dilation of the ventricular cavity with potential for subsequent systolic cardiac dysfunction. These states often lead to decreased cardiac function and heart failure over time. In contrast, exercise and pregnancy lead to a proportional increase in both wall thickness and chamber size [49]. Cardiac hypertrophy in pregnancy is mediated both by the increase in blood volume and circulating levels of sex steroid hormones [50]. Progesterone in particular tends to increase protein synthesis and thereby induce hypertrophy in cardiac muscle cells [51]. There is an increase in left ventricular wall thickness of up to 28% by the end of pregnancy, and an up to 52% increase in left ventricular wall mass [41,52]. Right ventricle similarly has been shown to undergo an increase in wall mass of up to 40% [5].

The effects of pregnancy on left ventricular function are not well understood. Both normal and decreased ventricular systolic function has been reported in the literature [53]. Mild LV diastolic dysfunction has also been reported during normal, otherwise uncomplicated pregnancies [54]. However, pregnancy-induced cardiac hypertrophy is similar to exercise-induced hypertrophy and differs from pathological hypertrophy in that it is reversible, with studies showing a normalization of heart size starting from 7–14 days up to 1 year postpartum [55].

The cardiac valves demonstrate effects of pregnancy as well. In animal studies, all four cardiac valves undergo remodeling throughout gestation, with increased leaflet size and a change in the biochemical composition to include a decrease in cell density and in collagen composition [56]. Valve area may increase dramatically, especially in the aortic and mitral valves, secondary to the increase in blood volume seen by the left ventricle [57]. This increase in valve annulus area with or without mild leaflet elongation can result in mild physiologic valvular insufficiency or regurgitation.

Clinical Implications

1. Pregnancy can expose undiagnosed cardiac pathology or it can cause cardiac pathology in otherwise healthy people.
2. Though the underlying etiology of peripartum cardiomyopathy is still a matter of investigation and is not the focus of this chapter, this condition illustrates the extent to which pregnancy functions as a cardiac stress model.
3. Peripartum cardiomyopathy, or heart failure near the end of pregnancy or within 5 months after delivery without any other identifiable cause, may represent a previously healthy cardiovascular system now unable to respond to the cardiac stress of pregnancy [48]. Alternately, it may reflect a heart with an underlying undiscovered insufficiency or be the result of unbalanced pregnancy hormones [58].

Intrapartum and Postpartum

The cardiovascular changes during labor and delivery are mediated by the autonomic nervous system. These changes occur more rapidly and have more pronounced effects than those that have been evolving gradually throughout pregnancy, and their clinical impact may be significant [59,60]. The blood loss experienced at time of delivery, as well as the contribution of anesthesia and surgical stress in patients who undergo cesarean section, also have profound effects on maternal hemodynamics. Though women with previously recognized cardiac disease require especially close monitoring in labor, even low-risk women can suffer adverse cardiovascular events during this time, and all obstetric providers should be familiar with the possible complications that can occur.

Hemodynamic Changes in Labor

An increase in cardiac output during labor has been long reported in the literature, dating back to the 1950s. In 1956, Hendricks and Quilligan studied changes in CO during late pregnancy, labor, and in the early postpartum period. They concluded that cardiac output increases by an average of 30.9% during contractions, with pain and anxiety contributing to this increase [61]. They additionally described a cumulative 35% increase in cardiac output over the course of prolonged labor. In 1958, Adams and Alexander used a dye-dilution technique to demonstrate that CO increases with each uterine contraction during labor and immediately after the uterus has been emptied, corresponding with an increase in heart rate. They also found that in patients whose heart rate decreased, or who had saddle block anesthesia (mitigation of pain in the sacral region, likely resulting in less increase in HR), CO decreased [62].

Subsequent investigations using various techniques of measuring cardiac output have shown similar findings [63,64].

A study by Robson et al. from 1987 showed an intrapartum increase in cardiac output from a pre-labor value of 6.99–7.88 L/min between contractions. This change was due entirely to an increase in stroke volume, as heart rate did not increase. During contractions, CO increased even more. The rate of increase was incremental as labor progressed, with higher CO demonstrated at more advanced stages of cervical dilation [65]. Autotransfusion of blood into the systemic circulation from the uterine sinuses during contractions may contribute to this increase, as may elevated HR from pain and anxiety [66]. However, even with good neuraxial analgesia and no pain, HR elevates during labor and delivery, indicating that autotransfusion and increase in preload likely contribute most to increased HR [67]. Increased CO also leads to an increase in both systolic and diastolic blood pressure during each contraction, as SVR changes only slightly in the intrapartum period [68].

As in the third trimester, maternal position has an impact on CO in labor, with CO between contractions is higher in the lateral position than supine [69]. Anesthesia also plays a critical role in intrapartum hemodynamics. Women with epidural anesthesia have been shown to have a significantly less dramatic increase in CO between contractions compared to those without regional anesthesia. The peak CO during contractions is not affected by epidural anesthesia. Regional anesthesia also has the potential to cause profound hypotension after placement, and this can in turn affect cardiac output [70].

Despite a multitude of evidence in older studies demonstrating an intrapartum increase in CO, newer data using more modern technologies have not consistently produced the same results. The LiDCOplus monitor calculates beat-to-beat stroke volume from the arterial pressure waveform obtained from an arterial line, and calibrates it using thermodilution; it can thus continuously calculate CO [71]. This method has been shown to be comparable to pulmonary artery catheter measurements in certain patient populations [72]. A 2017 study by Kuhn et al. used this technique for continuous monitoring of maternal hemodynamics in 20 healthy women with conflicting results in the first stage of labor. In the second stage, there was a decrease in CO and SVR and an increase in the remaining metrics for all patients [73].

Changes during the Second Stage

Bearing down to push during the second stage of labor has many similarities to the Valsalva maneuver, which is technically defined as expiration against a closed glottis after full inspiration. The Valsalva maneuver is commonly used in the assessment of patients with cardiovascular disorders. It can be divided into four phases:

- *Phase I*: Initial straining leads to increased intrathoracic pressure, followed by a transient increase in systemic blood pressure. HR remains stable.
- *Phase II*: A decrease in venous return which leads to a gradual decrease in right and left ventricular volumes, mean arterial pressure, pulse pressure, and stroke volume as well as reflex tachycardia.
- *Phase III*: Release of straining leads to an abrupt decrease in intrathoracic pressure and pooling of blood

in the expanded pulmonary bed, causing decreased blood pressure. HR remains stable.

- *Phase IV*: A systemic overshoot of blood pressure over baseline volume, likely due to return of left ventricular preload and reflex sympathetic activity in response to the hypotension of phase III [74].

In the second stage, bearing down while pushing causes changes to BP and HR that are comparable to those seen in the four phases of the Valsalva maneuver above. Active pushing has been associated with a 30% increase in HR, and 50% increase in CO [75]. Pushing in the left lateral position blunts these responses [76]. *It follows that in women with known or previously unrecognized cardiac disease, these fluctuations in hemodynamics could overwhelm the cardiovascular system.* Good-quality evidence proving this theory is lacking; for example, in a 2016 study that assessed the length of the second stage in 73 women with cardiac disease, 34% of women pushed longer than recommended, with no adverse cardiac events reported in the entire cohort [77]. Recommendations on whether a patient should be allowed to bear down or should have an assisted second stage must be individualized, and more evidence is needed before definitive guidelines can be put in place [75].

Clinical Implications

There are two main concerns with the cardiovascular changes during Valsalva maneuver.

1. Increase in arterial shear stress
2. Fluctuations in pre-load

The rapid rate of blood pressure increase from stage III to stage IV causes a great increase in momentary arterial shear stress which can be detrimental in patients with arterial pathology. Fluctuations in ventricular preload during Valsalva are especially worrisome in women with preload-dependent lesions.

Delivery and the Postpartum Period

The most marked hemodynamic changes occur at the moment of delivery itself and in the immediate postpartum period. CO increases up to 80% at delivery, then begins to decline to pre-labor values within approximately 1 hour following delivery [41]. Increased CO may be secondary to the return of blood supply from the uterus to the systemic circulation that leads to an increase in stroke volume [78]. Other factors that may contribute to this increase include increased venous return after relief of the weight of the gravid uterus and auto transfusion from uterine involution. An increase in CO may serve to combat the blood loss experienced at delivery. CO rapidly decreases for the first 2 weeks following delivery, and over the course of the postpartum period returns to pre-pregnancy values. Complete normalization of cardiac output can take up to 6 months postpartum [41].

Heart rate has been shown to decrease in the first 48 hours postpartum [9]. By 2 weeks after delivery, heart rate reaches its nadir and does not decrease further. In the 48 hours after delivery, stroke volume increases by 10% and then decreases steadily until up to 6 months postpartum. Blood pressure tends to remain stable throughout this period, except in those patients who have lost a clinically significant amount of blood [79].

Mode of delivery can have an impact on maternal hemodynamics. For example, blood volume decreases by 10% in the first 1–10 hours postpartum in women who had a vaginal delivery, but by 17%–29% in women who underwent cesarean section. Clinical significance of this difference is unclear as there is no difference in postoperative hematocrits between the two groups. Blood volume continues to decrease over the next 10 days in patients who had a vaginal delivery, but remains stable after the initial blood loss in those who have had a cesarean section. At 3 days postpartum, both groups tend to have an overall 10% lower blood volume than pre-delivery [69,80,81].

In more recent literature, CO was found to increase throughout cesarean section, peak within 2 minutes after delivery of newborn and placenta, and reach levels lower than baseline at 24–36 hours postoperatively [82]. This is likely secondary to the rapid increase in venous return and preload after delivery of the fetus and placenta. SVR and mean arterial pressures reach their lowest point immediately after delivery and return to their baseline levels by the time of fascial closure [83].

Analgesia (mild sensory block to prevent pain) and anesthesia (dense sensory and motor block to permit surgical stimulation) have known, relatively predictable influences on maternal hemodynamics. Spinal anesthesia for cesarean section, which creates a sensory and motor block to the level of T4, will lead to profound hypotension due to a decrease in SVR and a compensatory increase in CO; however, anesthesiologists routinely augment SVR with vasopressors (most commonly phenylephrine) to reverse this sympathetic block. Women who undergo cesarean section with an epidural already in place generally remain hemodynamically stable, with a slight decrease in BP that can be counteracted with phenylephrine; HR and CO generally remain unchanged [84]. It should be noted that slow neuraxial anesthesia via an epidural catheter allows time for the anesthesiologist to augment SVR with vasopressors so as to prevent significant maternal hemodynamic alterations due to anesthesia.

Distinguishing Physiology from Pathology

Many of the symptoms of normal pregnancy can mimic those of cardiovascular disease. A systematic approach to any pregnant or postpartum woman noting cardiac symptoms is essential so that symptoms of concern prompt appropriate workup, and normal findings do not lead to a barrage of unnecessary tests and procedures.

Symptoms

The common symptoms that can present in both normal pregnancy and in pregnancy affected by cardiac disease include decreased exercise tolerance, shortness of breath, fatigue, chest pain, and peripheral edema.

- *Shortness of breath*: Pregnant women will often complain of breathlessness or dyspnea and decreased exercise tolerance. While traditionally attributed to displacement of the diaphragm and chest wall by the growing uterus, some women experience breathlessness early in pregnancy. Hyperventilation seen in normal pregnancy may be perceived as shortness of breath by some women [85]. Older studies have found that up to 76% of women complain of dyspnea by the 31st week of pregnancy [86]. A low level of fatigue and decreased exercise tolerance are extremely common, though pregnant women should be able to perform their everyday activities and a low level of exercise without issue. Symptoms that should always prompt further investigation include additional symptoms listed in Table 3.1 [87].

- *Palpitations*: Heart palpitations are commonly experienced by women and may be due to an increase in heart rate, cardiac output, and stroke volume [88].
- *Chest pain*: Up to 15% of women report chest pain in the first trimester, increasing to 75% by the third trimester [86]. Pregnancy conditions such as gastroesophageal reflux are more common and can present as chest pain. Chest pain should have a low threshold for workup.

Physical Examination Findings

Some of the physical exam findings of normal pregnancy are similar to those of heart disease.

- Rales at the bases of the lungs that clear with cough or deep breathing can be a normal finding in pregnancy.

TABLE 3.1

Physiologic versus Pathologic Dyspnea

Favors Physiologic	Favors Pathologic
Gradual onset	Acute onset
No other symptoms	Presence of other symptoms
	Cough
	Chest pain
	Fever
	Hemoptysis
	Paroxysmal nocturnal dyspnea
	Orthopnea
	Wheezing
First or second trimester	Third trimester
Normal vital signs	Vital sign abnormalities
Clear lungs auscultation	Wheezes or crackles
Normal labs and imaging studies	Abnormalities in:
	BMP, LFTs, CBC
	BNP
	ECG
	Echocardiogram
	Chest x-ray
	CT angiogram

Abbreviations: BMP: basic metabolic panel; BNP: brain natriuretic peptide; CBC: complete blood count; CT: computed tomography; ECG: electrocardiogram; LFTs: liver function tests.

- Lower extremity edema is commonly present, particularly as pregnancy progresses, though rapid-onset edema should raise suspicion for a pathologic process.
- The jugular venous pulse can become more obvious after the 20th week despite normal jugular venous pressure.
- The heart will be shifted anteriorly and to the left as the uterus enlarges, and the point of maximal impulse will be displaced to the fourth intercostal space and lateral to the midclavicular line. Both the left and right ventricles may be hyper-dynamic and palpable because of increased CO and blood volume.
- Auscultatory changes present in the normal pregnant woman include wide splitting of S1 due to early closure of the mitral valve, soft systolic ejection murmurs or "flow murmurs" over the tricuspid valve, a third heart sound (S3) and a continuous murmur or "mammary soufflé" over the breast vasculature [89].
- Diastolic murmurs are not common in pregnant women and should prompt further evaluation for a pathologic condition.

Diagnostic Tests

Diagnostic tests may also appear abnormal in normal pregnancy.

- Chest x-ray may appear to show cardiomegaly due to the upward and lateral displacement of the heart and increased circulating blood volume. Prominent pulmonary vasculature may be a normal finding later in pregnancy.
- ECG changes are also common and likely reflect the changing position of the heart, changing blood volume, and hormonal variations. Left axis deviation, ST segment and T wave flattening, inverted T waves in lead III, V1–V3, and prominent Q waves in II, III, and aVF have all been reported [47,90,91].

Common Cardiac Complaints in Pregnancy

The basic systematic approach to any cardiac complaint in pregnancy is similar: elicit a thorough history including history of the patient's baseline function and exercise tolerance, current function, symptoms, and her obstetric and medical history, conduct a focused physical exam, and pursue the appropriate radiographic, electrocardiographic, and laboratory investigations. If cardiac disease is suspected, referral to a cardiologist should be pursued (see Chapter 6).

Conclusion

Pregnancy is itself a form of stress test and is uniquely the only non-pathologic state that causes dramatic alterations in physiology. The physiology of pregnancy is to promote fetal growth and development, and adaptations in the cardiovascular system are an integral part of this process. Because many of the cardiovascular adaptations to pregnancy are marked departures from the nonpregnant physiology, pregnancy may unmask previously unrecognized cardiac disease that can lead to significant morbidity and mortality. It is therefore essential for obstetric providers to be able to understand the physiologic changes of pregnancy, so that pathology can be recognized when it occurs and normal findings do not lead to a barrage of unnecessary tests and procedures.

Many of the symptoms of a healthy pregnancy can mimic those of cardiac disease; when a patient reports cardiovascular symptoms, a targeted and thorough workup must be undertaken to rule out either preexisting or new-onset disease. Consultation with a cardiologist should not be delayed. There is need for multidisciplinary care of any pregnant patient diagnosed with a cardiovascular condition. A systematic approach to the evaluation of any patient with suspected cardiovascular disease is critical in order to differentiate physiologic changes from a pathologic process.

REFERENCES

1. Hall ME, George EM, Granger JP. The heart during pregnancy. *Resp Esp Cardiol.* 2011;64(11):1045–50.
2. Mahendru AA et al. A longitudinal study of maternal cardiovascular function from preconception to the postpartum period. *J Hypertens.* 2014;32:849–56.
3. Creanga AA, Syverson C, Seed K, Callaghan WM. Pregnancy-related mortality in the United States, 2011–2013. *Obstet Gynecol.* 2017;130(2):366–73.
4. Chapman AB et al. Temporal relationships between hormonal and hemodynamic changes in early human pregnancy. *Kidney Int.* 1998;54(6):2056–63.
5. Hunter S, Robson SC. Adaptation of the maternal heart in pregnancy. *Br Heart J.* 1992;68:540–3.
6. Ouzounian JG, Elkayam U. Physiologic changes during normal pregnancy and delivery. *Cardiol Clin.* 2012;30:317–29.
7. Sanghavi M, Rutherford JD. Cardiovascular physiology of pregnancy. *Circulation.* 2014;130:1003–8.
8. Kinsella SM, Lohmann G. Supine hypotensive syndrome. *Obstet Gynecol.* 1994;83(5 pt 1):774–88.
9. Samways JW et al. Maternal heart rate during the first 48 h postpartum: A retrospective cross sectional study. *Eur J Obst Gynecol Repro Bio.* 2016;206:41–7.
10. Debrah DO et al. Relaxin is essential for systemic vasodilation and increased global arterial compliance during early pregnancy in conscious rats. *Endocrinology.* 2006;147(11):5126–31.
11. Weiner CP, Thompson LP. Maternal adaptations to pregnancy: Cardiovascular and hemodynamic changes. *Semin Perinatol.* 1997;21(5):367.
12. Gomez YH, Hudda Z, Mahdi N. Pulse pressure amplification and arterial stiffness in low-risk, uncomplicated pregnancies. *Angiology.* 2016;67(4):375–83.
13. O'Donnell E, Floras JS, Harvey PJ. Estrogen status and the renin angiotensin aldosterone system. *Am J Physiol Regul Integr Comp Physiol.* 2014;307(5):R498–500.
14. Meah VL et al. Cardiac output and related hemodynamics during pregnancy: A series of meta-analyses. *Heart.* 2016;102:518–26.
15. MacGillivray I, Rose GA, Rowe B. Blood pressure survey in pregnancy. *Clin Sci.* 1969;37(2):395–407.
16. Stander HJ, Cadden JF. The cardiac output in pregnant women. *Am. J. Obstet Gynecol* 1932;24;13.
17. Bernstein IM, Ziegler W, Badger GJ. Plasma volume expansion in early pregnancy. *Obstet Gynecol.* 2001;97(5 Pt 1):669.
18. Vricella LK. Emerging understanding and measurement of plasma volume expansion in pregnancy. *Am J Clin Nutr.* 2017;106(suppl 6):1620S–25S.
19. De Haas S et al. Physiological adaptation of maternal plasma volume during pregnancy: A systematic review and meta-analysis. *Ultrasound Obstet Gynecol.* 2017;49:177–87.
20. Lund CJ, Donovan JC. Blood volume during pregnancy. Significance of plasma and red cell volumes. *Am J Obstet Gynecol.* 1967;98:394–403.
21. Milman N et al. Serum erythropoietin during normal pregnancy: Relationship to hemoglobin and iron status markers and impact of iron supplementation in a longitudinal, placebo-controlled study on 118 women. *Int J Hematol.* 1997;66(2):159.
22. Hytten FE, Lind T. Indices of cardiovascular function. In: Hytten FE, Lind T, editors. *Diagnostic Indices in Pregnancy.* Basel: Documenta Geigy; 1973.
23. Chesley LC. Plasma and red cell volumes during pregnancy. *Am J Obstet Gynecol.* 1972;112:440–50.
24. Abbassi-Ghanavati M, Greer LG, Cunningham FG. Pregnancy and laboratory studies: A reference table for clinicians. *Obstet Gynecol.* 2009;114(6):1326–31.
25. Cao C, O'Brien KO. Pregnancy and iron homeostasis: An update. *Nutr Rev.* 2013;71:35–51.
26. Tabrizi FM, Barjasteh S. Maternal hemoglobin levels during pregnancy and their association with birth weight of neonates. *Iran J Ped Hematol Oncol.* 2015;5(4):211–17.
27. Stephansson O et al. Maternal hemoglobin concentration during pregnancy and risk of stillbirth. *JAMA.* 2000;284(20):2611.
28. Sala C et al. Atrial natriuretic peptide and hemodynamic changes during normal human pregnancy. *Hypertension.* 1995;25(4):631–36.
29. Maternal physiology. In: Cunningham FG, Leveno KJ, Bloom SL et al., editors. *Williams Obstetrics,* 24th ed. McGraw-Hill Education; 2014. p. 47.
30. Suranyi JM et al. Maternal haematological parameters and placental and umbilical cord histopathology in intrauterine growth restriction. *Med Prin and Prac.* 2019;28(2):101–108.
31. Duvekot JJ, Cheriex EC, Pieters FA. Maternal volume homeostasis in early pregnancy in relation to fetal growth restriction. *Obstet Gynecol.* 1995;85(3):361–67.
32. Boer P et al. Measurement of cardiac output by impedance cardiography under various conditions. *Am J Physiol.* 1979;237(4):H491–6.
33. Folland ED et al. Assessment of left ventricular ejection fraction and volumes by real-time, two-dimensional echocardiography. A comparison of cineangiographic and radionuclide techniques. *Circulation.* 1979;60(4):760–6.
34. Lee W, Rokey R, Cotton DB. Noninvasive maternal stroke volume and cardiac output determinations by pulsed Doppler echocardiography. *Am J Obstet Gynecol.* 1988;158(3 pt 1):505–10.
35. Mabie WC et al. A longitudinal study of cardiac output in normal human pregnancy. *Am J Obstet Gynecol.* 1994;170(3):849–56.
36. Robson SC et al. Serial study of factors influencing changes in cardiac output during human pregnancy. *Am J Physiol.* 1989;256(pt 2):H1060–65.

37. Kim YI, Chandra P, Marx GF. Successful management of severe aortocaval compression in twin pregnancy. *Obstet Gynecol.* 1975;46:362–4.

38. Kametas NA, McAuliffe F, Krampl E. Maternal cardiac function in twin pregnancy. *Obstet Gynecol.* 2003;102(4):806.

39. Vinayagam D et al. Maternal hemodynamics in normal pregnancy: Reference ranges and role of maternal characteristics. *Ultrasound Obstet Gynecol.* 2018;51:665–71.

40. Grindheim G, Estensen ME, Langesaeter E, Changes in blood pressure during pregnancy: A longitudinal cohort study. *J Hypertension* 2012:30;342–50.

41. Robson SC et al. Haemodynamic changes during the puerperium: A Doppler and M-mode echocardiographic study. *Br J Obstet Gynaecol.* 1987;94:1028–39.

42. Sufrin S et al. Blood pressure in the third trimester of pregnancy. *Mymensingh Med J.* 2016;25(1):18–22.

43. Iwasaki R et al. Relationship between blood pressure level in early pregnancy and subsequent changes in blood pressure during pregnancy. *Acta Obstet Gynecol Scand.* 2002;81(10):918–25.

44. Nama V et al. Midtrimester blood pressure drop in normal pregnancy: Myth or reality? *J Hpertension.* 2011;29:763–8.

45. Silva LM et al. No midpregnancy fall in diastolic blood pressure in women with a low educational level. *Hypertension.* 2008;52(4):645–51.

46. Pickering TG et al. Recommendations for blood pressure measurement in humans and experimental animals. Part 1. Blood pressure measurement in humans: A statement for professionals from the Subcommittee of Professional and Public Education of the American Heart Association Council on High Blood Pressure Research. *Circulation.* 2005;111:697–716.

47. Clark SL et al. Central hemodynamic assessment of normal term pregnancy. *Am J Obstet Gynecol.* 1989;161:1439.

48. Chung E, Leinwand LA. Pregnancy as a cardiac stress model. *Cardiovasc Res.* 2014;101:561–70.

49. McMullen JR, Jennings GL. Differences between pathological and physiological cardiac hypertrophy: Novel therapeutic strategies to treat heart failure. *Clin Exp Pharmacol Physiol.* 2007;34:255–62.

50. Souders CA et al. Pressure overload induces early morphological changes in the heart. *Am J Pathol.* 2012;181:1226–35.

51. Goldstein J, Sites CK, Toth MJ. Progesterone stimulates cardiac muscle protein synthesis via receptor-dependent pathway. *Fert Steril.* 2004;82:430–436.

52. Katz R, Karlner JS, Resnik R. Effects of a natural volume overload state (pregnancy) on left ventricular performance in normal human subjects. *Circulation.* 1978;58:434–41.

53. Diffee GM, Chung E. Altered single cell force-velocity and power properties in exercise-trained rat myocardium. *J Appl Physiol.* 2003;94:1941–8.

54. Schannwell CM et al. Left ventricular hypertophy and diastolic dysfunction in healthy pregnant women. *Cardiology.* 2002;97:73–8.

55. Umar S et al. Cardiac structural and hemodynamic changes associated with physiological heart hypertrophy of pregnancy are reversed postpartum. *J Appl Physiol.* 2012;113:1253–9.

56. Pierlot CM et al. Pregnancy-induced remodeling of heart valves. *Am J Physiol Heart Circ Physiol.* 2015;309:H1565–78.

57. Pierlot CM, Moeller AD, Lee JM et al. Biaxial creep resistance and structural remodeling of the aortic and mitral valves in pregnancy. *Ann Biomed Eng.* 2015;43:1772–85.

58. Sliwa K et al. Current state of knowledge on aetiology, diagnosis, management, and therapy of peripartum cardiomyopathy: A position statement from the Heart Failure Association of the European Society of Cardiology Working Group on peripartum cardiomyopathy. *Eur J Heart Fail.* 2010;12(8):767.

59. Reyes-Lagos JJ et al. A comparison of heart rate variability in women at the third trimester of pregnancy and during low-risk labour. *Physiol Behav.* 2015;149:255–61.

60. Musa SM et al. Maternal heart rate variability during the first stage of labor. *Front Physiol.* 2017;8:744.

61. Hendricks CH, Quilligan EJ. Cardiac output during labor. *Am J Obstet Gynecol.* 1956;71:953–72.

62. Adams JQ, Alexander AM. Alterations in cardiovascular physiology during labor. *Obstet Gynecol.* 1958;12(5):542–8.

63. Laird-Meter K et al. Cardiocirculatory adjustments during pregnancy—An echocardiographic study. *Clin Cardiol.* 1979:2(5);328–32.

64. Osofsky HJ, Williams JA. Changes in blood volume during parturition and the early postpartum period. *Am J Obstet Gynecol.* 1964;88(3):396–8.

65. Robson SC et al. Cardiac output during labor. *Brit Med Journal.* 1987;295:1169–72.

66. Lee W et al. Maternal hemodynamics effects of uterine contractions by M-mode and pulsed-Doppler echocardiography. *Am J Obstet Gynecol.* 1989;161:974–7.

67. Ueland K, Hansen JM. Maternal cardiovascular dynamics. III. Labor and delivery under local and caudal analgesia. *Am J Obstet Gynecol.* 1969;103:8–18.

68. Henricks CH. The hemodynamics of uterine contraction. *Am J Obstet Gynecol.* 1958;76:969–81.

69. Ueland K, Hansen JM. Maternal cardiovascular dynamics. II. Posture and uterine contractions. *Am J Obstet Gynecol.* 1969;103:1–7.

70. Ouzounian JG et al. Systemic vascular resistance index determined by thoracic electrical bioimpedance predicts the risk for maternal hypotension during regional anesthesia for cesarean delivery. *Am J Obstet Gynecol.* 1996;174:1019.

71. Langesaeter E, Gibbs M, Dyer RA. The role of cardiac output monitoring in obstetric anesthesia. *Curr Opin Anes.* 2015;28(3):247–53.

72. Dyer RA et al. Comparison between pulse waveform analysis and thermodilution cardiac output determination in patients with severe pre-eclampsia. *Br J Anaesth.* 2010;106:77–81.

73. Kuhn JC, Falk RS, Langesaeter E. Hemodynamic changes during labor: Continuous minimally invasive monitoring in 20 healthy parturients. *Int J Obstet Anesth.* 2017;31:74–83.

74. Nishmura RA, Tajik AJ. The Valsalva maneuver and response revisited. *Mayo Clin Proc.* 1986;61:211–17.

75. Regitz-Zagrosek V et al. ESC Guidelines on the management of cardiovascular diseases during pregnancy: The Task Force on the Management of Cardiovascular Diseases during Pregnancy of the European Society of Cardiology (ESC). *Eur Heart J.* 2011;32:3147–97.

76. Summers RL et al.: Theoretical analysis of the effect of positioning on hemodynamic stability during pregnancy, *Acad Emerg Med.* 2011;18:1094–8.

77. Cauldwell M et al. The management of the second stage of labour in women with cardiac disease: A mixed methods study. *Int J Cardiol.* 2016;222:732–6.

78. Elkayam U, Gleicher N. Hemodynamics and cardiac function during normal pregnancy and the puerperium. In: Elkayam U, Gleicher N, editors. *Cardiac Problems in Pregnancy*, 3rd ed. New York: Wiley-Liss; 1998, pp. 3–15.
79. Kjeldsen J. Hemodynamic investigations during labour and delivery. *Acta Obstet Gynecol Scand Suppl.* 1979;89:1.
80. Ueland K. Maternal cardiovascular dynamics VII. Intrapartum blood volume changes. *Am J Obstet Gynecol.* 1976;126:671–77.
81. Hansen JM, Ueland K. The influence of caudal analgesia on cardiovascular dynamics during normal labor and delivery. *Acta Anaesthesiol Scand.* 1966;23(suppl):449–52.
82. Tihtonen K et al. Maternal hemodynamics during cesarean delivery assessed by whole-body impedance cardiography. *Acta Obstet Gynecol Scan.* 2005;84(4):355–61.
83. Ram M et al. Cardiac hemodynamics before, during and after elective cesarean section under spinal anesthesia in low-risk women. *J Perinatol.* 2017;37(7):793–9.
84. Langesæter E, Dyer RA. Maternal haemodynamic changes during spinal anaesthesia for caesarean section. *Curr Opin Anaesthesiol.* 2011;24(3):242–8.
85. Prowse CM, Gaensler EA. Respiratory and acid-base changes during pregnancy. *Anesthesiology.* 1965;26:381–92.
86. Milne J, Howie A, Pack A. Dyspnea during normal pregnancy. *Br J Obstet Gynaecol.* 1978;85:260–63.
87. Monga M, Mastrobattista JM. Maternal cardiovascular, respiratory and renal adaptation to pregnancy. In: Creasy RK, Resnik R, Iams JD, Lockwood CJ, Moore TR, Greene MF, editors. *Creasy and Resnik's Maternal Fetal Medicine*, 7th ed. Philadelphia: Elsevier Saunders; 2014, pp. 93–99.
88. Choi, HS et al. Dyspnea and palpitation during pregnancy. *Korean J Int Med.* 2001;16(4):247–9.
89. Cutforth R, MacDonald CB. Heart sounds and murmurs in pregnancy. *Am Heart Journal.* 1966;71(6): 741–7.
90. M S, S C, Brid SV. Electrocradiographic QRS axis, Q wave and T-wave changes in 2nd and 3rd trimester of normal pregnancy. *J Clin Diagn Res.* 2014;8(9):BC17–21.
91. Oram S, Holt M. Innocent depression of the S-T segment and flattening of the T-wave during pregnancy. *J Obstet Gynaecol Br Emp.* 1961;68:765.

4

Preconception Care: Optimization of Cardiac Risk

Mary M. Canobbio

KEY POINTS

- Advances in medical and surgical arenas have created a larger pool of women of childbearing age with heart disease
- Congenital heart disease is the most frequently encountered type of cardiac disorder in pregnancy and must be managed by a multidisciplinary team with appropriate expertise in adult congenital heart disease

- The modified WHO risk classification is the more widely used and is the simplest risk scoring scale
- Pregnancy is not recommended for women in modified WHO risk category IV
- Contraceptive counseling should be an integral part of the clinical management of females with cardiac history who are of childbearing age

---

Introduction

The number of reproductive age women who are born with or develop heart disease is steadily growing, and with each decade the numbers continue to increase. While the exact numbers are unknown, advances in both medical and surgical arenas have created a larger pool of women of childbearing age with heart disease. Consequently, questions regarding pregnancy become an important issue for all providers who care for patients with heart disease, including congenital heart disease (CHD), acquired cardiac disorders, and those following cardiac transplant. In order to ensure their safety, it is imperative these patients undergo preconception counseling regardless of their desire to become pregnant; that they understand the actual or potential risk to them and to their fetus and the importance of avoiding an unplanned pregnancy. For cardiac and obstetrical providers, a number of risk scoring scales have been developed to help guide management. The importance of using risk assessment models to advise patients on the risk of pregnancy is reviewed.

Scope of the Problem

In the developed world, while prevalence rates are low, cardiovascular disease is the most common cause of maternal mortality [1–5]. CHD, which affects 0.8%–1.5% of the population, is the most frequently encountered cardiac disorder in obstetrics [6]. While the majority of women with simple CHD will tolerate pregnancy well, those with moderate to complex lesions that have been surgically repaired in childhood may present with residual effects of their surgical procedure as they grow older. It is therefore difficult to categorize these patients based solely on

their primary defect, because many may be at risk for developing complications such as ventricular dysfunction, arrhythmias, or thromboembolic events. For women with complex CHD who have undergone surgical repair, such as univentricular circulation (Fontan palliation) or transposition of great arteries (Mustard, Senning), or those with cyanotic heart disease, the risk of developing complications during and after delivery is higher [7–13]. *For women who remain cyanotic (O_2 saturation $\leq 85\%$), with or without pulmonary hypertension, or those with critical left ventricular outflow tract obstruction (gradients >60 mmHg) or severe ventricular function pregnancy is not advisable* [7].

While CHD is more prevalent, those with acquired heart disease carry a higher risk of mortality during childbirth [7,14]. These include women with ischemic heart disease, aortopathies, various cardiomyopathies, hypertensive disorders, and valvular heart disease, particularly requiring anticoagulation. In addition, over the past 2–3 decades, the number of children undergoing heart transplant has risen and consequently the number of these young women now and in future will be seeking to become pregnant. Today, transplanted female patients represent approximately 20% of overall cardiac transplants population, 25% of which are reported to be between the ages of 18–39 years [15,16]. While successful pregnancies have been reported, the majority experience complications such as hypertensive disorders of pregnancy, prematurity, graft rejection, and/or infection [17,18].

Preconception Counseling

The task of advising females regarding the safety of pregnancy has been challenging until recently. After almost three decades, the body of literature in this field has moved from expert opinion and case reporting to cumulative data reported from multicenter studies and international registries [8,19]. As result, we now have growing evidence-based data that permits us to advise patients regarding the safety of carrying a pregnancy. Less clear is the potential risk pregnancy poses to long-term survival of patients with complex cardiac lesions. Reports regarding long-term outcomes in patients with CHD indicate that for the majority of patients, the effects of pregnancy resolve within the first year after delivery, while for others it may be longer, but may not have a lasting effect on long-term survival [7,9].

Estimating Maternal and Fetal Risk

While the information regarding pregnancy outcomes across the spectrum of various cardiac disorder is growing, it remains a challenge to assign risk solely on the basis of their cardiac lesion. Therefore, in order to determine maternal risk, the patients must be evaluated against a number of parameters (Table 4.1) that include not only maternal primary disorder, but also any residual effects associated with the primary defect, such as diminished ventricular function, history of arrhythmias, and any prior surgical or procedural interventions [47]. A thorough review of the past medical history should also include the presence of any noncardiac comorbidities that may influence pregnancy, such as thyroid disease, diabetes, and history of use of recreational drugs, alcohol, and cannabis products, particularly those with tetrahydrocannabinol (THC), which passes through the placenta [20]. The history must also take into account a number of social factors such as history of medical compliance, geographical distance to doctor's office and hospital as well the patient's spousal and extended family support. The latter is of particular concern for the patient considered high risk in the event that post-delivery clinical problems arise making it difficult for the patient to care for her infant.

TABLE 4.1

Maternal Factors to Assess in Estimating Pregnancy Risk

- *Primary cardiac defect* (acyanotic vs. cyanotic)
- *Genetic disorder* (22q deletion, Turner syndrome, Marfan syndrome)
- *Surgical intervention*
  - Palliative
  - Corrective
    - Integrity of prosthetic valves
    - Patency of baffles/conduits
- *Medications* (e.g., ACE inhibitors, anticoagulants)
- *Comorbidities* (e.g., diabetes, thyroid dysfunction)
- *Presence of devices* (pacemaker, internal defibrillator)
- *Residual and/or sequelae associated with the lesion/surgery*
  - Cyanosis   Arrhythmias
  - Pulmonary hypertension Systemic hypertension
  - Obstruction   Ventricular dysfunction
- *Social factors*
  - Access to medical center with experience in managing cardiac patients
  - Geographical distance
  - History of compliance

Source: Adapted from Canobbio MM. *Prog Pediatr Cardiol.* 2004; 19:1–3.

Maternal Risk Assessment

Maternal risk assessment is based on several factors as outlined above. Several predictors have been described and more recently various risk assessment models have been validated for use in pregnancy.

1. *Functional capacity*: Maternal functional capacity using the New York Heart Association (NYHA) classification has traditionally been used as a predictor of maternal and fetal prognosis. Thus women who enter the pregnancy in NYHA class I and II were reported to have a maternal mortality rate of less than 1% (0.4%) while class III–IV patients could have a rate that ranged from 5%–15%. A major limitation of this system, however, is that assessments are based upon subjective assessment rather than clinical data.

2. *Risk scoring scales*: Over the last two decades, a number of pregnancy risk scoring scales have been developed to better predict the likelihood of developing cardiac complications during pregnancy.

   a. *CARPREG*: The first risk scoring system for women with various forms of heart disease was the Cardiac Disease in Pregnancy risk index (CARPREG), a population-based study that assesses the risk of an adverse maternal event on the basis of four specific indicators (Table 4.2) [19]. Each indicator is awarded one point each for poor functional status (NYHA >II), cyanosis (<90%), left ventricular (LV) systolic dysfunction, left heart obstruction, and history of cardiac events prior to pregnancy including arrhythmias, stroke, or pulmonary edema [19]. Thus a risk index score of 0 is estimated at a 5% risk, but a risk index of 1 rises to 27%, and at a risk index of >1, the likelihood of adverse event is 75%. For the past two decades this has been the most widely used index despite reported limitations, including that it was event-directed versus lesion-specific, thus excluding patients born with congenital heart disease, with pulmonary hypertension, and prosthetic valves [21].

   b. *ZAHARA*: The ZAHARA (Zwangerschap bij vrouwen met een Aangeboredn HARtAfwijking-II) classification, a second retrospective study, was designed for patients with CHD, but also included patients with mechanical prosthetic valves. In addition, it identified additional predictors, such as use of cardiac medications before pregnancy, and unrepaired cyanotic heart disease, to develop a pregnancy risk score [22] (Table 4.2).

   While both CARPREG I and ZAHARA, have been recognized as important risk assessment systems, they each are limited to their study population, and the retrospective and small sample size nature of the study, but have identified significant predictors for maternal and fetal risk that can impact pregnancy outcomes. These include prior

TABLE 4.2

Pregnancy Risk Stratification Methods

Risk Stratification Index	Categories/Predictors	Risk Score
WHO classification: Index score in 4 areas for women with heart disease includes acquired and congenital	I. No detectable increase of maternal mortality and no/mild increase in morbidity II. Small increase of maternal mortality or moderate increase in morbidity III. Significant increased risk of maternal mortality or morbidity IV. Pregnancy contraindicated	WHO categories range from very low risk (Class I) to highest risk (Class IV)
CARPREG I: Index score for women with heart disease	Pre-pregnancy history of cardiac events (heart failure, stroke) or arrhythmias: 1 point Baseline NYHA functional class >II or cyanosis: 1 point Left heart obstruction: 1 point Mitral valve area: <2 cm^2 Aortic valve area: <1.5^2 Reduced systemic ventricular function (ejection fraction <40%): 1 point	CARPREG I risk score for each CARPREG predictor: 0 point: 5% 1 point: 27% >1 point: 75%
ZAHARA: Index score for congenital heart disease	Prior arrhythmias: 1.5 NYHA class >II: 0.75 Left heart obstruction: 2.5 (Peak aortic gradient >50 mmHG, aortic valve area <1.0 cm^2) Cardiac medications before pregnancy: 1.5 Moderate/severe systemic AV valve regurgitation: 0.75 Moderate/severe subpulmonary regurgitation: 0.75 Mechanical valve prosthesis: 4.5 Cyanotic heart disease: 1.0	ZAHARA: Highest number of the 8 risk factors/or total number of points: 13 Each factor is individually weighted from 0.75 to 4.5 points. A score of >3.51 points carries the highest risk category of 70% risk of developing a cardiac event

cardiac events, left heart obstruction (mitral valve area <2 cm^2, aortic valve area <1.5 cm^2, peak left ventricular outflow tract gradient >30 mmHg), and reduced systemic ventricular systolic function and baseline NYHA functional class >II [14,23].

   c. *Modified World Health Organization (WHO) risk classification*: The modified WHO risk classification is the more widely used and simplest risk scoring scale being used. A large validated prospective study, it integrates all known maternal cardiovascular risk predictors plus varying forms of heart disease, and takes into account medical history that includes comorbidities as well as functional class [25]. Recommended by the European Society of Cardiology (ESC) as the most reliable method of risk assessment to determine pregnancy risk of women with heart disease, it is made up of four categories, the WHO class I, which indicates low risk, WHO class II, intermediate risk, WHO class III, high risk, and WHO class IV, indicates pregnancy is contraindicated because of extreme high risk (Table 4.3) [6,7,21,24,26].

   d. CARPREG II: Recognizing the limitations of CARPREG's original scoring system that excluded prosthetic heart valves and aortopathies, as well as the emergence of additional factors that could influence pregnancy outcomes, such as smoking, as well as factors related to patient management, a more comprehensive risk stratification index has been developed [27]. Silversides et al. have identified 10 predictors of maternal complications, which now make up the updated risk index, CARPREG

II [28]. Summarized in Table 4.4. CARPREG II includes five general predictors that include patient history such as arrhythmias, physical examination, four specific lesions including mechanical valves, aortopathy, and one for delivery of care. CARPREG II also recognizes and allows for the inclusion of other factors that may directly or indirectly impact pregnancy outcomes including patient compliance and access to care. The addition of these factors along with the patient's cardiac condition permits us to determine a more comprehensive level of risk to avoid the likelihood of poor outcomes. It further emphasizes the importance of developing an individualized risk assessment that includes not only clinical predictors but other maternal comorbidities and lifestyle.

Fetal/Neonatal Risk Assessment

Maternal functional class is a major determinant of fetal mortality, with an incremental risk ranging from zero for gravidas who are asymptomatic to a 20%–30% fetal mortality rate in women who fall into NYHA and WHO class III and IV [29,30]. Perinatal complications occur in 34% of women with heart disease compared to 15% of the control population. The most frequent complication, accounting for 61%, is prematurity and small for gestational age; both average birth weight and birth weight percentile in the maternal heart disease group were significantly lower than in the control population [31].

Maternal cyanosis, reduced cardiac output, threatens the growth development and viability of the fetus. Infants born to cyanotic mothers are typically small for gestational age, and premature

TABLE 4.3

Modified WHO Classification of Maternal Cardiovascular Risk

Pregnancy Risk Category	Risk Description	Maternal Risk Factors
WHO I	No detectable increase in maternal mortality and no/mild increase in morbidity risk Maternal cardiac event rate 5.7%–10.5%	Uncomplicated small/mild pulmonary stenosis, PDA, mitral valve prolapse Successfully repaired simple lesions (ASD, VSD, PDA, anomalous pulmonary venous drainage) Atrial or ventricular ectopic beats, isolated
WHO II	Small increase in maternal mortality and moderate increase in morbidity risk Maternal cardiac event rate 2.5%–5%	(If otherwise well and uncomplicated) Unoperated ASD, VSD Repaired TOF Most arrhythmias
WHO II–III	Moderate increase in maternal mortality morbidity risk Maternal cardiac event rate 10%–19%	Mild LV impairment Hypertrophic cardiomyopathy Native or tissue valvular disease (not considered risk category I or IV) Marfan syndrome without aortic dilation Aortic dilation <45 mm in bicuspid aortic valve aortopathy Repaired coarctation
WHO III	Significantly increased maternal mortality or severe morbidity risk Expert counseling required In the event of pregnancy, intensive specialist cardiac and obstetric monitoring needed throughout pregnancy, childbirth and the puerperium Maternal cardiac event rate 9%–27%	Mechanical valve Systemic RV Fontan circulation Cyanotic heart disease (unrepaired) Other complex CHD Aortic dilation 40–45 mm in Marfan syndrome Aortic dilation 45–50 mm in bicuspid aortic valve aortopathy
WHO IV	Extremely high maternal mortality or severe morbidity risk Pregnancy is contraindicated In the event of pregnancy, termination should be discussed If pregnancy continues, care should follow class III recommendations Maternal cardiac event rate 40–100%	Pulmonary arterial hypertension (of any cause) Severe systemic ventricular dysfunction (LV ejection fraction <30%, NYHA class III–IV) Previous peripartum cardiomyopathy with any residual impairment of LV function Severe mitral stenosis, severe symptomatic aortic stenosis Aortic dilation >45 mm in Marfan syndrome Aortic dilation >50 mm in bicuspid aortic valve aortopathy Native severe coarctation

Source: Modified from Regitz-Zagrosek V et al. *Eur Heart J Eur Heart J.* 2018;39:3165–241; Canobbio MM et al. *Circulation.* 2017;135:e50–8; Thorne S et al. *Heart.* 2006;92:1520–5; Jastrow N et al. *Int J Cardiol.* 2011;151(2):209–13.

Abbreviations: AS, aortic stenosis; ASD, atrial septal defect; LV, left ventricle; NYHA, New York Heart Association; PDA, patient ductus arteriosus; RV, right ventricle; TOF, tetralogy of Fallot; VSD, ventricular septal defects; WHO, World Health Organizations.

(see later). The rate of spontaneous abortion is high, and the rate increases roughly in parallel to maternal hypoxemia [32].

Additional risk takes the form of recurrence of CHD in the offspring. It is generally agreed that the risk for CHD increases tenfold over the general population if the mother is affected [19,33]. The exact risk of inheritance varies but it is generally agreed that recurrent risk of any defect is between 3%–7% [34,35]; however, patients with left heart obstructive lesions have a reportedly higher rate [36].

Genetic screening is recommended for patients with confirmed or suspected fetal chromosomal abnormalities [37,38]. Autosomal dominant conditions including 22q11 deletion, Marfan, Noonans, and Holt–Oram syndromes confer a 50% risk of recurrence. Preconception genetic counseling, particularly in those patients with a history of multiple cases of congenital heart lesions, should also be offered to ensure a fully informed decision to proceed with pregnancy. For patients with autosomal dominant conditions such as Turner's, 22q deletion syndrome, a history of familial recurrence of heart defects, or concern for drug exposures, consultation with a geneticist is equally important to determine risk of recurrence or fetal abnormalities. For patients who are already pregnant, genetic counseling beginning at 12–16 weeks can provide parents guidance in deciding whether to proceed or terminate a pregnancy.

Preconception Counseling: Understanding the Short-Term and Long-Term Risks

Beginning in adolescence and continuing throughout their reproductive years, females with heart disease should understand that while for the majority of women with structural or acquired heart disease pregnancy is possible at a low to moderate risk, it remains important to plan all pregnancies, and that she discuss her specific pregnancy risk with her cardiology team on a regular basis. It should be further explained that, regardless of whether she is contemplating a pregnancy, for the majority of women with cardiac disorders, pregnancy is possible, and therefore precautions in terms of contraception must be taken in order to avoid an unplanned pregnancy.

TABLE 4.4a

CARPREG II Predictors of Adverse Events in Pregnant Women with Heart Disease

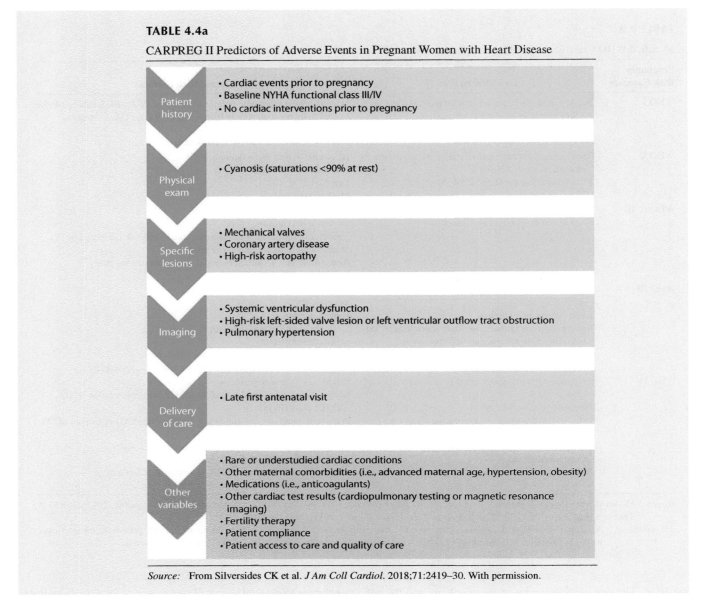

Patient history
- Cardiac events prior to pregnancy
- Baseline NYHA functional class III/IV
- No cardiac interventions prior to pregnancy

Physical exam
- Cyanosis (saturations <90% at rest)

Specific lesions
- Mechanical valves
- Coronary artery disease
- High-risk aortopathy

Imaging
- Systemic ventricular dysfunction
- High-risk left-sided valve lesion or left ventricular outflow tract obstruction
- Pulmonary hypertension

Delivery of care
- Late first antenatal visit

Other variables
- Rare or understudied cardiac conditions
- Other maternal comorbidities (i.e., advanced maternal age, hypertension, obesity)
- Medications (i.e., anticoagulants)
- Other cardiac test results (cardiopulmonary testing or magnetic resonance imaging)
- Fertility therapy
- Patient compliance
- Patient access to care and quality of care

Source: From Silversides CK et al. *J Am Coll Cardiol.* 2018;71:2419–30. With permission.

It is important to counsel the patient about the appropriate choice of contraception, regardless of whether she is in a sexual relationship. For adolescents, these discussions should include her parents so they can not only continue to stress and explain the importance of pregnancy planning, but encourage their daughter to ask questions as she gets older.

Regardless of whether she is considering a pregnancy, each female should be counseled about the potential problems, such as arrhythmias and ventricular dysfunction, that may occur as a result of her heart defect/disorder, as well as any risks that the medications she takes may have on fetal development. Patients at higher risk need to be aware of the increased risk for obstetrical complications including preterm delivery, premature rupture of membranes (PROM), and intrauterine growth retardation (IUGR). The patient should also understand that at the time she begins to contemplate pregnancy, she will undergo a diagnostic evaluation to determine her underlying clinical status and pregnancy risk. It also provides an opportunity to identify and correct any unrepaired or residual heart defects as well as treat any complications such as arrhythmias to improve cardiac function prior to conception.

Multidisciplinary Team

Once the patient has made the decision to become pregnant, she along with her spouse/partner should meet with her cardiologist to once again review the risk of pregnancy and determine the level of obstetrical care she will require. For the woman who falls into WHO II–III, discussion on what degree of level of care is required, and it will be determined what if any noncardiac factors will hinder her access to the availability of an experienced multidisciplinary team required to manage the patient throughout her pregnancy (Table 4.5). In areas where a multidisciplinary team is not available, a model of shared care with a tertiary center prepared to manage high-risk cardiac patients can be initiated.

TABLE 4.4b

CARPREG II Risk Prediction Index: Incidence of Adverse Cardiac Events

Predictor	Points
Prior cardiac event	3
Baseline NYHA III–IV	3
Mechanical valve	3
Ventricular dysfunction	2
High-risk left-sided valve disease	2
Pulmonary hypertension	2
Coronary artery disease	2
High-risk aortopathy	2
No prior cardiac intervention	1
Late pregnancy assessment	1

Risk Prediction Index for Primary Cardiac Events
0–1 points (5%)
2 points (10%)
3 points (15%)
4 points (22%)
>4 points

Source: From Silversides CK et al. *J Am Coll Cardiol.* 2018;71:2419–30. With permission.

TABLE 4.5

Multidisciplinary Approach to Managing Patients with Heart Disease[a]

WHO I Low risk	
Cardiologist (general)	
Obstetrician (general or high risk)	
Anesthesiologist (obstetrical)	
Geneticist	
WHO II Intermediate risk	
Cardiologist (general and/or consultation with ACHD specialist)	
Obstetrician (general or high risk)	
Anesthesiologist (obstetrical)	
Geneticist	
WHO III Moderate high risk	
Cardiologist (specialist: ACHD, HF, HTX, EP)	
Obstetrician (high risk)	
Anesthesiologist (obstetrical or cardiac)	
Genetic	
Neonatologist	
WHO IV Extremely high risk	
Cardiologist (Specialist: ACHD, HF, HTX, EP)	Other
Obstetrician (high risk)	Intensivist
Anesthesiologist (cardiac)	Cardiac surgery
Geneticist	Specialist
Neonatologist	Pulmonary
Social services	Hematologist

Abbreviations: ACHD, adult congenital heart disease; HF, heart failure; HTX, cardiac transplant; EP, electrophysiologist.
[a] Team is individualized to needs of patient.

Diagnostic Testing

Ideally, the diagnostic evaluation is carried out prior to pregnancy, but often it is carried out in a patient with an unplanned pregnancy. Diagnostic testing is individualized; however, most patients will require a minimum of electrocardiogram (ECG), echocardiogram, and exercise stress test. Pregnancy exercise capacity >80% is considered a favorable prognostic indicator for successful pregnancy outcomes [30].

Routine laboratory assays (complete blood count, serum electrolytes, and urinalysis), renal and liver function tests, and thyroid function tests (thyroid-stimulating hormone) should be measured as a baseline, particularly in patients suspected of depressed ventricular function. In addition, during pregnancy the level of B-type natriuretic peptide (BNP) is known to rise to twice the level of non-pregnancy women [39]. In pregnant women with heart disease, however, BNP has been shown to be a predictive of adverse maternal cardiovascular events [40,41].

Additional investigations, such a magnetic resonance imaging (MRI) or computed tomography (CT) are indicated for a comprehensive evaluation of aortic pathology (Table 4.6).

Medication Review

At this time, any medications that have teratogenic effect on the fetus such as warfarin, ACE inhibitors, or ARBs can be discontinued and/or changed.

Long-Term Implications

Finally, for the prospective mother who is at high risk, it is important that she, her partner, and family be made aware not only of the risks of a pregnancy on the cardiovascular system, but also understand the uncertainty of her functional capacity that may be affected as a result of the pregnancy as well as a potentially shortened life span.

TABLE 4.6

Preconception Diagnostic Testing

Diagnostic Test	All Patients	Select patients
Electrocardiogram	♥	
Echocardiogram	♥	
Exercise stress test	♥	
Complete blood count; electrolytes, kidney, liver function, TSH; BNP	♥	
Chest radiograph		♥ Shortness of breath
Holter monitor or prolonged cardiac monitoring		♥ Palpitations, syncope
CT angiogram		♥ Aortic pathology, atherosclerosis
MR imaging/MR angiogram		♥ Cardiomyopathies, aortic pathology
Right/left heart catheterization		♥ Pulmonary hypertension, coronary artery disease

TABLE 4.7

WHO Risk of Combined Hormonal Contraceptives for Various Cardiac Conditions

WHO 1 Always Usable	WHO 2 Broadly Usable	WHO 3 Caution in Use		WHO 4 Do Not Use
Minor valve lesions; mitral valve prolapse with trivial mitral regurgitation; bicuspid aortic valve with normal function	Tissue prosthetic valve lacking any WHO 3 or 4 features	Thrombotic risk, even on warfarin	Mechanical valves: bileaflet valve	Mechanical valves Bjork Shiley, Starr Edwards, any tricuspid valve
	Uncomplicated mild native mitral and aortic valve disease	Risk paradoxical embolism	Previous thromboembolism	Ischemic heart disease
Mild pulmonary stenosis	Most arrhythmias other than atrial fibrillation or flutter		Atrial arrhythmia	Pulmonary hypertension any cause
Repaired coarctation with no hypertension or aneurysm	Hypertrophic cardiomyopathy lacking any WHO 3 or 4 features		Dilated left atrium (0.4 cm)	Dilated cardiomyopathy and LV dysfunction any cause
	Past cardiomyopathy, fully recovered, including peripartum cardiomyopathy		Potential reversal of left to right shunt: unoperated ASD	LVEF, 30% Fontan circulation
Simple congenital lesions successfully repaired in childhood and with no sequelae	Uncomplicated Marfan syndrome			Previous arteritis involving coronary arteries, e.g., Kawasaki disease
	Congenital heart disease lacking any WHO 3 or 4 features; small left to right shunt not reversible with physiological maneuvers, e.g., small VSD			Cyanotic heart disease; pulmonary AVM

Source: From Thorne S et al. *Heart.* 2006;92:1520–5. With permission.

Abbreviations: ASD, atrial septal defect; AVM, arteriovenous malformation; LV, left ventricular; LVEF, left ventricular ejection fraction; VSD, ventricular septal defect.

Depending on the complexity of the heart condition, the decision to permit and/or manage a pregnancy should be a collaborative effort that includes the patient and her spouse/partner as well as input from a multidisciplinary team consisting of a cardiologist, an obstetrician trained in maternal-fetal medicine, an anesthesiologist, and geneticist as indicated, all of whom have knowledge and experience in managing the cardiac patient. A team approach from the beginning ensures an informed decision from the prospective parent(s).

Contraception

Contraceptive counseling should be an integral part of the clinical management of females with cardiac history who are of childbearing age. Regardless of whether the patient is known to be sexually active, she should be instructed on the types of contraceptive that are safe given her heart history. Because there is no contraceptive that is both completely effective and completely free from side effects, the selection of a contraceptive method must be individualized, taking into account the primary cardiac defect, related surgical interventions, associated complications she may have experienced, and medications [24,42,43].

For women who fall into WHO I classification, most contraceptive methods may be used. For women in WHO II, III, IV, the risk varies based on their defect or presence of complications. Tables 4.7 and 4.8 outline the cardiovascular risks for various cardiac conditions.

TABLE 4.8

Cardiovascular Risk of Progestogen-Only Contraceptive Methods

Method	Cardiac Condition	WHO Risk
Progesterin-only pill (POP) minipill	All cardiac patients	1 (but not recommended if pregnancy high risk)
Cerazette	All cardiac patients	1 (but caution if taking warfarin)
Levonelle emergency contraception	All cardiac patients	1
Depo Provera	All cardiac patients unless: High endocarditis risk	3
Mirena IUD	Pulmonary hypertension, Fontan or other condition where vagal reaction would be poorly tolerated	3
Implanon	All cardiac patients	1

Source: From Thorne S et al. *Heart.* 2006;92:1520–5. With permission.

Alternative Options for Pregnancy

A number of patients will be advised against pregnancy, and for others conception may be difficult, which raises the possibility of seeking alternative ways to have children.

For couples having difficulty in conceiving, assisted reproductive technology (ART) including in vitro fertilization and related intracytoplasmic sperm injection, intrauterine insemination, or ovulation induction alone have become widespread, accounting for ~2% of all births worldwide [44]. While ART is becoming more widely used among childless couples, it is not without its side effects and complications for mother and potentially her off-spring, including multi-fetal pregnancies. In one study, the risk of severe maternal morbidity included severe postpartum hemorrhage, ICU admission, and sepsis. In vitro fertilization carried the greatest risk of severe maternal morbidity or maternal death, whereas such increased risks were not evident for noninvasive infertility treatment [44].

In addition, there is concern for an increased prevalence of CHDs [45]. While recent studies indicate no clear evidence of increased CHD risk associated with ART treatment, another study reported in vitro fertilization to be the independent risk factor of CHD [46].

For women with CHD or other acquired heart conditions, there are no guidelines or recommendations on the safety of utilizing ART. For women with complex CHD, the use of hormone injections to stimulate egg production raises concern of thrombotic risk; therefore it is essential that couples discuss the potential risk of ART with their cardiologist, the fertility specialist, and for women with CHD or other autosomal dominant conditions, a geneticist, to determine what risks may be incurred because of her heart condition and her medications, as well as risk to the infant, prior to beginning any treatments.

For those women who have been told the risk of pregnancy is too high, an alternative option may include surrogacy where a gestational carrier, a woman, often a sister, who has an embryo produced from her egg and the sperm of the patient's husband is implanted in her uterus.

Lastly, adoption may be an option. Over time, the laws restricting adoption in couples where one parent has a chronic disease have lifted, and private adoption agencies have also made this a more viable option.

REFERENCES

1. Cantwell R et al. Saving Mothers' Lives: Reviewing maternal deaths to make motherhood safer: 2006–2008. The Eighth Report of the Confidential Enquiries into Maternal Deaths in the United Kingdom. *BJOG*. 2011;118(Suppl. 1):1–203.
2. Szamotulska K, Zeitlin J. What about the mothers? An analysis of maternal mortality and morbidity in perinatal health surveillance systems in Europe. *BJOG*. 2012;119:880–9.
3. Khairy P et al. Changing mortality in congenital heart disease. *J Am Coll Cardiol*. 2010;56:1149–57.
4. Knight M et al. (eds.) on behalf of MBRRACE-UK. *Saving Lives, Improving Mothers' Care—Surveillance of Maternal Deaths in the UK 2012–14 and Lessons Learned to Inform Maternity Care from the UK and Ireland Confidential Enquiries into Maternal Deaths and Morbidity 2009–2014*. Oxford: National Perinatal Epidemiology Unit, University of Oxford; 2016.
5. van Hagen IM et al. Global cardiac risk assessment in the registry of pregnancy and cardiac disease: Results of a registry from the European Society of Cardiology. *Eur J Heart Fail*. 2016;18:523–33.
6. Greutmann M, Pieper PG. Pregnancy in women with congenital heart disease. *Eu Heart J*. 2015;36:2491–9.
7. Regitz-Zagrosek V et al. 2018 ESC guidelines on the management of cardiovascular diseases during pregnancy. *Eur Heart J*. 2018;39:3165–241.
8. Roos-Hesselink JW et al., on behalf of the ROPAC Investigators. Outcome of pregnancy in patients with structural or ischaemic heart disease: Results of a registry of the European Society of Cardiology. *Eur Heart J*. 2013;34:657–65.
9. Canobbio MM et al. Management of pregnancy in patients with complex congenital heart disease. A scientific statement for healthcare professionals from the American Heart Association. *Circulation*. 2017;135:e50–8.
10. Drenthan W et al. Pregnancy and delivery in women after Fontan palliation. *Heart*. 2006;92:1290–4.
11. Gouton M et al. Maternal and fetal outcomes of pregnancy with Fontan circulation: A multicentric observational study. *Int J Cardiol*. 2015;187:84–9.
12. Canobbio MM, Morris CD, Graham TP, Landzberg MJ. Pregnancy outcomes after atrial repair for transportation of the great arteries. *Am J Cardiol*. 2006;98:668–72.
13. Trigas V et al. Pregnancy-related obstetric and cardiologic problems in women after atrial switch operation for transposition of the great arteries. *Circ J*. 2014;78:443–9.
14. Ruys TEP, Cornette J, Roos-Hesselink JW. Pregnancy and delivery in cardiac disease. *J Cardiol*. 2013;61:107–12.
15. Lund LH et al. The Registry of the International Society for Heart and Lung Transplantation: Thirtieth official adult heart transplant report—2013; focus theme: Age. *J Heart Lung Transplant*. 2013;32(10):951–64.
16. McKay DB et al. Reproduction and transplantation: Report on the AST Consensus Conference on Reproductive Issues and Transplantation. *Am J Transpl*. 2005;5(7):1592–9.
17. Armenti VT, Constantinescu S, Moritz MJ, Davison JM. Pregnancy after transplantation. *Transplant Rev*. 2008;22:223–40.
18. Armenti VT et al. Report from the National Transplantation Pregnancy Registry (NTPR): Outcomes of pregnancy after transplantation. *Clin Transplants*. 2004:103–14.
19. Siu SC et al. Prospective multicenter study of pregnancy outcomes in women with heart disease. *Circulation*. 2001;104:515–21.
20. American College of Obstetricians and Gynecologists. Marijuana Use During Pregnancy and Lactation. *ACOG Committee Opinion Number 722*, October 2017.
21. Balci A et al. Prospective validation and assessment of cardiovascular and offspring risk models for pregnant women with congenital heart disease. *Heart*. 2014;100(17):1373–81.
22. Elkayam U. How to predict pregnancy risk in an individual woman with heart disease. *J Am Coll Cardiol*. 2018;71:2431–3.
23. Drenthen W et al. ZAHARA Investigators: Predictors of pregnancy complications in women with congenital heart disease. *Eur Heart J*. 2010;31:2124–32.
24. Thorne S, MacGregor A, Nelson-Piercy C. Risks of contraception and pregnancy in heart disease. *Heart*. 2006;92:1520–5.
25. Khairy P et al. Pregnancy outcomes in women with congenital heart disease. *Circulation*. 2006;113:517–24.
26. Jastrow N et al. Prediction of complications in pregnant women with cardiac diseases referred to a tertiary center. *Int J Cardiol*. 2011;151(2):209–13.
27. Elkayam U, Goland S, Pieper PG, Silverisde CK. High-risk cardiac disease in pregnancy: Part I. *J Am Coll Cardiol*. 2016;68(4):396–410.
28. Silversides CK et al. Pregnancy outcomes in women with heart disease. The CARPREG II study. *J Am Coll Cardiol*. 2018;71:2419–30.

29. Wada H et al. analysis of maternal and fetal risk in 584 pregnancies with heart disease. *Nippon Sanka Fuminka Gakkai Zasshi.* 1996;48:255–62.
30. Drenthen W et al. Outcome of pregnancy in women with congenital heart disease: A literature review. *J Am Coll Cardiol.* 2007;49:2303–11.
31. Gelson E et al. Effect of maternal heart disease on fetal growth. *Obstet Gynecol.* 2011;117:886–91.
32. Presbitero P et al. Pregnancy in cyanotic congenital heart disease: Outcome of mother and fetus. *Circulation.* 1994;89:2673–76.
33. Siu SC et al. Adverse neonatal and cardiac outcomes are more common in pregnant women with heart disease. *Circulation.* 2002;105:2179–84.
34. Pierpont ME, Basson CT, Benson DW et al. Genetic basis for congenital heart defects: Current knowledge: A scientific statement from the American Heart Association Congenital Cardiac Defects Committee, Council on Cardiovascular Disease in the Young: Endorsed by the American Academy of Pediatrics. *Circulation.* 2007;115:3015–38.
35. Øyen N et al. Recurrence of congenital heart defects in families. *Circulation.* 2009;120:295–301.
36. Gill HK, Splitt M, Sharland GK, Simpson JM. Patterns of recurrence of congenital heart disease: An analysis of 6640 consecutive pregnancies evaluated by detailed fetal echocardiography. *J Am Coll Cardiol.* 2003;42:923–9.
37. ACOG Practice Bulletin No.77: Screening for fetal chromosomal abnormalities. *Obstet Gynecol.* 2007;109:217–27.
38. Siu SC et al. Genetic counseling in the adult with congenital heart disease: What is the role? *Curr Cardiol Rep.* 2011;13: 347.
39. Hameed AB, Chan K, Ghamsary M, Elkayam U. Longitudinal changes in the B-type natriuretic peptide levels in normal pregnancy and postpartum. *Clin Cardiol.* 2009;32:60–2.
40. Kampman MA et al.; ZAHARA II investigators. N-terminal pro-B-type natriuretic peptide predicts cardiovascular complications in pregnant women with congenital heart disease. *Eur Heart J.* 2014;35:708–15.
41. Tanous D et al. B-type natriuretic peptide in pregnant women with heart disease. *J Am Coll Cardiol.* 2010;56:1247–53.
42. American College Obstetrics Gynecology (ACOG) Practice Bulletin #121. Long-acting reversible contraceptives: Implants and intrauterine devices. *Obstet Gynecol.* 2011;118: 184–96.
43. Miner PA et al. Contraceptive practices of women with complex congenital heart disease. *Am J Cardiol.* 2017;119: 911–5.
44. Dayan N et al. Infertility treatment and risk of severe maternal morbidity: A propensity score-matched cohort study. *CMAJ.* 2019;191:E118–27.
45. Iwashima S, Ishikawa T, Itoh H. Reproductive technologies and the risk of congenital heart defects. *Human Fertility.* 2016;20:1–8.
46. Pavlicek J et al. Congenital heart defects according to the types of the risk factors—A single center experience. *J Matern Fetal Neo Med.* 2019;32:3606–11.
47. Canobbio MM. Pregnancy in congenital heart disease: Maternal risk. *Prog Pediatr Cardiol.* 2004;19:1–3.

5

Termination and Contraceptive Options for the Cardiac Patient

Blake Zwerling and Rachel Perry

KEY POINTS

- Reproductive age women with cardiac disease must have access to contraception and preconception counseling
- Considerations for contraception in a cardiac patient include its thrombogenic potential, effect on blood pressure, fluid balance, glucose, lipids, drug metabolism, potential risk of bacteremia, and vasovagal reaction

- Progestin-only contraceptives do not increase risk of hypertension, stroke, myocardial infarction, or venous thromboembolism
- A multidisciplinary approach with the heart team is essential for patients with complex cardiac disease seeking pregnancy termination

Introduction

All patients of reproductive age should be counseled on family planning and contraception as part of routine health care. This is particularly crucial for women* with cardiac conditions given their potentially heightened risk of pregnancy-associated morbidity and mortality. When a patient with a cardiac condition is faced with an unintended pregnancy, clinicians are tasked with risk assessment and subsequent options counseling, including pregnancy continuation and induced abortion. This chapter explores contraception and induced abortion options for women with cardiac conditions.

Contraception Considerations for Women with Cardiac Disease

The U.S. Medical Eligibility Criteria (MEC) for Contraception Use details the recommendations from the U.S. Centers for Disease Control and Prevention (CDC) on contraceptive choices for various medical conditions. These classifications are referenced in this chapter for select cardiac conditions. Noncardiac contraindications to methods are not addressed here; however, the MEC (available online and in a mobile application) should be referenced for women with other medical comorbidities or special considerations such as the postpartum period or during concomitant breastfeeding. (See Box 5.1).

---

* Of note, although the term "woman" is used throughout this chapter with female pronouns for simplicity, these recommendations refer to all people with uteruses of reproductive age. This includes intersex, gender nonconforming, and trans individuals at risk of pregnancy.

BOX 5.1   UNITED STATES MEDICAL ELIGIBILITY CRITERIA (MEC) FOR CONTRACEPTIVE USE [1]

U.S. MEC Category	Description
1	No restrictions for a contraceptive method for the medical condition
2	Benefits of the contraceptive method generally outweigh the risks
3	Theoretical or proven risks generally outweigh the benefits
4	Unacceptable health risk

How Do You Counsel Women of Reproductive Age with Cardiac Conditions about Contraception?

Despite increased risks of pregnancy, many women with cardiac disease do not receive adequate contraceptive counseling. Over half of patients with congenital heart disease report receiving no cardiac-specific contraception counseling [4], and many leave medical visits with unanswered questions about contraception and pregnancy [5]. One study found that 63% of women reported no knowledge of contraindications to particular contraceptive methods specific to their heart disease [4].

Building a trusting, nonjudgmental dynamic is key: observational studies have shown that the interpersonal quality of family planning counseling is associated with higher patient satisfaction in their contraceptive method as well as overall contraceptive use [6]. More effective forms of contraception should be emphasized while still respecting patient autonomy. In addition, women should be counseled on dual protection for sexually transmitted infections (STIs), and clinicians may offer advance provision of emergency contraception [6].*

Ideally, patients with cardiac conditions should receive joint counseling with their cardiologists and obstetrician-gynecologists to streamline recommendations for contraceptive methods along with information on maternal and fetal prognosis during pregnancy. This multidisciplinary approach prevents conflicting advice from different providers and patient concerns can be answered simultaneously [2].

For hormonal methods of contraception, unique considerations include:

- Does the method have thrombogenic potential?
- Could it affect blood pressure, volume status, blood glucose levels, or lipid profiles?
- Does it affect metabolism of anticoagulants or cardiac medications?

For contraceptive methods requiring procedures such as permanent surgical contraception or intrauterine devices, considerations include [3]:

- Potential risk of bacteremia/endocarditis
- Anesthesia risk
- Risk of Vasovagal reaction

All of these possibilities must be weighed against the potential risk of pregnancy.

Contraceptive Methods

Highly Effective Methods

Intrauterine Devices

Intrauterine devices (IUDs) are a highly effective form of long-acting reversible contraception (LARC) that include hormonal (levonorgestrel) and nonhormonal (copper) options.

- *Mechanism of action*: Multiple mechanisms of action contribute to the effectiveness of IUDs. The levonorgestrel in hormonal IUDs thickens cervical mucus, which acts as a barrier to sperm. Secondary progestin effects include slowed tubal motility and endometrial decidualization and atrophy [7]. Copper impairs sperm migration, viability, and the acrosomal reaction, thereby preventing fertilization.†
- *Efficacy*: All IUDs boast high efficacy. With typical use, first-year pregnancy rates are 0.1%–0.2% for the 52 mg levonorgestrel IUD and 0.5%–0.8% for the copper IUD [8].
- *Benefits*: include safety,‡ quick return of fertility, and ease of use. The 52 mg levonorgestrel IUD causes amenorrhea in 20%–40% of patients. For those who

continue to have menses, most report a reduction in menstrual flow and dysmenorrhea. Therefore, hormonal IUDs may be a particularly good choice for women on anticoagulation or with bleeding diatheses (see "Anticoagulation" section). Unscheduled bleeding may occur with any of the devices, though it generally improves with time [9]. The copper IUD does not affect ovulation but may cause increased menstrual flow and dysmenorrhea and therefore should be avoided with those patients at risk for hemorrhage, including women on therapeutic anticoagulation. It is approved for longer term use in the United States (up to 10 years) and acts as a very effective form of emergency contraception if inserted within 5 days of unprotected intercourse.

- Risks of IUDs include infection, uterine perforation, vasovagal reaction during placement, and a theoretical risk of endocarditis [10]. Large epidemiological studies have not identified an increased risk of stroke, myocardial infarction (MI), or venous thromboembolism (VTE) for progestin-only contraceptives such as the hormonal IUD [1]. For Fontan-type circulation, IUDs should be avoided due to the risk of cardiovascular collapse with a vasovagal reaction, which occurs in approximately 2% of patients undergoing IUD insertion [12]. The theoretical concern for endocarditis has not been demonstrated (see section "Pregnancy Contraindicated [WHO Class IV], Endocarditis"). The American Heart Association guidelines do not recommend antibiotic prophylaxis for genitourinary procedures, including IUD insertion [13].

Contraceptive Implant

- The etonogestrel contraceptive implant is a radio-opaque single-rod progestin implant that is placed subdermally in the inner arm. It contains 68 mg of etonogestrel and provides highly effective contraception for at least 3 years with a pregnancy rate of only 0.05% in the first year [8]. Its primary mechanism of action is suppression of ovulation. Secondary progestin mechanisms are similar to the hormonal IUD [14].
- Benefits include reduced dysmenorrhea. Some users report irregular bleeding, which may or may not improve with continued use [14].
- Bosentan—a dual endothelin receptor antagonist commonly used in the treatment of pulmonary artery hypertension—interacts with etonogestrel, reducing its efficacy (see section "Pregnancy Contraindicated [WHO Class IV], Pulmonary Artery Hypertension").

Permanent Surgical Sterilization

- Female permanent contraception (tubal sterilization) is highly effective, with a 10-year pregnancy risk of less than 1% [15]. It requires a surgical procedure that may involve general anesthesia and therefore risks of anesthesia should be considered when counseling patients.
- Vasectomy (male permanent contraception) is the most cost-effective and safest method of permanent

---

* Of note, it is also best practice to screen patients for intimate partner violence, including reproductive coercion and contraception sabotage.
† There is no evidence that IUDs disrupt an implanted pregnancy [91].
‡ Though previous IUDs like the Dalkon shield carried an increased infectious risk due to braided strings, modern IUDs use monofilament strings.

sterilization. It should be recommended to women with cardiac conditions who are monogamous with a male partner. Male sterilization can be performed in the out-patient setting [16].

Moderately Effective Methods

Estrogen-Containing Combined Hormonal Contraceptives: Contraceptive Pill, Patch, and Ring

Combined hormonal contraception (CHC) contains both synthetic estrogen and progestin. Ethinyl estradiol is the estrogen in most CHCs in the United States, but various progestins are used depending on the product formulation. CHCs are available as oral contraceptive pills, contraceptive patches, and contraceptive vaginal rings.

- *Mechanism of action*: CHCs function by preventing ovulation. Secondary progestin effects also contribute to the mechanism of action.
- *Efficacy*: The typical use failure rate is 9% in the first year, largely due to inconsistent use [17–19].
- *Benefits*: Include cycle regularity and decreased dysmenorrhea.
- *Side effects*: Include irregular bleeding, nausea, bloating, breast tenderness, and headaches, though these often resolve in the first 3 months [20]. The synthetic estrogen component of CHCs increases the production of hepatic pro-coagulation factors (VII, VIII, and X) while simultaneously decreasing the production of fibrinolytic factors (tissue plasminogen activator and antiplasmin), which can result in increased thrombo-embolic events [3]. However, the risk of venous thromboembolic or arterial thrombotic events are lower with CHCs than during pregnancy or the immediate post-partum period [21,22]. CHC users are at an increased risk of MI and cerebrovascular accident (CVA) [23]. Some progestins are associated with a slight decrease in HDL and increase in LDL cholesterol [24]. Oral, but not transdermal estrogens are associated with an increase in serum triglycerides [25,26]. Potential fluid retention may exacerbate cardiac conditions [3]. Studies in both normotensive and chronic hypertensive patients have shown a small increase in systolic blood pressure of 7–8 mmHg for women using CHCs [27,28].
- *Contraindications*: CHCs should not be given to smokers over the age of 35, those with known thrombophilias, or a history of VTE or stroke [1]. Other contraindications include those with multiple risk factors for arterial cardiovascular disease (older age, smoking, diabetes, and hypertension), known ischemic heart disease, complicated valvular disease, and migraine with aura (due to increased stroke risk) [1]. The patch (applied weekly) and vaginal ring (inserted monthly) are thought to confer similar benefits and risks as the contraceptive pill but have been less well studied. Patients with contraindications to estrogen should also avoid these methods.

Progestin-Only Oral Contraceptive Pills

The primary mechanism of progestin-only pills (POPs) is thought to be cervical mucus thickening; they do not reliably inhibit ovulation. The effectiveness of POPs is lower than other progestin-only contraceptives as they require daily dosing. National survey data do not distinguish between CHCs and POPs, but the typical failure rate within the first year is likely higher than the 9% cited due to the necessity for strict dosing timing (pills should be considered skipped if they are taken more than 3 hours late) [17]. Studies have not identified an increased risk of MI, CVA, or VTE with the use of POPs [29,30]. They are therefore a safe contraceptive option for a wide range of cardiac patients.

Depot Medroxyprogesterone Acetate Injections

Depot medroxyprogesterone acetate (DMPA) is an injectable intramuscular progestin-only contraceptive dosed every 3 months. It works primarily by suppressing ovulation [31]. The unintended pregnancy rate in the first year of typical use is 6%, with most failures associated with late injections [17].

DMPA can reduce or eliminate menstrual bleeding [32]. Side effects of DMPA include irregular menstrual bleeding, injection site reactions, headache, mood changes, and weight gain [33]. A 2016 systematic review found the mean weight gain for DMPA users was less than 2 kg for most studies, and generally comparable to users of other contraceptive methods [34]. Though DMPA can induce bone mineral density loss, best available data indicate that DMPA does not reduce peak bone mass or increase the risk of osteoporotic fractures later in life for women at average risk of osteoporosis [35]. There may be a delay in return in fertility for up to 1 year after cessation of DMPA use [1].

DMPA should not be used for those with ischemic heart disease as it can decrease HDL levels. It should be used with caution for women with hypertension given concern for increased risk of cardiovascular events (see section "Hypertension") [1].

Least Effective Methods

Barrier Methods and Pericoital Contraceptives

Barrier and pericoital methods include male and female/receptive condom, the cervical diaphragm, spermicidal agents, and the contraceptive sponge. These methods must be used with each act of intercourse. Therefore, they are prone to reduced effectiveness due to inconsistent or incorrect use. There are few contraindications to the use of barrier methods.

Condoms are the only form of contraception that can help prevent or reduce the risk of transmission of STIs. Given their user-dependent nature, unintended pregnancy with typical use is 18% and 21% for male and female condoms, respectively, within the first year [17].

The diaphragm, contraceptive sponge, and cervical cap function by maintaining a reservoir of spermicide against the cervix. Spermicide creates a chemical barrier by immobilizing sperm. All have high failure rates, making them less optimal choices for women with cardiac conditions for whom pregnancy carries high risk [17].

Fertility Awareness–Based or "Natural Family Planning" Methods

Fertility awareness–based methods of contraception are based on avoiding intercourse on the fertile days of a woman's cycle [36]. These methods have a 24% pregnancy rate in the first year with typical use [17].

Emergency Contraception

Emergency contraception (EC) is used to prevent pregnancy after unprotected intercourse* and includes the copper IUD and oral medications. EC does not disrupt an implanted pregnancy [37].

The copper IUD is the most effective form of emergency contraception. When inserted within 72 hours, it prevents over 95% of expected pregnancies [38,39]. In addition, it has the advantage of providing ongoing contraception.

Oral EC functions primarily by delaying ovulation [40]. In the United States, two formulations are available: ulipristal and levonorgestrel. Of these, ulipristal prevents two-thirds and levonorgestrel one-half of expected pregnancies [38].† Ulipristal is a selective progesterone receptor modulator taken as a single pill within 120 hours of unprotected intercourse, though efficacy is higher with earlier dosing. Levonorgestrel EC (available over the counter), is either a single dose or two tablets taken 12 hours apart. There are no cardiovascular conditions for which the risks of EC outweigh potential benefits [1]. (See Box 5.2).

Contraceptive Considerations by Cardiac Disease

Risk of Pregnancy by Cardiac Condition

See Box 5.3.

Low Risk (WHO Class I) Conditions

Small Shunts (ASD, VSD, PDA, PFO)

Women with repaired shunts have no increased thrombogenic risk and therefore are candidates for all forms of contraception. Atrial septal defects confer a risk of paradoxical thromboembolism and stroke, making CHCs Category 3 [42]. However, VSDs and small PDAs do not carry the same risk, so CHCs are not contraindicated [41].‡ Two community-based studies have failed to find a consistent independent association between asymptomatic PFOs and thromboembolic events [43,44]. Therefore, CHC use is permissible for women with asymptomatic PFOs, and screening is not indicated prior to initiation [42]. CHCs are Category 3 for those with a previous thromboembolic event [1].

Mitral Valve Prolapse/Mild Pulmonary Stenosis

The MEC does not distinguish between valvular defects: CHCs are Category 2 for all of them [1]. However, other schema that

parse out types of valvular defects note that women with mitral valve prolapse and minimal to no regurgitation have no contraindication to CHC use [3].

Isolated Premature Atrial or Ventricular Contractions

All methods of contraception are considered appropriate for isolated premature atrial or ventricular contractions if no underlying structural abnormality exists [3].

Moderate Risk (WHO Class II)

Repaired Tetralogy of Fallot

In the absence of right-to-left shunting, CHCs are safe for women with repaired tetralogy of Fallot. There is a theoretical risk of endocarditis from the copper IUD (Category 2, see section "Endocarditis"), but there are no further restrictions on the forms of contraception these women can receive [3].

Arrhythmia

While CHCs are appropriate for many of women with arrhythmias, they should be avoided for those with atrial fibrillation or flutter due to increased thromboembolic risk [3].

Mild Left Ventricular Dysfunction (Left Ventricular Ejection Fraction 40%–50%)

The risks of thrombosis, fluid retention, and hypertension must all be considered for women with mild left ventricular dysfunction. Recommendations for women in this category are largely based on expert opinion and vary widely. Whereas the MEC rates CHCs as absolutely contraindicated (Category 4), other schema do not rate the risk as highly. Progestin-only methods and IUDs are considered safe [1].

Hypertrophic Cardiomyopathy

Data are very limited on contraceptive safety for patients with hypertrophic cardiomyopathy [45–48]. Classification of contraceptive options is largely based on potential sequalae, including arrhythmias, thromboembolism, and endocarditis. For uncomplicated cases, CHCs are generally considered Category 2, but should be considered Category 3 if sequalae of the disease are present.

Marfan Syndrome

The risk of aortic dissection for patients with Marfan syndrome is proportional to the aortic root diameter, with morbidity increasing sharply with dilatation >4 cm (see section "Aortic Root Dilatation >4 cm") [3]. Without aortic root dilatation, there are no specific recommendations for contraceptives by the MEC [1].

Ehlers-Danlos and Other Connective Tissue Disorders

There are no specific recommendations for women with Ehlers-Danlos regarding contraception, therefore recommendations are the same as for Marfan syndrome [3].

Repaired Aortic Coarctation

Due to the potential of exacerbating hypertension, CHCs are Category 3 for women with a known aortic aneurysm or persistent hypertension [1].

---

* Including failure of another method.
† It should be noted that the efficacy of oral emergency contraception may be reduced for overweight and obese women and they should be counseled appropriately [11].
‡ This recommendation includes those with unrepaired defects or uncomplicated repairs.

BOX 5.2   CONTRACEPTIVE METHOD CONTRAINDICATIONS [1]

Method of Contraception	Cardiac Contraindications	Noncardiac Contraindications
IUDs	• Care should be taken with those with contraindications to Valsalva such as those who have had a Fontan procedure	• Severe distortion of the uterine cavity due to difficulty of insertion and increased risk of expulsion • Active pelvic infection • Cervical cancer awaiting treatment (initiation) • Gestational trophoblastic disease • Immediate post-septic abortion or postpartum sepsis • Current purulent cervicitis or known chlamydia or gonorrhea infection • Pelvic TB • Endometrial cancer (initiation, though hormonal IUD may be used as treatment in poor surgical candidates) • Unexplained vaginal bleeding suspicious for serious condition (initiation, continuation) Hormonal IUDs • Breast cancer • Cirrhosis Copper IUDs • Wilson disease or a copper allergy
Implant	• Ischemic heart disease (continuation) • History of CVA (continuation) • SLE with antiphospholipid antibodies (or unknown)	• Known or suspected breast cancer • Cirrhosis • Unexplained vaginal bleeding • Benign or malignant liver tumors • Bosentan—a dual endothelin receptor antagonist commonly used in the treatment of pulmonary artery hypertension—interacts with etonogestrel, reducing its efficacy
CHCs	• Personal history of DVT/PE • Migraine with aura • Hypertension • Ischemic heart disease • Known thrombogenic mutation • History of CVA • Peripartum cardiomyopathy • <21 days postpartum or 21–45 days postpartum with VTE risk factors • Smokers age >35 • Diabetes >20 years or with microvascular disease • Major surgery with prolonged immobilization • SLE with antiphospholipid antibodies (or unknown) • Complicated valvular heart disease • Multiple risk factors of atherosclerotic disease	• Known or suspected breast cancer • Benign or malignant liver tumors • Acute liver disease • Cirrhosis • Malabsorptive bariatric surgeries may interfere with efficacy, as can some anticonvulsants • Medically treated or current gallbladder disease • History of CHC-related cholestasis • Complicated solid organ transplant • Select antiretroviral, anticonvulsant, and antiparasitic therapy
POPs	• History of CVA (continuation) • Ischemic heart disease (continuation) • SLE with antiphospholipid antibodies (or unknown)	• Known or suspected breast cancer • Benign or malignant liver tumors • Cirrhosis • Malabsorptive bariatric surgeries may interfere with efficacy, as can some anticonvulsants • Select anticonvulsant therapy • Rifampin or rifabutin therapy
DMPA	• Diabetes >20 years or with microvascular disease • Uncontrolled hypertension • Multiple risk factors of atherosclerotic disease • SLE with antiphospholipid antibodies or severe thrombocytopenia (or unknown)	• Known or suspected breast cancer • Undiagnosed abnormal uterine bleeding • Malignant liver tumors • Cirrhosis • High risk for nontraumatic fractures

Abbreviations: IUD, intrauterine device; TB, tuberculosis; CVA, cerebrovascular accident; SLE, systemic lupus erythematosus; DVT/PE, deep vein thrombosis/pulmonary embolism; CHC, combined hormonal contraceptive; VTE, venous thromboembolism; POP, progestin-only pill; DMPA, depo-medroxyprogesterone acetate contraceptive injection.

BOX 5.3   MODIFIED WHO PREGNANCY RISK CLASSIFICATION SYSTEM BY CARDIAC CONDITION

WHO Category	Description	Conditions
I	No detectable increased risk of mortality and no or mild increased morbidity	• Small shunts (ASD, VSD, PDA, PFO) • Mitral valve prolapse/mild pulmonary stenosis • Isolated premature atrial or ventricular contractions
II	Small increased risk of maternal mortality or moderate increased risk of morbidity (presuming the patient is otherwise well)	• Repaired tetralogy of Fallot • Arrhythmia • Mild left ventricular dysfunction (left ventricular ejection fraction 40%–50%) • Hypertrophic cardiomyopathy • Marfan syndrome • Ehlers-Danlos and connective tissue disorders • Repaired aortic coarctation
III	Significantly increased risk of maternal mortality or severe morbidity	• Ischemic cardiovascular disease • Mechanical prosthetic valve • Complex congenital heart disease • Aortic root dilatation >4 cm
IV	Extremely high risk of maternal mortality or severe morbidity; pregnancy is contraindicated	• Severe pulmonary hypertension • Significant left ventricular dysfunction • Severe or complicated mitral or aortic stenosis (coexisting atrial fibrillation, pulmonary hypertension, or history of endocarditis) • Peripartum cardiomyopathy with any residual impairment of left ventricular function • Fontan-type circulation

Source: Adapted from Thorne S et al. *J Fam Plan Reprod Heal Care.* 2006;32(2):75–81.

High Risk (WHO Class III)

Ischemic Cardiovascular Disease

Given its rarity, little data exist on the risks of contraception and pregnancy for women with a history of MI. Those with significant residual left ventricular dysfunction or NYHA class III or IV symptoms should be considered WHO class IV risk [3]. CHCs are generally contraindicated due to concern for thrombosis, hypertension, hyperlipidemia, and glucose derangements [1,42]. DMPA is Category 3 due to reduction in HDL [1]. The MEC labels progestin-only contraceptive methods Category 2 for continuation and Category 3 for initiation due to theoretical concern for lipid profile effects. For women with ischemic heart disease generally, the copper IUD is the ideal method of contraception. However, if this method is not an option, other LARC methods should be encouraged [1].

Mechanical Prosthetic Valve

Women with mechanical prosthetic valves carry an increased risk of thromboembolic events [49]. However, the risk will vary depending on the type of valve, how long it has been in place, and which valvular position it is in. In addition, these patients are often on anticoagulation (see "Women on Anticoagulation"). Overall, CHCs are Category 3–4 [1]. Progestin-only methods are safe for women with mechanical prosthetic valves [1]. LARC methods are preferred. The MEC rates IUDs as Category 4 due to concern for infective endocarditis with insertion, but newer data including a prospective trial of 20 anticoagulated women demonstrated improved bleeding profiles, higher hemoglobin, and no cases of endocarditis for hormonal IUD users, suggesting this method may be safe for use [50].

Complex Congenital Heart Disease

CHCs should be avoided in women with complex congenital heart disease due to risk of pulmonary artery thrombosis and pulmonary emboli [41,51].

Aortic Root Dilatation >4 cm

CHCs are Category 3 for patients with aortic root dilatation >4 cm due to concern for exacerbation of hypertension and potential aortic dissection [1].

Pregnancy Contraindicated (WHO Class IV)*

Severe Pulmonary Hypertension

CHCs are Category 4 for women with severe pulmonary hypertension due to thrombotic and hypertensive risk [1]. Of note, bosentan—a dual endothelin receptor antagonist—can reduce the effectiveness of ethinyl estradiol as well as several progestin-only methods (contraceptive implant and POP). DMPA does not interact with bosentan, but women with pulmonary hypertension are often anticoagulated, which carries the theoretical concern of hematoma. IUDs may be contraindicated due to the potentially fatal consequences of a vasovagal reaction during placement. In cases where no other acceptable method is available, this risk may be mediated with the use of a paracervical block or epidural anesthesia [3].

---

* Given high risk of pregnancy-associated morbidity, highly effective contraception is recommended, making POPs and less effective methods relatively contraindicated [1].

Significant Left Ventricular Dysfunction

Considerations for contraceptives for women with significant left ventricular dysfunction are the same as for those with mild to moderate dysfunction (see "Mild Left Ventricular Dysfunction"), but with higher risk of morbidity.

Severe or Complicated Mitral or Aortic Stenosis (Coexisting Atrial Fibrillation, Pulmonary Hypertension, or History of Endocarditis)

The MEC lumps valvular heart defects into a single category, considering CHCs "broadly useable" for uncomplicated lesions without sequalae [1,3]. CHCs are Category 4 for those with complicated lesions. Progestin-only methods and IUDs are Category 1 [1], though there is a theoretical concern for infective endocarditis for IUDs [3].

Peripartum Cardiomyopathy with Any Residual Impairment of Left Ventricular Function

A systematic review revealed no primary research articles that addressed the safety of any contraceptive method among women with peripartum cardiomyopathy [45]. The patient's functional status and time since delivery (less than 6 months vs. greater than 6 months) aids in classifying contraceptive methods. Depending on the time since delivery, CHCs are Category 3 or 4 for women with normal cardiac function. POPs, DMPA, and the implant are all Category 1 with normal or mildly impaired cardiac dysfunction, but Category 2 for women with moderate to severe cardiac dysfunction. Regardless of functional status, all IUDs are Category 2. Though no direct evidence on the safety of IUDs exists, there is theoretical concern for the induction of arrhythmias during IUD insertion. Limited evidence did not demonstrate any cases of arrhythmia or infective endocarditis in women with cardiac disease who received IUDs [1].

Fontan-Type Circulation

Though not specifically mentioned in the WHO classification system, Fontan-type circulation is considered a contraindication to pregnancy [41,52,53]. Contraceptive recommendations are the same as for others with complex congenital heart disease (see "Complex Congenital Heart Disease").

Hypertension

Estrogen-containing methods may affect blood pressure. Estrogen stimulates angiotensinogen production by the liver and simultaneously increases activation of the renin-angiotensin system [54]. Given the cardiovascular risks of pregnancy, elevated blood pressure reading should not delay the initiation of contraception, though it may affect the choice of method.

CHCs increase systolic blood pressure an average of 8 mmHg and diastolic 6 mmHg [27]. The effect is dose-dependent and increases with age and BMI [55]. The increase in blood pressure is small, but it does confer an increased risk of MI and CVA, particularly for women with preexisting hypertension [56]. CHCs are Category 3 for women with moderate hypertension (140–159/90–99) or adequately treated hypertension. If estrogen-containing methods are used, the lowest possible estrogen dose should be chosen [29]. CHCs are Category 4 for women with severe hypertension >160/100 [1]. Given these risks, blood pressure measurement is recommended before the initiation of CHCs [57].

The MEC does not distinguish between estrogen-containing hormonal contraceptive methods in its recommendations for women with hypertension [1]. There is a paucity of data for the effect of other estrogen-containing contraceptive methods. Systemic estrogen levels for the ring are 50% that of CHCs, but evidence suggests the ring still confers an increased risk of CVA [29,58]. In contrast, the patch has been shown to result in higher estrogen levels than CHCs and is assumed to confer similar risk.

Progestin-only methods do not affect blood pressure [59]. POPs are Category 1 for women with mild or well-controlled hypertension, and Category 2 for women with severe hypertension citing "Limited evidence suggest[ing] that among women with hypertension, those who used POPs or progestin-only injectables had a small increased risk for cardiovascular events" [1].

DMPA is Category 2 for women with moderate or well-controlled hypertension and Category 3 for women with severe hypertension [3].

No studies exist exploring the relationship between progestin-containing implants and IUDs on blood pressure. There is little biological plausibility that the hormonal IUDs would increase blood pressure [3]. The MEC therefore gives these methods the same ratings as POPs: Category 1 for moderate or well-controlled hypertension and Category 2 for severe. There are no limitations on the use of copper IUDs [1].

Multiple Risk Factors for Atherosclerotic Disease

For women with multiple risk factors for atherosclerotic disease (e.g., age >35, smoking, diabetes, hypertension, low HDL, high LDL, or high triglycerides), the copper IUD is Category 1. POPs, the implant, and the hormonal IUD are all Category 2, DMPA Category 3, and CHCs Category 3/4. Evidence backing the recommendation is sparse. Given these women might have a substantially increased risk of cardiovascular disease, CHCs represent an unacceptable risk. DMPA is rated Category 3, as it persists for some time after discontinuation in the case of adverse effects. The MEC states that simple addition of categories for multiple risk factors is not intended (e.g., two Category 2 risk factors does not make a Category 4), however it does not delineate specific guidelines for how many risk factors need be present and to what severity [1].

Known Thrombogenic Mutations

Women with known thrombogenic mutations (e.g., factor V Leiden; prothrombin mutation; or protein S, protein C, or antithrombin deficiencies) can freely use the copper IUD. Progestin-only methods are Category 2. CHCs are Category 4 due to increased risk of thrombosis. Routine screening for these mutations is not appropriate as it is not cost-effective due to the rarity of mutations and the cost of screening [1].

Women on Anticoagulation

CHCs should generally be avoided in women requiring anticoagulation. Beyond prothrombotic effect, CHCs can also interfere with hepatic metabolism of anticoagulants like warfarin, and therefore INR should be closely monitored if CHCs are

BOX 5.4   MEDICAL ELIGIBILITY CRITERIA FOR CONTRACEPTIVE USE IN CARDIAC PATIENTS

Condition	Cu-IUD	LNG-IUD	Implants	DMPA	POP	CHCs
Multiple risk factors for atherosclerotic cardiovascular disease (e.g., older age, smoking, diabetes, hypertension, low HDL, high LDL, or high triglyceride levels)	1	2	2	3	2	3/4
Hypertension						
a. Adequately controlled hypertension	1	1	1	2	1	3
b. Elevated blood pressure levels (properly taken measurements)						
i. Systolic 140–159 mmHg or diastolic 90–99 mmHg	1	1	1	2	1	3
ii. Systolic $\geq$160 mmHg or diastolic $\geq$100 mmHg	1	2	2	3	2	4
c. Vascular disease	1	2	2	3	2	4
History of high blood pressure during pregnancy (when current blood pressure is measurable and normal)	1	1	1	1	1	2
Deep venous thrombosis/Pulmonary embolism						
a. History of DVT/PE, not receiving anticoagulant therapy						
i. Higher risk for recurrent DVT/PE (one or more risk factors)	1	2	2	2	2	4
• History of estrogen-associated DVT/PE						
• Pregnancy-associated DVT/PE						
• Idiopathic DVT/PE						
• Known thrombophilia, including antiphospholipid syndrome						
• History of recurrent DVT/PE						
ii. Lower risk for recurrent DVT/PE (no risk factors)	1	2	2	2	2	3
b. Acute DVT/PE	2	2	2	2	2	2
c. DVT/PE and established anticoagulant therapy for at least 3 months						
i. Higher risk for recurrent DVT/PE (one or more risk factors)	2	2	2	2	2	4
• Known thrombophilia, including antiphospholipid syndrome						
• History of recurrent DVT/PE						
ii. Lower risk for recurrent DVT/PE (no risk factors)	2	2	2	2	2	3
d. Family history (first-degree relatives)	1	1	1	1	1	2
e. Major surgery						
i. With prolonged immobilization	1	2	2	2	2	4
ii. Without prolonged immobilization	1	1	1	1	1	2
f. Minor surgery without immobilization	1	1	1	1	1	1
Known thrombogenic mutations (e.g., factor V Leiden; prothrombin mutation; protein S, protein C, and antithrombin deficiencies)	1	2	2	2	2	4

Condition	Cu-IUD	LNG-IUD		Implants	DMPA		POP	CHCs	
Current and history of ischemic heart disease		Initiation	Continuation	Initiation	Continuation			Initiation	Continuation
	2	3	2	3	3		2	3	4
Stroke (history of cerebrovascular accident)				Initiation	Continuation			Initiation	Continuation
	2	2		3	3		2	3	4
Valvular Heart Disease									
a. Uncomplicated	1	1		1	1		1	2	

(Continued)

BOX 5.4 (*CONTINUED*) MEDICAL ELIGIBILITY CRITERIA FOR CONTRACEPTIVE USE IN CARDIAC PATIENTS

Condition	Cu-IUD	LNG-IUD	Implants	DMPA	POP	CHCs
b. Complicated (pulmonary hypertension, risk for atrial fibrillation, or history of subacute bacterial endocarditis)	1	1	1	1	1	4
Peripartum Cardiomyopathy						
a. Normal or mildly impaired cardiac function (New York Heart Association Functional Class I or II: Patients with no limitation of activities or patients with slight, mild limitation of activity) [1]						
i. <6 months	2	2	1	1	1	4
ii. ≥6 months	2	2	1	1	1	3
b. Moderately or severely impaired cardiac function (New York Heart Association Functional Class III or IV: Patients with marked limitation of activity or patients who should be at complete rest) [1]	2	2	2	2	2	4

Source: Data from https://www.cdc.gov/reproductivehealth/contraception/mmwr/mec/appendixk.html#cardio

used [60]. There is a theoretical risk of intramuscular hematoma formation with DMPA injection. Though no studies have specifically looked at this concern, a prospective series of women taking anticoagulation with a history of bleeding complications did not report any intramuscular hematomas [32]. It is thought that subdermal implants carry a lower risk, as hematomas would be more superficial and therefore easier to detect and monitor [3]. (See Box 5.4.)

Considerations for Induced Abortion in Women with Cardiac Disease

In 2011, 45% of all pregnancies in the United States were unplanned. Of these, approximately 40% ended in induced abortion [61]. Approximately 1 in 4 women will have an abortion in the United States by age 45 [62].* One study found 12% of women cited health concerns as a reason for their abortion [63].

Induced abortion is safe and effective [64]. The majority of abortions in the United States occur at early gestations, with over 90% performed at less than 13 weeks' gestation. In general, induced abortion is safer than carrying a pregnancy to term. It has a lower risk of complications at earlier gestations. In the United States between 1998 and 2005, the pregnancy-associated mortality rate was 8.8 deaths per 100,000 live births, which represents an approximately 14-fold increase over the mortality rate related to induced abortion (0.6 deaths per 100,000 abortions) [65]. The risk of maternal death increases by 38% for each additional week of gestation. Cardiac events account for 17% of abortion-related mortality [66]. Major complications (those requiring hospital stay,

surgery, or blood transfusion) occur in less than 0.5% of induced abortions [64]. There are no high-quality studies on the safety of abortion for women with preexisting medical conditions.

Most patients with cardiac disease presenting for induced abortion will be aware of their cardiac diagnosis. Routine questions detailing functional status should be asked of the patient regarding her ability to climb stairs, whether she experiences angina at rest or with exercise, or paroxysmal nocturnal dyspnea [67]. A comprehensive consultation including cardiac testing and risk assessment with Maternal Fetal Medicine and Cardiology is advised.

The American College of Cardiology and American Heart Association emphasize the importance of a team approach for complex cardiovascular patients given increasing evidence-based data, new technologies, and improved survivorship for complex congenital heart disease. This is particularly important in the setting of decisions regarding mode of induced abortion and preoperative planning for surgical abortion. For complex cardiac patients, the heart team may comprise obstetrician-gynecologists (possibly including subspecialists in maternal-fetal medicine and family planning), cardiology, anesthesia (or cardiac anesthesia), and social work [68].

First Trimester Abortion

First trimester abortion is among the safest medical procedures. It may be performed in one of two ways: surgical abortion via dilation and aspiration (D&A, also called dilation and suction curettage [D&C]) or medication abortion with mifepristone and misoprostol.

First Trimester Surgical Abortion

During a D&A, the cervix is dilated with sequentially increasing dilators to allow passage of a suction curette into the uterus and removal of the pregnancy. Surgical abortion affords multiple advantages—particularly active monitoring and options for

---

* Per ACOG guidelines, all health care providers must provide accurate and unbiased reproductive health information to allow patients to make informed decisions. Physicians have a duty to refer patients in a timely manner to other providers if they cannot provide standard reproductive services due to conscientious objection [71].

anesthesia (local, regional, sedation, or general anesthesia). In addition, it is predictable in timing and there is immediate confirmation of completion [69]. Surgical abortion in the first trimester has a lower average blood loss and lower rate of delayed hemorrhage compared to medication abortion [70]. A surgical approach is preferred for most patients with cardiac conditions, particularly those who are sensitive to changes in intravascular volume that could occur with bleeding during a medication abortion, or who would benefit from cardiac monitoring. Major complications are rare at <0.01% of procedures [64], and include uterine or cervical injury, hemorrhage, and sepsis. Minor complications such as minor infection, incomplete abortion requiring repeat procedure, or seizure due to local anesthetic occur in <1% of procedures [72].

First Trimester Medication Abortion

Mifepristone, a progesterone modulator, is approved in the United States for medical abortion up to 10 weeks' gestation in conjunction with the prostaglandin misoprostol. The success rate is 95%–98%, with 2%–5% requiring repeat misoprostol or D&A for retained products of conception [73]. Medication abortion avoids a surgical procedure and anesthesia for the majority of patients. Patients may feel greater agency over the process as they manage it privately at home [74].

Bleeding and cramping will be experienced by most women. Other side effects of medication abortion include nausea, vomiting, diarrhea, headache, vertigo, and thermoregulatory effects [75].

Contraindications to medication abortion related to cardiac disease include severe anemia (<9.5 g/dL), bleeding diatheses, and anticoagulation. Most trials have excluded women with uncontrolled hypertension or cardiovascular disease, therefore scant data exist on the risks for women with cardiac disease. Prostaglandins are vasoactive with variable vasodilatory and vasoconstrictive actions depending on the target organ. A small study demonstrated that 600 μg intravaginal misoprostol in the second trimester does not alter maternal cardiac function as measured by transthoracic electrical bioimpedance [76]. A case study in developing countries with heterogenous cardiac conditions likewise demonstrated no adverse effects to mifepristone or misoprostol in the first or second trimester [77]. Concomitant use of medications that induce cytochrome P450 may reduce the effectiveness of mifepristone [75]. For critically ill intubated patients who cannot be placed in lithotomy or for whom surgical risks are too great, medication abortion may provide a safer alternative and can be induced with intramuscular methotrexate and misoprostol [69].

Second Trimester Abortion

In the United States, 7.6% of abortions are performed between 14 and 20 weeks' gestation, with even fewer (1.3%) at ≥21 weeks' gestation. Of these, 95% are performed by the surgical technique dilation and evacuation (D&E) [78].

Second Trimester Surgical Abortion

D&E generally requires cervical preparation (preoperative "ripening" and/or dilation of the cervix) in order to avoid trauma to the cervix. This can be achieved with osmotic dilators, prostaglandins, or mifepristone. Evacuation of the pregnancy is then performed with specialized forceps and suction. The difficulty of the procedure is commensurate with gestational age of the pregnancy and requires a skilled provider. Many women may not have access due to paucity of providers or state-specific legal restrictions [79].

Major complications of D&E are uncommon at <0.1% (though somewhat more frequent than D&A procedures) [79,80] and include hemorrhage, cervical lacerations, infection, and uterine perforation.

Second Trimester Medication Abortion

Medical abortion via induction of labor generally involves the use of prostaglandin analogues to cause uterine contractions and expulsion of the products of conception. Mifepristone—which increases misoprostol efficacy and shortens induction time—may be administered 24–48 hours prior to misoprostol [79]. In the United States, second trimester medical abortion is generally performed in an inpatient setting, often on the labor and delivery unit.

Compared with D&E, medical abortion in the second trimester is less cost effective and more time consuming. It is also associated with a slightly higher risk of complications, particularly retained products of conception (20% of cases), which may require subsequent D&E or curettage for retained placental tissue [81,82]. Other complications include uterine rupture, cervical lacerations, hemorrhage, and infection. Hemorrhage rates are comparable between D&E and second trimester medical abortion.

Referral Centers for Family Planning

Women with stable, chronic medical conditions are often candidates for outpatient abortion, but hospital referral may be appropriate for some patients. The operating room affords several advantages, including improved lighting; access to specialized instruments, monitoring equipment, and anesthesia services; specialized medications and blood products; more intensive levels of care; and a variety of support staff and other specialists [69]. However, hospital-based abortion may introduce additional barriers to care, including increased costs, travel, and potential lack of hospital-based providers or trained/willing support staff [69].

Preexisting conditions that may warrant hospital-based referral or referral to a family planning specialist include uncontrolled hypertension (systolic blood pressures >160, or diastolic >105); congenital cardiac defects including cyanotic disease, right or left ventricular dilation, and uncontrolled tachyarrhythmias; coronary artery disease including history of angina or myocardial infarction; current or historic cardiomyopathies; valvular disease including aortic stenosis peak gradient equal or greater to 60 mmHg, mitral stenosis valve area less than 1.5 cm², and mitral or aortic regurgitation with left ventricular dilation; as well as pulmonary hypertension [67].

Special Considerations for Pregnancy Termination for Cardiac Patients

Anesthesia Considerations

Cardiac anesthesiologists are preferred for surgical abortion in women with high risk cardiac conditions. Preoperative anesthesiology consultation along with multidisciplinary planning should be considered for these patients.

Hypertensive and Thrombotic Disorders

Women with poorly controlled hypertension should receive treatment prior to surgical abortion, which may be accomplished with beta-blockers or a vasodilator [67]. Those with a history of MI should be carefully monitored in a hospital environment with attention to rate control with a beta-blocker as well as pain management. Aspirin should be continued [67]. Cardiomyopathy with left ventricular dilation or compromise poses the risk of acute hemodynamic decompensation and arrhythmia. Those with a normal echocardiogram will likely tolerate the procedure well but should be monitored afterward for decompensation. During the procedure, attention should be paid to rate control, and diuretics and afterload reduction considered. Volume management is particularly important for those with hypertrophic cardiomyopathy who will have poor tolerance of hemorrhage with hypovolemia [67]. For women with pulmonary hypertension, even modest volume shifts may result in right heart decompensation. Invasive hemodynamic monitoring and aggressive diuresis both during and after the procedure is recommended [67]. Pregnancy termination with these cases should be planned with a multidisciplinary team, otherwise known as the heart team.

Anticoagulation

For patients who are already anticoagulated or on antiplatelet therapy and seeking an abortion, clinicians must weigh the procedural bleeding risk versus the thromboembolic risk if the medications are discontinued. Reversal can take several days, which may delay abortion and extend the period of increased thromboembolic risk. Sparse data exist exploring the effect of anticoagulation on blood loss during abortion. For first trimester procedures, a case series of women on heterogenous anticoagulation therapies (both prophylactic and therapeutic) found anticoagulated women had a higher mean procedural and postoperative blood loss compared to controls. However, differences in postoperative hemoglobin were not significant and no blood transfusions occurred, so the clinical implications are unclear [83]. A second study found that continuation of anticoagulation for planned first trimester surgical abortion under 14 weeks does not appear to be associated with heavy bleeding [84]. Another case series of D&Es at 16–22 weeks for women on low molecular weight heparin found only one case of greater-than-expected bleeding and overall suggested the procedure may be safe for women with recent or current low molecular weight heparin use [85].

For these patients, the surgeon may consider uterine massage or prophylactic agents to prevent hemorrhage like misoprostol or methylergonovine [86]. Some providers may still briefly stop anticoagulation or transition to heparin [67]. Decisions regarding continuation or interruption of anticoagulation should be in conjunction with the multidisciplinary team, the heart team, including cardiology, and anesthesia. Low dose unfractionated heparin (e.g., 5000 units subcutaneously every 8 hours) or low molecular weight heparin (e.g., enoxaparin 40 mg subcutaneously daily) can be considered for those taking a recess from therapeutic anticoagulation.

No modern study exists exploring the risk of bleeding for women on antiplatelet therapy undergoing abortion. In general, antiplatelet therapy should ideally be discontinued 5 days prior to surgery, but the decision must be individualized. Clopidogrel should not be discontinued within 12 months of placement of a drug-eluting stent [87]. Low-dose aspirin does not appear to increase the perioperative bleeding complication or mortality rate [88], but patients on combined therapy (e.g., aspirin and clopidogrel) do incur an increased bleeding risk [89].

Other Medications

Ergot alkaloids like carboprost that may be used in cases of hemorrhage should be avoided in patients with hypertension or a history of MI. NSAIDs should also be avoided for pain control for those with significant preexisting cardiac disease. Lidocaine for local anesthesia can generally be used safely in patients with cardiac conditions [69].

Infective Endocarditis Prophylaxis

The Society for Family Planning recommends routine antibiotic administration for all patients undergoing surgical or medical abortion to reduce pelvic infection risk, but the American Heart Association does not recommend additional medications as infective endocarditis prophylaxis [13,90]. Therefore, no additional antibiotics are warranted for patients at risk for endocarditis [69].

REFERENCES

1. Curtis KM et al. U.S. Medical eligibility criteria for contraceptive use, 2016. *MMWR Recomm Reports.* 2016;65(3): 1–103. Accessed November 22, 2018.
2. Chor J, Oswald L, Briller J, Cowett A, Peacock N, Harwood B. Reproductive health experiences of women with cardiovascular disease. *Contraception.* 2012;86(5):464–9.
3. Allen RH, Cwiak CA, eds. *Contraception for the Medically Challenging Patient.* New York: Springer-Verlag. 2014.
4. Hinze A, Kutty S, Sayles H, Sandene EK, Meza J, Kugler JD. Reproductive and contraceptive counseling received by adult women with congenital heart disease: A risk-based analysis. *Congenit Heart Dis.* 2013;8(1):20–31.
5. Simko LC, McGinnis KA, Schembri J. Educational needs of adults with congenital heart disease. *J Cardiovasc Nurs.* 21(2):85–94.
6. Dehlendorf C, Krajewski C, Borrero S. Contraceptive counseling: Best practices to ensure quality communication and enable effective contraceptive use. *Clin Obstet Gynecol.* 2014;57(4):659–73.
7. Ortiz ME, Croxatto HB, Bardin CW. Mechanisms of action of intrauterine devices. *Obstet Gynecol Surv.* 1996;51(12 Suppl):S42–51.
8. Effectiveness of Family Planning Methods. US Department of Health and Human Services; Center for Disease Control and Prevention. https://docs.google.com/viewer?url=https%3A%2 F%2Fwww.cdc.gov%2Freproductivehealth%2Fcontracep tion%2Funintendedpregnancy%2Fpdf%2FContraceptive_ methods_508.pdf. Accessed January 4, 2019.

9. Villavicencio J, Allen RH. Unscheduled bleeding and contraceptive choice: Increasing satisfaction and continuation rates. *Open Access J Contracept.* 2016;7:43–52.

10. Jatlaoui TC, Riley HEM, Curtis KM. The safety of intrauterine devices among young women: A systematic review. *Contraception.* 2017;95(1):17–39.

11. Jatlaoui TC, Curtis KM. Safety and effectiveness data for emergency contraceptive pills among women with obesity: A systematic review. *Contraception.* 2016;94(6):605-11.

12. Farmer M, Webb A. Intrauterine device insertion-related complications: Can they be predicted? *J Fam Plan Reprod Heal Care.* 2003;29(4):227–31.

13. Wilson W et al. Prevention of infective endocarditis. *Circulation.* 2007;116(15):1736–54.

14. Nexplanon- etonogestrel implant. US Food and Drug Administration (FDA) approved product information. https://dailymed.nlm.nih.gov/dailymed/drugInfo.cfm?setid=b03a3917-9a65-45c2-bbbb-871da858ef34. Accessed January 4, 2019.

15. Peterson HB, Xia Z, Hughes JM, Wilcox LS, Tylor LR, Trussell J. The risk of pregnancy after tubal sterilization: Findings from the U.S. Collaborative Review of Sterilization. *Am J Obstet Gynecol.* 1996;174(4):1161–8; discussion 1168–70.

16. Trussell J. Update on and correction to the cost-effectiveness of contraceptives in the United States. *Contraception.* 2012;85(6):611.

17. Trussell J. Contraceptive failure in the United States. *Contraception.* 2011;83(5):397–404.

18. Sober SP, Schreiber CA. Controversies in family planning: Are all oral contraceptive formulations created equal? *Contraception.* 2011;83(5):394–6.

19. Generic OCs bioequivalent, but much maligned. *Contracept Technol Update.* 1989;10(6):77–81.

20. Brynhildsen J. Combined hormonal contraceptives: Prescribing patterns, compliance, and benefits versus risks. *Ther Adv Drug Saf.* 2014;5(5):201–13.

21. Trussell J, Jordan B. Reproductive health risks in perspective. *Contraception.* 2006;73(5):437–9.

22. Gardner J, Miller L. Promoting the safety and use of hormonal contraceptives. *J Womens Health (Larchmt).* 2005;14(1):53–60.

23. Roach REJ, Helmerhorst FM, Lijfering WM, Stijnen T, Algra A, Dekkers OM. Combined oral contraceptives: The risk of myocardial infarction and ischemic stroke. *Cochrane Database Syst Rev.* 2015;(8):CD011054.

24. Endrikat J et al. An open label, comparative study of the effects of a dose-reduced oral contraceptive containing 20 μg ethinyl estradiol and 100 μg levonorgestrel on hemostatic, lipids, and carbohydrate metabolism variables. *Contraception.* 2002;65(3):215–21.

25. Foulon T et al. Effects of two low-dose oral contraceptives containing ethinylestradiol and either desogestrel or levonorgestrel on serum lipids and lipoproteins with particular regard to LDL size. *Contraception.* 2001;64(1):11–6.

26. Kiriwat O, Petyim S. The effects of transdermal contraception on lipid profiles, carbohydrate metabolism and coagulogram in Thai women. *Gynecol Endocrinol.* 2010;26(5):361–5.

27. Cardoso F, Polónia J, Santos A, Silva-Carvalho J, Ferreira-de-Almeida J. Low-dose oral contraceptives and 24-hour ambulatory blood pressure. *Int J Gynecol Obstet.* 1997;59(3):237–43.

28. Narkiewicz K, Rocco Graniero G, D'Este D, Mattarei M, Zonzin P, Palatini P. Ambulatory blood pressure in mild hypertensive women taking oral contraceptives a case-control study. *Am J Hypertens.* 1995;8(3):249–53.

29. Lidegaard Ø, Løkkegaard E, Jensen A, Skovlund CW, Keiding N. Thrombotic stroke and myocardial infarction with hormonal contraception. *N Engl J Med.* 2012;366(24):2257–66.

30. Tepper NK, Whiteman MK, Marchbanks PA, James AH, Curtis KM. Progestin-only contraception and thromboembolism: A systematic review. *Contraception.* 2016;94(6):678–700.

31. Kaunitz AM. Long-acting injectable contraception with depot medroxyprogesterone acetate. *Am J Obstet Gynecol.* 1994;170(5 Pt 2):1543–9.

32. Sönmezer M, Atabekoğlu C, Cengiz B, Dökmeci F, Cengiz S. Depot-medroxyprogesterone acetate in anticoagulated patients with previous hemorrhagic corpus luteum. *Eur J Contracept Reprod Heal Care.* 2005;10(1):9–14.

33. *DEPO-PROVERA - medroxyprogesterone acetate injection, suspension.* Pharmacia and Upjohn Company LLC. http://labeling.pfizer.com/ShowLabeling.aspx?id=522. Accessed January 4, 2019.

34. Lopez LM et al. Progestin-only contraceptives: Effects on weight. *Cochrane Database Syst Rev.* 2016;(8):CD008815.

35. Kaunitz AM, Arias R, McClung M. Bone density recovery after depot medroxyprogesterone acetate injectable contraception use. *Contraception.* 2008;77(2):67–76.

36. Gribble JN, Lundgren RI, Velasquez C, Anastasi EE. Being strategic about contraceptive introduction: The experience of the Standard Days Method. *Contraception.* 2008;77(3):147–54.

37. Practice bulletin no. 152: Emergency contraception. *Obstet Gynecol.* 2015;126(3):e1–11.

38. Cheng L, Che Y, Gülmezoglu AM. Interventions for emergency contraception. Cheng L, ed. *Cochrane Database Syst Rev.* 2012;(8):CD001324.

39. Cleland K, Zhu H, Goldstuck N, Cheng L, Trussell J. The efficacy of intrauterine devices for emergency contraception: A systematic review of 35 years of experience. *Hum Reprod.* 2012;27(7):1994–2000.

40. Gemzell-Danielsson K. Mechanism of action of emergency contraception. *Contraception.* 2010;82(5):404–9.

41. Thorne S et al. Pregnancy and contraception in heart disease and pulmonary arterial hypertension. *J Fam Plan Reprod Heal Care.* 2006;32(2):75–81.

42. Thorne S, MacGregor A, Nelson-Piercy C. Risks of contraception and pregnancy in heart disease. *Heart.* 2006;92(10):1520–5.

43. Di Tullio MR, Sacco RL, Sciacca RR, Jin Z, Homma S. Patent foramen ovale and the risk of ischemic stroke in a multiethnic population. *J Am Coll Cardiol.* 2007;49(7):797–802.

44. Meissner I et al. Patent foramen ovale: Innocent or guilty? *J Am Coll Cardiol.* 2006;47(2):440–5.

45. Tepper NK, Paulen ME, Marchbanks PA, Curtis KM. Safety of contraceptive use among women with peripartum cardiomyopathy: A systematic review. *Contraception.* 2010;82(1):95–101.

46. Taurelle R, Ruet C, Jaupart F, Magnier S. [Contraception using a progestagen-only minipill in cardiac patients]. *Arch Mal Coeur Vaiss.* 1979;72(1):98–106.

47. Suri V, Aggarwal N, Kaur R, Chaudhary N, Ray P, Grover A. Safety of intrauterine contraceptive device (copper T 200 B) in women with cardiac disease. *Contraception.* 2008;78(4):315–8.

48. Avila WS, Grinberg M, Melo NR, Aristodemo Pinotti J, Pileggi F. [Contraceptive use in women with heart disease]. *Arq Bras Cardiol.* 1996;66(4):205–11.

49. North RA, Sadler L, Stewart AW, McCowan LM, Kerr AR, White HD. Long-term survival and valve-related complications in young women with cardiac valve replacements. *Circulation.* 1999;99(20):2669–76.

50. Kilic S et al. The effect of levonorgestrel-releasing intrauterine device on menorrhagia in women taking anticoagulant medication after cardiac valve replacement. *Contraception.* 2009;80(2):152–7.

51. Silversides CK, Colman JM, Sermer M, Siu SC. Cardiac risk in pregnant women with rheumatic mitral stenosis. *Am J Cardiol.* 2003;91(11):1382–5.

52. European Society of Gynecology (ESG), Association for European Paediatric Cardiology (AEPC), German Society for Gender Medicine (DGesGM) et al. ESC Guidelines on the management of cardiovascular diseases during pregnancy: The Task Force on the Management of Cardiovascular Diseases during Pregnancy of the European Society of Cardiology (ESC). *Eur Heart J.* 2011;32(24):3147–97.

53. Uebing A, Steer PJ, Yentis SM, Gatzoulis MA. Pregnancy and congenital heart disease. *BMJ.* 2006;332(7538):401–6.

54. August P. Hypertension in Women. *Adv Chronic Kidney Dis.* 2013;20(5):396–401.

55. Chasan-Taber L et al. Prospective study of oral contraceptives and hypertension among women in the United States. *Circulation.* 1996;94(3):483–9.

56. Farley TM, Collins J, Schlesselman JJ. Hormonal contraception and risk of cardiovascular disease. An international perspective. *Contraception.* 1998;57(3):211–30.

57. Steenland MW, Zapata LB, Brahmi D, Marchbanks PA, Curtis KM. Appropriate follow up to detect potential adverse events after initiation of select contraceptive methods: A systematic review. *Contraception.* 2013;87(5):611–24.

58. Timmer CJ, Mulders TMT. Pharmacokinetics of etonogestrel and ethinylestradiol released from a combined contraceptive vaginal ring. *Clin Pharmacokinet.* 2000;39(3):233–42.

59. Hussain SF. Progestogen-only pills and high blood pressure: Is there an association? *Contraception.* 2004;69(2):89–97.

60. Zingone MM, Guirguis AB, Airee A, Cobb D. Probable drug interaction between warfarin and hormonal contraceptives. *Ann Pharmacother.* 2009;43(12):2096–102.

61. Finer LB, Zolna MR. Declines in unintended pregnancy in the United States, 2008–2011. *N Engl J Med.* 2016;374(9):843–52.

62. Jones RK, Jerman J. Population group abortion rates and lifetime incidence of abortion: United States, 2008–2014. *Am J Public Health.* 2017;107(12):1904–9.

63. Finer LB, Frohwirth LF, Dauphinee LA, Singh S, Moore AM. Reasons U.S. women have abortions: Quantitative and qualitative perspectives. *Perspect Sex Reprod Health.* 2005;37(3):110–8.

64. White K, Carroll E, Grossman D. Complications from first-trimester aspiration abortion: A systematic review of the literature. *Contraception.* 2015;92(5):422–38.

65. Raymond EG, Grimes DA. The comparative safety of legal induced abortion and childbirth in the United States. *Obstet Gynecol.* 2012;119(2, Part 1):215–9.

66. Bartlett LA et al. Risk factors for legal induced abortion–related mortality in the United States. *Obstet Gynecol.* 2004;103(4):729–37.

67. Paul M. *Management of Unintended and Abnormal Pregnancy: Comprehensive Abortion Care.* Wiley-Blackwell; 2009. https://www.wiley.com/en-us/Management+of+Unintended+and+Abnormal+Pregnancy%3A+Comprehensive+Abortion+Care+-p-9781405176965. Accessed December 20, 2018.

68. Holmes DR, Rich JB, Zoghbi WA, Mack MJ. The heart team of cardiovascular care. *J Am Coll Cardiol.* 2013;61(9):903–7.

69. Guiahi M, Davis A, Society of Family Planning. First-trimester abortion in women with medical conditions: Release date October 2012 SFP guideline #20122. *Contraception.* 2012;86(6):622–30.

70. Allen RH, Westhoff C, De Nonno L, Fielding SL, Schaff EA. Curettage after mifepristone-induced abortion: Frequency, timing, and indications. *Obstet Gynecol.* 2001;98(1):101–6.

71. American College of Obstetricians and Gynecologists. *ACOG Committee Opinion.* American College of Obstetricians and Gynecologists. https://www.acog.org/Clinical-Guidance-and-Publications/Committee-Opinions/Committee-on-Ethics/The-Limits-of-Conscientious-Refusal-in-Reproductive-Medicine?IsMobileSet=false. Accessed March 5, 2019.

72. Hakim-Elahi E, Tovell HM, Burnhill MS. Complications of first-trimester abortion: A report of 170,000 cases. *Obstet Gynecol.* 1990;76(1):129–35.

73. Gatter M, Cleland K, Nucatola DL. Efficacy and safety of medical abortion using mifepristone and buccal misoprostol through 63 days. *Contraception.* 2015;91(4):269–73.

74. Robson SC et al. Randomised preference trial of medical versus surgical termination of pregnancy less than 14 weeks' gestation (TOPS). *Health Technol Assess.* 2009;13(53):1–124, iii–iv.

75. American College of Obstetricians and Gynecologists. Practice bulletin no. 143. *Obstet Gynecol.* 2014;123(3):676–92.

76. Ramsey PS, Hogg BB, Savage KG, Winkler DD, Owen J. Cardiovascular effects of intravaginal misoprostol in the mid trimester of pregnancy. *Am J Obstet Gynecol.* 2000;183(5):1100–2.

77. Bagga R, Choudhary N, Suri V et al. First and second trimester induced abortions in women with cardiac disorders: A 12-year analysis from a developing country. *J Obstet Gynaecol (Lahore).* 2008;28(7):732–7.

78. O'Connell K, Jones HE, Lichtenberg ES, Paul M. Second-trimester surgical abortion practices: A survey of National Abortion Federation members. *Contraception.* 2008;78(6):492–9.

79. Practice bulletin no. 135. *Obstet Gynecol.* 2013;121(6):1394–406.

80. Grossman D, Blanchard K, Blumenthal P. Complications after second trimester surgical and medical abortion. *Reprod Health Matters.* 2008;16(sup31):173–82.

81. Bryant AG, Grimes DA, Garrett JM, Stuart GS. Second-trimester abortion for fetal anomalies or fetal death. *Obstet Gynecol.* 2011;117(4):788–92.

82. Autry AM, Hayes EC, Jacobson GF, Kirby RS. A comparison of medical induction and dilation and evacuation for second-trimester abortion. *Am J Obstet Gynecol.* 2002;187(2):393–7.

83. Kaneshiro B, Bednarek P, Isley M, Jensen J, Nichols M, Edelman A. Blood loss at the time of first-trimester surgical abortion in anticoagulated women. *Contraception.* 2011;83(5):431–5.

84. Kaneshiro B, Tschann M, Jensen J, Bednarek P, Texeira R, Edelman A. Blood loss at the time of surgical abortion up to 14 weeks in anticoagulated patients: A case series. *Contraception.* 2017;96(1):14–8.

85. Tschann M, Edelman A, Jensen J, Bednarek P, Kaneshiro B. Blood loss at the time of dilation and evacuation at 16 to 22 weeks of gestation in women using low molecular weight heparin: A case series. *Contraception*. 2018;97(1):54–6.

86. Kerns J, Steinauer J. Management of postabortion hemorrhage. *Contraception*. 2013;87(3):331–42.

87. Johnson BE, Porter J. Preoperative evaluation of the gynecologic patient. *Obstet Gynecol*. 2008;111(5):1183–94.

88. Burger W, Chemnitius J-M, Kneissl GD, Rucker G. Low-dose aspirin for secondary cardiovascular prevention—Cardiovascular risks after its perioperative withdrawal versus bleeding risks with its continuation—Review and meta-analysis. *J Intern Med*. 2005;257(5):399–414.

89. Squizzato A, Keller T, Romualdi E, Middeldorp S. Clopidogrel plus aspirin versus aspirin alone for preventing cardiovascular disease. *Cochrane Database Syst Rev*. 2011;(1):CD005158.

90. Achilles SL, Reeves MF, Society of Family Planning. Prevention of infection after induced abortion. *Contraception*. 2011;83(4):295–309.

91. Videla-Rivero L, Etchepareborda JJ, Kesseru E. Early chorionic activity in women bearing inert IUD, copper IUD and levonorgestrel-releasing IUD. *Contraception*. 1987;36(2):217–26.

6

Cardiovascular Symptoms: Is It Pregnancy or the Heart?

Melissa Perez and Afshan B. Hameed

KEY POINTS

- Obstetric care providers should be able to differentiate common complaints of pregnancy from those of cardiovascular disease
- Cardiovascular disease typically manifests with a combination of moderate to severe symptoms, vital sign abnormalities, and/or physical examination findings

- All self-reported cardiac symptoms in a pregnant patient should be fully evaluated
- Palpitations are the most common cardiac symptom encountered during pregnancy in women with or without structural heart disease
- New-onset asthma or bilateral pulmonary infiltrates may be indicative of heart failure in pregnancy

---

Introduction

Cardiovascular disease (CVD) has emerged as the leading cause of maternal mortality in the United States, accounting for over one-third of all pregnancy-related deaths. A significant proportion of these deaths are preventable [1]. One of the key elements in CVD-related deaths is the inability of the health care provider to identify the presenting symptoms as markers for CVD, thus causing delays or missed diagnosis [2]. Pregnancy is a state of hemodynamic overload that may result in signs and symptoms similar to those of cardiovascular disease. It is often challenging to distinguish physiologic symptoms of pregnancy from heart disease. Common symptoms include palpitations, shortness of breath (SOB), fatigue, chest pain, and dizziness. It is imperative that the obstetrics care provider be able to differentiate benign pregnancy symptoms from those of potentially life-threatening causes. This chapter provides an overview of the common cardiovascular symptoms of pregnancy and the California Maternal Quality Care Collaborative Cardiovascular (CMQCC) disease in pregnancy toolkit designed to identify pregnant women who are at increased risk of CVD requiring further cardiovascular evaluation [3].

Basic Approach to a Symptomatic Patient

Cardiac symptoms in pregnancy and during the postpartum period, particularly if they are self-reported, require further workup. The basic systematic approach to any cardiac complaint in pregnancy follows three general principles (Figure 6.1):

1. A thorough history including the patient's baseline exercise capacity, New York Heart Association functional status, detailed symptoms, prior cardiac history, pregnancy outcomes, and underlying medical issues.
2. Focused physical examination of the cardiovascular system.
3. Appropriate radiographic, imaging, electrocardiographic, and laboratory investigations as indicated.

If cardiac disease is high in the differential diagnosis, the goal is to refer the patient to a cardiologist for further evaluation. For the purposes of this discussion, we will focus on approach to the common cardiovascular symptoms of pregnancy.

The Cardiovascular Toolkit (CMQCC)

Maternal mortality reviews indicate that most mothers who died of CVD during pregnancy or the postpartum period had presented to the health care provider with signs and symptoms on more than one occasion that were not recognized. There is a need to maintain an index of suspicion for cardiac disease in women presenting with cardiac complaints, and to have a low threshold for further workup. The CMQCC Cardiovascular Disease in Pregnancy and Postpartum Task Force developed a toolkit that includes an overview of clinical assessment and management strategies based on risk factors and presenting signs and symptoms [3]. In this regard, it contains two algorithms designed to guide stratification and initial evaluation of symptomatic or high-risk pregnant or postpartum women (Figures 6.2 and 6.3).

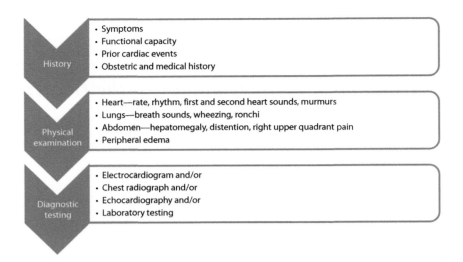

FIGURE 6.1   Basic approach to cardiac symptoms.

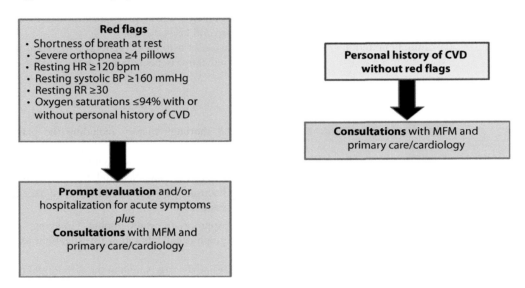

FIGURE 6.2   Cardiovascular disease assessment in women presenting with red flags (severe signs and symptoms or personal history of CVD). (Adapted from CMQCC.com, with permission.)

The first algorithm identified women who exhibit "red flags" and must get prompt evaluation and appropriate consultations. The second algorithm addresses women who are stable and without evidence of red flags or personal history of CVD. Among the 64 CVD-related maternal deaths in California between 2002–2006, the algorithms would have identified 93% of these women as high risk for CVD, with a significant potential for saving lives.

In general, global cardiovascular risk assessment should be obtained in all pregnant women, with or without symptoms (Figure 6.2). Providers can screen women any time in pregnancy, postpartum, and/or if any new or concerning symptoms arise. Providers can begin screening women at their prenatal appointments, on admission to an antepartum or postpartum unit, or for those patients who have not received care from the provider before their admission or delivery. This implementation strategy is currently underway at the University of California, Irvine and Einstein/Montefiore, Bronx, New York.

Common Cardiac Symptoms in Pregnancy

Physiologic changes in pregnancy most often lead to signs and symptoms that may mimic cardiac disease. Common complaints include nausea, fatigue, back pain, lower extremity swelling, SOB, palpitations, and chest pain (Table 6.1).

Palpitations

Palpitations—"awareness of the heart beat"—is the most common cardiac complaint encountered in pregnancy [5]. An increase in heart rate is a normal physiologic adaptation of pregnancy [6,7]; however, palpitations may also be due to serious underlying arrhythmia and/or cardiac dysfunction [8,9]. Heart rate begins to increase as early as 5 weeks of gestation, which may be perceived as palpitations that continue throughout

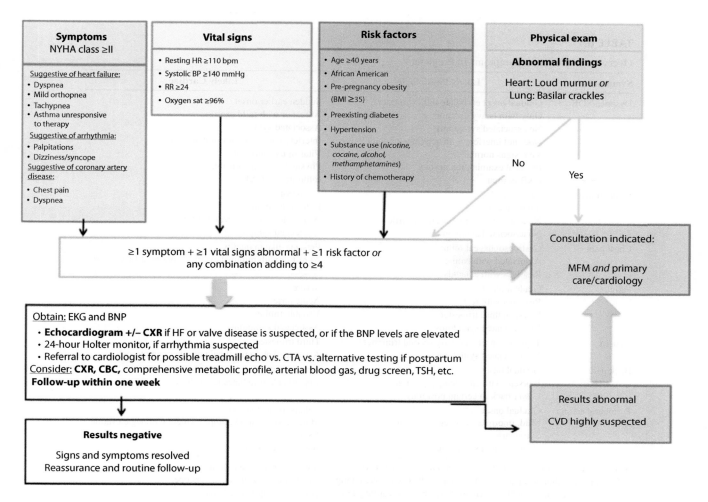

Symptoms
NYHA class ≥II

Suggestive of heart failure:
- Dyspnea
- Mild orthopnea
- Tachypnea
- Asthma unresponsive to therapy

Suggestive of arrhythmia:
- Palpitations
- Dizziness/syncope

Suggestive of coronary artery disease:
- Chest pain
- Dyspnea

Vital signs
- Resting HR ≥110 bpm
- Systolic BP ≥140 mmHg
- RR ≥24
- Oxygen sat ≥96%

Risk factors
- Age ≥40 years
- African American
- Pre-pregnancy obesity (BMI ≥35)
- Preexisting diabetes
- Hypertension
- Substance use (*nicotine, cocaine, alcohol, methamphetamines*)
- History of chemotherapy

Physical exam

Abnormal findings

Heart: Loud murmur *or*
Lung: Basilar crackles

No   Yes

≥1 symptom + ≥1 vital signs abnormal + ≥1 risk factor *or* any combination adding to ≥4

Consultation indicated:

MFM *and* primary care/cardiology

Obtain: EKG and BNP
- **Echocardiogram +/– CXR** if HF or valve disease is suspected, or if the BNP levels are elevated
- 24-hour Holter monitor, if arrhythmia suspected
- Referral to cardiologist for possible treadmill echo vs. CTA vs. alternative testing if postpartum

Consider: **CXR, CBC,** comprehensive metabolic profile, arterial blood gas, drug screen, TSH, etc.

Follow-up within one week

Results abnormal

CVD highly suspected

Results negative

Signs and symptoms resolved
Reassurance and routine follow-up

FIGURE 6.3 Cardiovascular disease assessment in women without red flags. (Adapted from CMQCC.com, with permission.)

pregnancy. The propensity to arrhythmias in pregnancy is likely due to (i) the atrial and/or ventricular stretch caused by increased blood volume which may occur in patients with or without structural heart disease, or (ii) prolongation of QT interval by the high estrogen levels in pregnancy. Estrogen effects on cardiac arrhythmia may explain why arrhythmias are seen more frequently in females than their male counterparts [5,10]. Fortunately, most rhythm disorders seen in pregnancy are limited to sinus tachycardia or atrial/ventricular ectopic beats, both of which are considered benign. On the other hand, life-threatening arrhythmias may manifest for the first time in pregnancy [11]. Complaints of palpitations should always be taken seriously and not dismissed as a symptom of physiologic increase in heart rate. Palpitations may be the first presenting sign of a previously undiagnosed cardiac condition. The most common new-onset arrhythmia during pregnancy is supraventricular tachycardia [5,12], followed by atrial fibrillation, which may be associated valve stenosis with or without a history of rheumatic heart disease [13]. See Figure 6.4.

Potentially life-threatening diagnoses such as sustained arrhythmias and cardiomyopathy must be ruled out in a patient presenting with palpitations.

The initial workup of a pregnant patient with palpitations follows the same principles as the nonpregnant patient (Box 6.1).

1. *History*: Patients history may help identify the etiology. Onset of palpitations at an early age may be suggestive of congenital heart defect or an underlying metabolic disorder. Certain features may be indicative of a specific etiology, such as "flip-flopping" encountered in premature atrial or ventricular contractions, and "pounding in the neck" being associated with atrioventricular dissociation. As a general rule, pre-syncope should never be considered normal for pregnancy and should prompt a workup [5,12]. Medical conditions that can precipitate arrhythmias are thyroid disorders, diabetes, and anxiety or panic attacks. Many medications, such as sympathomimetic agents, vasodilators, and anticholinergic drugs, can lead to the sensation of palpitations, or may cause arrhythmias. Beta-blocker withdrawal, herbal medication, or illicit drug use may be the etiology.

2. *Physical examination*: Heart rate may be irregular in a patient with current arrhythmia with or without symptoms. Diagnosis of arrhythmia on physical exam can be difficult if the arrhythmia is not occurring at the time of the examination. However, the physical exam may lead to suspicion of a structural cardiac defect, i.e., cardiac auscultation findings may be suggestive of heart failure or valve disease.

TABLE 6.1

Overview of Common Symptoms in Pregnancy

Symptoms	Likely Physiologic	Likely Cardiac
Dyspnea/SOB	Gradual onset early/late third trimester	Sudden earlier onset
	Only with heavy exertion	At rest or with mild exertion
	No associated symptoms[a]	Associated symptoms[a]
	Does not interfere with activities of daily living	Interfere with activities of daily living
	Vital signs normal	Vital signs abnormal
	Physical examination normal	Physical examination abnormal[b]
	CXR normal	Infiltrates on CXR
Palpitations	Self-limited	Persistent
	Short duration	Longer durations
	No association with physical exertion	Worsening with physical exertion
	No associated symptoms[a]	Associated symptoms[a]
Chest pain	Gastroesophageal reflux	Pressure-like in quality
	Associated with eating	At rest or with minimal exertion abnormal ECG
	Resolves with antacids	
Fatigue	Gradual onset	Severe
	Resolves with rest	Acute onset
	Worse in third trimester	Variable timing
	No associated symptoms[a]	Associated symptoms[a]
Nausea	Typically in first or early second trimester	Third trimester
	No associated symptoms[a]	Associated abdominal pain or other symptoms[a]
Back pain	Gradual onset	Acute onset
	Worsens with advancing gestation	Upper back or radiates from chest
	Lower back in certain positions	
Peripheral edema	Gradual onset	Relatively acute onset
	Mild, improves with leg elevation	Marked with minimal improvement with leg elevation
	Symmetric	Asymmetric
	No associated symptoms[a]	Associated symptoms[a]

Source: Adapted from *ACOG Practice Bulletin 212, 201*; CMQCC Cardiovascular disease toolkit.

[a] Chest pain, orthopnea, paroxysmal nocturnal dyspnea, cough, fatigue, palpitations, dizziness, or syncope.

[b] Murmur, wheezing, crackles, decreased breath sounds at lung bases, significant peripheral edema.

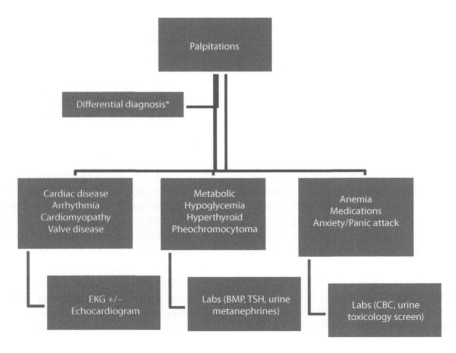

FIGURE 6.4 Palpitations in pregnancy. *Differential diagnosis: Physiologic, anemia, thyrotoxicosis, sympathomimetic medications, anxiety, panic attacks, sinus tachycardia, premature atrial or ventricular contractions, supraventricular tachycardia, atrial fibrillation, or ventricular tachycardia.

BOX 6.1   APPROACH TO A PATIENT WITH PALPITATIONS

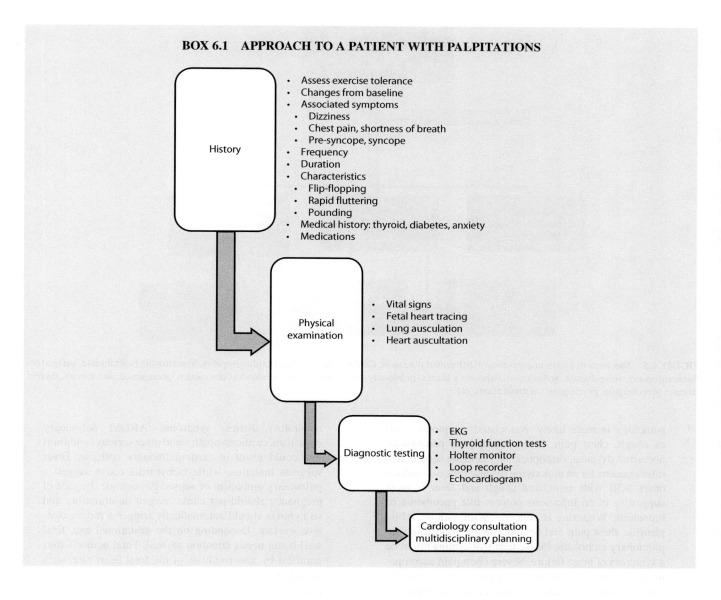

History
- Assess exercise tolerance
- Changes from baseline
- Associated symptoms
  - Dizziness
  - Chest pain, shortness of breath
  - Pre-syncope, syncope
- Frequency
- Duration
- Characteristics
  - Flip-flopping
  - Rapid fluttering
  - Pounding
- Medical history: thyroid, diabetes, anxiety
- Medications

Physical examination
- Vital signs
- Fetal heart tracing
- Lung ausculation
- Heart auscultation

Diagnostic testing
- EKG
- Thyroid function tests
- Holter monitor
- Loop recorder
- Echocardiogram

Cardiology consultation multidisciplinary planning

3. *Diagnostic testing*: A 12-lead EKG is a standard test in a patient with palpitations. If EKG is normal but clinical suspicion for an arrhythmia remains high, the next step is to obtain 24–48 hours of Holter monitoring. A continuous loop recorder may be indicated if the palpitations are infrequent. Once arrhythmia is confirmed, an echocardiogram should be obtained to assess for structural malformations. There are no laboratory investigations specific for arrhythmias, but thyroid function tests and complete blood count to rule out anemia should be obtained in pregnant women with palpitations [14,15]. See Chapter 16 for further details.

Shortness of Breath

Dyspnea or shortness of breath (SOB) is a common complaint encountered in up to 75% of pregnant patients. The perception of SOB in pregnancy is due to the progesterone-mediated increased drive for ventilation exacerbated in the later part of pregnancy due to the elevation of the diaphragm [7]. Approximately 15% of pregnant women in the first trimester have SOB, which increases to 75% in the third trimester. Classically, the physiologic breathlessness is present at rest or while talking and may paradoxically improve during mild activity [7]. SOB related to pregnancy physiology gradually improves postpartum and returns to normal within 4–6 weeks after delivery [16]. Significant SOB may be due to an underlying cardiac disease [17]. See Figure 6.5.

Potentially life-threatening diagnoses such as pulmonary embolism, pulmonary edema, and cardiomyopathy must be ruled out in a patient presenting with SOB.

Basic Approach:

1. *History*: The first step in assessing SOB is to take a detailed history. The components of the history of present illness may help distinguish physiologic from pathologic SOB [4,18,19]. Physiologic SOB is usually gradual in onset, begins in the first or second trimester, and has no other associated symptoms. When dyspnea is sudden in onset and occurs close to term,

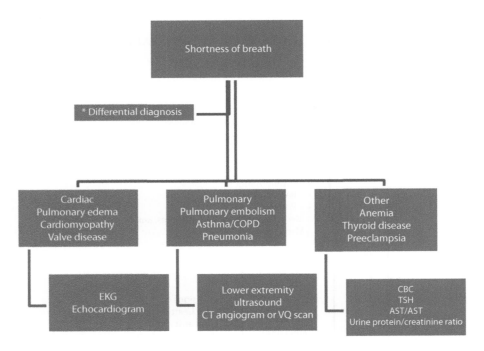

FIGURE 6.5 Shortness of breath in pregnancy. *Differential diagnosis: Cardiac causes (dilated cardiomyopathy, hypertrophic heart disease, peripartum cardiomyopathy, valve disease, arrhythmia), Pulmonary causes (pulmonary embolism, asthma, mechanical obstruction, pneumonia), and anemia, thyroid disease, preeclampsia, psychogenic, or medications, etc.

pathology is more likely. Associated symptoms, such as cough, chest pain, fever, hemoptysis, paroxysmal nocturnal dyspnea, orthopnea, or wheezing should also raise concern for an underlying disease process. Sudden onset SOB with associated cough and fever is most suggestive of an infectious process like pneumonia or bronchitis. Wheezing is concerning for asthma, while pleuritic chest pain and hemoptysis are concerning for pulmonary embolism. Please note that asthma might be a symptom of heart failure. Severe chest pain accompanying sudden onset SOB should prompt a workup for coronary artery ischemia or dissection, and orthopnea is more suggestive of pulmonary edema, valve disease, and possibly cardiomyopathy. Past medical history, family history, including family members with congenital heart disease, sudden death, or thromboembolic disease, are important components of evaluation. Certain medications can cause SOB, either as a side effect of the drug itself or secondary to an adverse effect caused by the drug. For example, nonselective beta-blockers can lead to bronchoconstriction and therefore SOB; terbutaline may lead to pulmonary edema and SOB. A recent travel history, in addition to eliciting the patient's country of origin, can help to determine if there is a need to broaden the search to diseases not typically encountered in the United States. (See further Box 6.2.)

2. *Physical examination*: Physiologic dyspnea typically has normal vital signs, while pathologic dyspnea may be associated with significant vital sign abnormalities. Hypertension with SOB would suggest preeclampsia with resultant pulmonary edema. Hypotension, on the other hand, should raise alarm for sepsis, acute

respiratory distress syndrome (ARDS), pulmonary embolism, cardiomyopathy, and other serious conditions that could result in cardiopulmonary collapse. Fever suggests infection, while tachycardia could suggest a pulmonary embolism or sepsis. Physiologic dyspnea of pregnancy should not cause oxygen desaturation, and so hypoxia should automatically trigger a more extensive workup. Depending on the gestational age, fetal well-being needs attention as well. Fetal acidosis may manifest by abnormalities of the fetal heart rate, such as minimal or absent variability and late decelerations, and therefore this information can be used as a supplemental "vital sign," as it indicates maternal perfusion and oxygenation. Lungs should be clear to auscultation in women with physiologic SOB. Wheezing on lung exam suggests an asthma exacerbation or acute bronchitis. Rales or crackles occur when the lung parenchyma are involved, as in pulmonary edema or interstitial lung disease. Common causes of pulmonary edema in pregnancy include preeclampsia, often secondary to magnesium sulfate exposure, tocolytics, and cardiac disease. ARDS due to sepsis or an amniotic fluid embolism can also cause rales on lung exam. A consolidation as from pneumonia would lead to focal crackles. In addition, while some degree of pedal edema is present in up to 80% of pregnant women, an increased amount of edema beyond what is normal for pregnancy should prompt a workup for heart failure [17,20].

3. *Diagnostic testing*: A chest radiograph (CXR) should be considered for patients in whom pneumonia or pulmonary edema is suspected. The amount of fetal radiation exposure from CXR is minimal and any fetal risk is

BOX 6.2 APPROACH TO A PATIENT WITH SHORTNESS OF BREATH

History
- Description of symptoms: factors more concerning for pathology over physiology are listed in Table 6.1
- Assess exercise tolerance
- Changes from baseline
- Medical history: lung disease, asthma, VTE, heart murmurs
- Obstetric history: preeclampsia or cardiomyopathy in a prior pregnancy
- Family history: structural malformations, VTE, sudden death at a young age
- Medications
- Travel history

Physical examination
- Vital signs
- Fetal heart tracing
- Lung auscultation
- Heart auscultation
- Pedal edema

Diagnostic testing
- CXR
- CT angiography if high suspicion for PE (alternately V/Q scan or LE Dopplers)
- Echocardiogram
- Laboratory testing
  - CBC
  - Kidney/liver function tests
  - LDH for preeclampsia
- BNP
- ABG

Referral to cardiologist multidisciplinary team planning

clearly outweighed by the benefit of a correct diagnosis [21]. If pulmonary embolism (PE) is high on the differential diagnosis, the workup may include lower extremity Doppler studies, a ventilation perfusion (V/Q) scan, and/or computed tomography (CT) scan [22]. Although CT scan carries with it more radiation exposure than an x-ray or V/Q scan, the risks associated with radiation outweigh the risks of an undiagnosed or incorrectly diagnosed PE [23,24]. If dyspnea is more suggestive of a cardiac etiology, an echocardiogram is performed. Laboratory investigations include a complete blood count, renal and liver function tests, as well as lactic dehydrogenase to assess for hemolysis if preeclampsia

or pulmonary edema are suspected. A brain natriuretic peptide (BNP) or a pro-NT BNP level is important when cardiomyopathy is suspected [25,26]. Arterial blood gas may be useful to determine acid base balance and alveolar to arterial oxygen gradient.

Chest Pain

Chest pain is a less common complaint in pregnancy than SOB but may be represent a life-threatening emergency. Fortunately, a vast majority of chest pains in pregnancy are due to benign causes. Gastroesophageal reflux disease (GERD) is one of the top causes of chest pain seen in 40%–85% of pregnant women

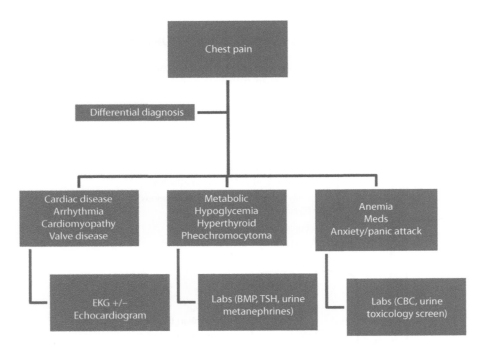

FIGURE 6.6 Chest pain in pregnancy.

[27,28]. It typically begins in the late first trimester and worsens with advancing gestational age as the uterus displaces the diaphragm upward. In addition, hormones decrease the tone in the lower esophageal sphincter, promoting acid reflux. Worsening of the pain with lying down and relief with sitting up is suggestive of GERD. Musculoskeletal pain or costochondritis may occur in normal pregnancy and are not a cause for alarm. Regardless, a workup for more concerning diagnoses should always be undertaken. The differential diagnosis for chest pain in pregnancy is similar to that outside of pregnancy, including myocardial ischemia/infarction (MI), PE, aortic dissection, and pregnancy-specific conditions such as peripartum cardiomyopathy (PPCM), especially if in the third trimester. See further Figure 6.6.

Potentially life-threatening diagnoses such as myocardial infarction, pulmonary embolism, and aortic dissections must be ruled out in a patient presenting with chest pain.

The evaluation of chest pain in pregnancy (Box 6.3) begins with:

1. *History*: The quality of the pain, duration and time of onset, alleviating or exacerbating factors, and radiation are important factors to elicit when taking a history. Pain that is relieved with cessation of exercise is more concerning for cardiac ischemia, while pain that is relieved by sitting up from a lying down position or by taking antacids is more suggestive of GERD. The presence of associated symptoms, such as SOB or dizziness, is suggestive of a more serious etiology. An obstetric history of any cardiovascular complications, history of murmurs, coronary artery disease, hypertension, venous thromboembolic disease, and vascular disease or connective tissue disorder such as Marfan syndrome should be reviewed. As with SOB, a comprehensive family history, medications, and travel history are obtained. Family history significant for arrhythmia—or use of arrhythmia-provoking medications—should prompt an EKG to assess for arrhythmia.

2. *Physical examination*: Vital sign abnormalities in the context of chest pain should prompt expedited evaluation. In the outpatient setting, hypo- or hypertension, tachycardia, tachypnea, hypoxia, or an abnormal fetal heart tracing should lead to immediate hospital transfer. The characteristics of chest pain may lead to more specific etiology; for example, in a patient with tearing chest pain and a history suggestive of Marfan or similar connective tissue disorder, blood pressure should be checked in both arms to assess for aortic dissection. A physical exam should focus on the cardiopulmonary examination, wide splitting of S1, and S3, and systolic murmurs can be part of a normal cardiac examination in pregnancy. On the other hand, diastolic murmurs are almost always pathologic. As in the workup for dyspnea, the fetal heart tracing can be used as another marker for maternal perfusion and oxygenation.

3. *Diagnostic testing*: In patients with chest pain, an EKG is an initial test to rule out myocardial ischemia. EKG may indicate rhythm abnormality, ischemic changes, atrial enlargement, or ventricular hypertrophy, which should be followed by an echocardiogram for confirmation. If clinical suspicion is high for cardiac ischemia, cardiac enzymes are obtained and the patient is put on continuous EKG monitoring. CXR may be an initial test for a suspected pulmonary etiology. Consultation with a cardiologist should be prompt if suspicion for cardiac pathology is high to ensure appropriate testing and follow-up.

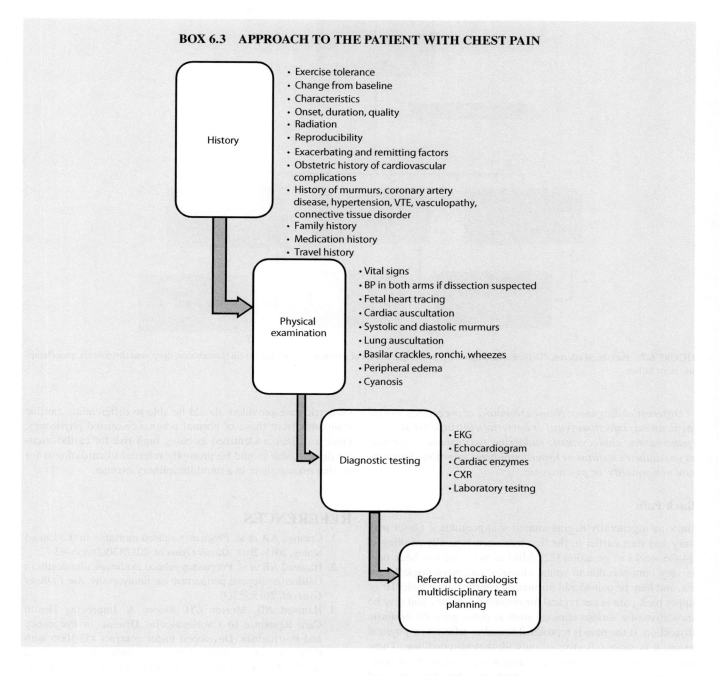

BOX 6.3   APPROACH TO THE PATIENT WITH CHEST PAIN

History
- Exercise tolerance
- Change from baseline
- Characteristics
- Onset, duration, quality
- Radiation
- Reproducibility
- Exacerbating and remitting factors
- Obstetric history of cardiovascular complications
- History of murmurs, coronary artery disease, hypertension, VTE, vasculopathy, connective tissue disorder
- Family history
- Medication history
- Travel history

Physical examination
- Vital signs
- BP in both arms if dissection suspected
- Fetal heart tracing
- Cardiac auscultation
- Systolic and diastolic murmurs
- Lung auscultation
- Basilar crackles, ronchi, wheezes
- Peripheral edema
- Cyanosis

Diagnostic testing
- EKG
- Echocardiogram
- Cardiac enzymes
- CXR
- Laboratory tesitng

Referral to cardiologist multidisciplinary team planning

Peripheral Edema

Peripheral edema is a very common finding in pregnancy. It is due to a combination of decreased systemic vascular resistance, increased blood volume, and compression of inferior vena cava with advancing gestation. In addition, saphenous veins of the lower extremity contain progesterone and estrogen receptors, which contribute to the venous dilation and valve failure during pregnancy, thereby worsening lower extremity edema [29]. See Figure 6.7.

Fatigue

Fatigue is a common complaint in up to 44% of pregnant women, and the symptom presentation is extremely variable throughout pregnancy. However, it is more widely accepted that fatigue worsens in the third trimester, as the burden of carrying increased weight from the pregnancy is at the maximum.

Differential diagnosis: Normal variant versus anemia, cardiac disease, i.e., PPCM, congestive heart failure, electrolyte imbalance.

Nausea

Nausea is a common complaint of pregnancy most prevalent in the first trimester that generally subsides by 12 weeks of pregnancy [30] however, it may persist into the late second trimester in patients with severe hyperemesis. Nausea can occur during labor, especially with use of analgesia; however, it should completely resolve within a few days postpartum [31].

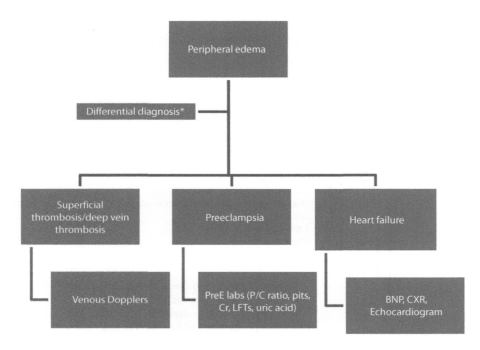

FIGURE 6.7 Peripheral edema. *Differential diagnosis: Physiologic edema of pregnancy, superficial vein thromboses, deep vein thrombosis, preeclampsia, heart failure.

Differential diagnosis: Nausea/vomiting of pregnancy, drugs/ medications, infectious (viral or bacterial), intrinsic GI disorder (pancreatitis, cholecystitis), endocrine (gastroparesis secondary to diabetes mellitus or hyperthyroidism), migraine, intracranial abnormality, or psychogenic.

Back Pain

Back pain generally begins around mid-pregnancy. Onset may vary and start earlier in the first trimester, typically peaking at 24–36 weeks of gestation [32]. Mild to moderate low back pain is very common due to spinal changes, i.e., physiologic lordosis, and may be considered normal. In contrast, midclavicular or upper back pain is not typical for normal pregnancy and may be indicative of a serious etiology such as pulmonary PE or aortic dissection. If the pain is reproducible and/or relieved on physical exam, it is more reflective of musculoskeletal condition. There are a few case series suggestive of an association between neuraxial anesthesia and interscapular back pain, but this is not well studied [33].

Differential diagnosis: Normal due to musculoskeletal changes in pregnancy, asthma, aortic dissection, PE.

Conclusion

Pregnancy mimics cardiac disease. Symptoms of palpitations and shortness of breath are common in pregnant women. Maternal mortality reviews indicate that the most important driving factors are delays in diagnosis and treatment of heart disease in pregnancy and a lack of recognition by the health care provider. All self-reported symptoms in pregnancy should be thoroughly evaluated in a manner similar to that of the nonpregnant state.

Obstetric care providers should be able to differentiate cardiac symptoms from those of normal pregnancy-related physiology. Once a patient is identified as being high risk for cardiovascular disease, she should be promptly referred to cardiologist for further management in a multidisciplinary manner.

REFERENCES

1. Creanga AA et al. Pregnancy-related mortality in the United States, 2011–2013. *Obstet Gynecol.* 2017;130(2):366–73.
2. Hameed AB et al. Pregnancy-related cardiovascular deaths in California: Beyond peripartum cardiomyopathy. *Am J Obstet Gynecol.* 2015;213(3).
3. Hameed AB, Morton CH, Moore A. Improving Health Care Response to Cardiovascular Disease in Pregnancy and Postpartum. Developed under contract #11-1006 with California Department of Public Health, Maternal Child and Adolescent Health Division. Published by the California Department of Public Health. http://www.CMQCC.org. 2017.
4. Hollier LM et al. Pregnancy and heart disease. *Obstet Gynecol.* 2019;133(5):E320–56.
5. Shotan A et al. Incidence of arrhythmias in normal pregnancy and relation to palpitations, dizziness, and syncope. *Am J Cardiology.* 1997;79(8):1061–4.
6. Robson SC et al. Hemodynamic-changes during early human-pregnancy—An M-mode and Doppler echocardiographic study. *Br Heart J.* 1987;57(6):584–5.
7. Soma-Pillay P et al. Physiological changes in pregnancy. *Cardiovasc J Afr.* 2016;27(2):89–94.
8. Drenthen W et al. Predictors of pregnancy complications in women with congenital heart disease. *Eur Heart J.* 2010;31(17):2124–32.

9. Li JM et al. Frequency and outcome of arrhythmias complicating admission during pregnancy: Experience from a high-volume and ethnically-diverse obstetric service. *Clin Cardiol.* 2008;31(11):538–41.

10. Yarnoz MJ, Curtis AB. More reasons why men and women are not the same (gender differences in electrophysiology and arrhythmias). *Am J Cardiol.* 2008;101(9):1291–6.

11. Knotts RJ, Garan H. Cardiac arrhythmias in pregnancy. *Seminars Perinatol.* 2014;38(5):285–8.

12. Vaidya VR et al. Burden of arrhythmia in pregnancy. *Circulation.* 2017;135(6):619–21.

13. Vaidya VR et al. P6055 Impact of atrial fibrillation in pregnancy: An analysis from the nationwide inpatient sample. *Eur Heart J.* 2017;38(Suppl 1):1273–1273.

14. Joglar JA, Page RL. Management of arrhythmia syndromes during pregnancy. *Curr Opin Cardiol.* 2014;29(1):36–44.

15. Adamson DL, Nelson-Piercy C. Managing palpitations and arrhythmias during pregnancy. *Heart.* 2007;93(12):1630–6.

16. Czerwinski EM. Case report postpartum cough and dyspnea. *Adv Emerg Nurs J.* 2016;38(3):190–8.

17. Goland S et al. Shortness of breath during pregnancy: Could a cardiac factor be involved? *Clin Cardiol.* 2015;38(10):598–603.

18. Wagner S et al. The impact of pregnancy on the work-up of chest pain and shortness of breath in the emergency department. *Obstet Gynecol.* 2017;129:176s–7s.

19. Varnier N et al. All that wheezes is not asthma: A cautionary case study of shortness of breath in pregnancy. *Obstet Med.* 2015;8(3):149–51.

20. Prasad M. Shortness of breath in pregnancy. *J General Internal Med.* 2015;30:S453–S453.

21. Copel J et al. Guidelines for diagnostic imaging during pregnancy and lactation. *Obstet Gynecol.* 2017;130(4):E210–16.

22. Wan T et al. Guidance for the diagnosis of pulmonary embolism during pregnancy: Consensus and controversies. *Thromb Res.* 2017;157:23–8.

23. Shahir K et al. Pulmonary embolism in pregnancy: CT pulmonary angiography versus perfusion scanning. *Am J Roentgenol.* 2010;195(3):W214–20.

24. Scarsbrook AF, Bradley KM, Gleeson FV. Perfusion scintigraphy: Diagnostic utility in pregnant women with suspected pulmonary embolic disease. *Eur Radiol.* 2007;17(10):2554–60.

25. Wei T et al. Systolic and diastolic heart failure are associated with different plasma levels of 13-type natriuretic peptide. *Int J Clin Pract.* 2005;59(8):891–4.

26. Grewal J et al. BNP and NT-proBNP predict echocardiographic severity of diastolic dysfunction. *Eur J Heart Fail.* 2008;10(3):252–9.

27. Ali RAR, Egan LJ. Gastroesophageal reflux disease in pregnancy. *Best Pract Res Clin Gastroenterol.* 2007;21(5):793–806.

28. Body C, Christie JA. Gastrointestinal diseases in pregnancy nausea, vomiting, hyperemesis gravidarum, gastroesophageal reflux disease, constipation, and diarrhea. *Gastroenterol Clin North Am.* 2016;45(2):267–83.

29. Smyth RMD, Aflaifel N, Bamigboye AA. Interventions for varicose veins and leg oedema in pregnancy. *Cochrane Database Syst Rev.* 2015(10):CE001066.

30. Bai GN et al. Associations between nausea, vomiting, fatigue and health-related quality of life of women in early pregnancy: The generation R study. *PLOS ONE.* 2016;11(11).

31. Kirshon B, Lee W, Cotton DB. Prompt resolution of hyperthyroidism and hyperemesis gravidarum after delivery. *Obstet Gynecol.* 1988;71(6):1032–4.

32. Vermani E, Mittal R, Weeks A. Pelvic girdle pain and low back pain in pregnancy: A review. *Pain Practice.* 2010;10(1):60–71.

33. Klumpner TT et al. Interscapular pain associated with neuraxial labour analgesia: A case series. *Can J Anesth.* 2016;63(4):475–9.

7

Cardiac Diagnostic Testing in Pregnancy

Edlira Tam and Cynthia Taub

KEY POINTS

- Cardiac complications in pregnant women with heart disease occur in 16% of pregnancies and are primarily related to maternal arrhythmias and heart failure
- The most sensitive period for embryopathy is between 5–12 weeks of gestation, and non-urgent radiological testing should be avoided during this time

- The accepted cumulative dose of ionizing radiation during pregnancy is 50 mGy
- Echocardiography should be obtained in pregnant women who complain of chest pain, syncope, shortness of breath out of proportion to pregnancy, and palpitations
- Cardiac MRI can be especially helpful in the assessment of complex congenital heart disease and aortic pathology

---

Introduction

Maternal heart disease, although it complicates a small percentage of all pregnancies in developed countries, is a major cause of non-obstetric maternal morbidity and mortality. *Cardiac complications in pregnant women with heart disease occur in 16% of pregnancies and are primarily related to maternal arrhythmias and heart failure.* The majority of cardiac complications are seen in the antepartum period, followed by the postpartum period, with the fewest occurring at the time of labor and delivery [1]. Maternal mortality continues to rise, and cardiovascular death is one of the main driving factors. Between 2011 and 2013, cardiovascular disease accounted for approximately 15% of maternal mortality in America [2]. Congenital heart disease is the most common form of heart disease complicating pregnancy in the United States, whereas rheumatic heart disease remains the most common form of heart disease in developing countries.

Pregnant women with known or suspected cardiovascular disease often require cardiovascular diagnostic testing during their pregnancy. There are multiple testing modalities available that can be used in pregnant women with suspected cardiac disease to confirm the diagnosis, risk stratify, treat, and assess response to therapy. The imaging modalities used for these purposes include electrocardiogram (ECG), x-ray (which encompasses chest radiography, computed tomographic pulmonary angiography [CTPA], coronary computed tomographic angiography [CCTA], fluoroscopy, and invasive angiography), echocardiography, cardiac magnetic resonance imaging (MRI), and nuclear techniques [3].

Special Considerations in Pregnancy

Normal cardiovascular changes in pregnancy such as increased cardiac output, volume overload, and reduced systemic vascular resistance may lead to significant changes in physical examination findings, laboratory changes, and imaging findings that often mimic cardiac pathology. A detailed exam should be performed in all women with signs and symptoms of cardiovascular disease, such as dyspnea, fatigue, palpitations, low oxygen level, and changes in blood pressure [2].

Imaging studies are important adjuncts in the diagnostic evaluation of cardiovascular disease in pregnancy. Poor understanding about the safety of imaging modalities in pregnancy and lactating women often results in unnecessary avoidance of useful diagnostic tests. Thus, it is important that the physician understand the indications for, limitations of, and potential harms or benefits of tests ordered during pregnancy. Appropriate counseling of patients before radiological studies are performed is critical, and informed consent should always be obtained. Risk to the embryo or fetus depends on the type and amount of radiation and gestational age of the fetus. Reports vary, but the most sensitive period for CNS teratogenicity seems to be between 8–17 weeks of gestation, with a higher threshold dose at more advanced gestational ages. Based on dose-response calculations, diagnostic procedures involving radiation do not pose a risk to the fetus unless the cumulative dose to the uterus is greater than 10 cGy; conservative guidelines suggest that non-urgent radiological testing should be avoided during this time and cumulative exposure to the uterus during pregnancy be kept below 5 cGy [3–5].

TABLE 7.1

Effects of Radiation on the Fetus (Gestational Age, Dose, and Effects)

Gestational Age	Estimated Threshold Dose	Effect
Before implantation (0–2 weeks)	50–100 mGy	Death of embryo or no consequence
Organogenesis (2–8 weeks after fertilization)	200 mGy 200–250 mGy	Congenital anomalies (skeleton, eyes, genitals) Growth restrictions
8–15 weeks	60–310 mGy 200 mGy	Severe intellectual disability (high risk) Microcephaly
16–25 weeks	250–280 mGy	Severe intellectual disability (low risk)

Source: Adapted from Patel SJ et al. *Radiographics.* 2007;27(6): 1705–22.

Pregnancy may limit the diagnostic accuracy of various imaging modalities. For instance, the appearance of cardiomegaly on chest x-ray, QRS axis changes in electrocardiogram, or exaggerated transvalvular gradient on echocardiogram can be due to the normal structural, physiological, and hemodynamic changes in pregnancy [2,6].

Radiation Exposure in Pregnancy

It is estimated that a fetus will be exposed to 1 mGy of background radiation in pregnancy [7]. The risk to the fetus from ionizing radiation is dependent on gestational age at the time of exposure and dose of radiation. The accepted cumulative dose of ionizing radiation during pregnancy is 50 mGy (equal to 50 mSv or 5 rads). If extremely high-dose exposure (in excess of 1 Gy) occurs during early embryogenesis, it will most likely be lethal to the embryo. The most common adverse effects seen with high-dose radiation exposure in humans beyond the period of early embryogenesis are growth restriction, microcephaly, and intellectual disability. However, for the development of these adverse effects the radiation exposure has to be sufficiently high. Fetal anomalies, growth restrictions, and miscarriages have not been reported with radiation exposure of less than 50 mGy (see Table 7.1) [4]. The estimated minimal threshold for an adverse effect is thought to be in the range of 60–310 mGy; however, the lowest clinically documented dose to produce severe intellectual disability has been reported to be 610 mGy [8]. Cardiovascular diagnostic imaging does not reach these levels, therefore these effects are rarely of concern for patients.

Laboratory Tests in Pregnancy

Laboratory tests should be the initial screening modality in women presenting with chest pain and shortness of breath out of proportion to pregnancy. Serum biomarkers can be used as screening tests to aid in diagnosis of cardiovascular disease.

TABLE 7.2

Laboratory Tests

Laboratory Test	Indications
BNP/NT-proBNP	Assess for cardiomyopathy, women with congenital heart disease, severe preeclampsia
Troponin	Assess for acute coronary syndromes or pulmonary embolism
D-dimer	High negative predicative value for pulmonary embolism May be even less sensitive in pregnancy, as level increases progressively throughout gestation
CBC	Assess for anemia: differential diagnosis of dyspnea out of proportion to pregnancy

B-type natriuretic peptides (BNP or its inactive amino terminal fragment NT-proBNP) are important biomarkers used in diagnosis and management of heart failure. Levels of natriuretic peptides may be elevated based on stage of pregnancy, preeclampsia, preexisting cardiomyopathies, congenital heart disease, or peripartum cardiomyopathy. Furthermore, BNP can be elevated in noncardiac conditions such as sepsis, kidney disease, and anemia [9,10]. A complete blood count (CBC) would aid in diagnosing anemia or an active infection. High levels of natriuretic peptides are associated with increased risk of cardiovascular events and should raise suspicion for cardiac disease and lead to careful supervision during pregnancy and postpartum period [10]. Troponin is another serum biomarker used to diagnose cardiovascular disease, particularly acute coronary syndrome (ACS) and massive PE with hemodynamic compromise. Pregnant women with ACS present similar to their female counterparts. Coronary artery disease (CAD), and in particular ACS, during pregnancy are associated with high risk of mortality and significant morbidity. A low threshold to investigate women with chest pain is paramount. Elevated troponin level in pregnant women with chest pain should be investigated seriously [11].

The plasma level of D-dimer is nearly always increased in the presence of acute pulmonary embolism (PE). It is a commonly used test with high sensitivity for ruling out venous thromboembolism (VTE) in nonpregnant patients [12]. The diagnosis of PE in pregnancy poses a challenge to physicians. Signs and symptoms of PE such as dyspnea, lower extremity edema, and tachycardia occur as part of normal pregnancy, and diagnostic tests such as the D-dimer can be unreliable because the level steadily rises throughout pregnancy [13]. A negative D-dimer is still reliable in pregnant patients with low pretest probability, and especially in the first trimester. However, if suspicion for VTE and pretest probability is high, further workup with imaging modalities is necessary. See Table 7.2.

Chest Radiograph

The chest radiograph is a commonly used diagnostic modality in pregnancy and it provides important information about the lungs, airways, blood vessels, and size of the heart and bones of the spine and chest.

Indications for obtaining a chest radiograph in pregnancy are no different from those in nonpregnant patients and should be considered in any pregnant patient who presents with new-onset dyspnea to evaluate for pulmonary edema, cardiomegaly, and atrial enlargement [8,14]. A review of 200 chest radiographs from pregnant women analyzed lung parenchyma, cardiac contour, and vascular markings and found no characteristic changes in pregnancy [15]. Thus, abnormal findings in pregnancy should be investigated just as they are in nonpregnant patients. Medically indicated chest radiograph can be safely performed in pregnancy provided that fetal (abdominal) shielding is used.

Electrocardiogram

The electrocardiogram (ECG) is often one of the initial diagnostic modalities performed in pregnant women with suspected heart disease. The ECG is helpful in identifying conditions such as myocardial infarction, arrhythmia, and PE. During normal pregnancy there may be some subtle changes in the ECG, such as shortening of the PR and QT intervals, left axis deviation [5], and nonspecific ST-T wave changes in the left precordial leads [16].

Rhythm Monitors

Palpitations, dizziness, and syncope are common complaints in pregnancy and are among the most frequent causes of referral to high-risk obstetric clinics [17]. According to the 2018 guidelines by the American College of Cardiology, American Heart Association, and Heart Rhythm Society, the presence of unexplained palpitations, syncope, or dizziness is considered a class 1 indication for ambulatory electrocardiogram monitoring [18].

Several types of ambulatory cardiac rhythm monitoring are available. For symptoms frequent enough to be detected within a short period, Holter monitoring can be used, which is a continuous recording for 24–72 hours but can be as long as 2 weeks in the newest models. External patch recorders continuously record and store rhythms for up to 14 days and have patient-trigger capability to allow for symptom rhythm correlation. The patch is leadless, can be easily self-applied, and is largely water resistant, making it more comfortable and less cumbersome, potentially improving patient compliance. In high-risk patients, mobile cardiac outpatient monitoring should be considered. This device records and transmits data for up to 30 days. If significant arrhythmias are detected, the data is automatically transmitted to a live central monitoring station, allowing for real-time and immediate feedback to a health care provider [18].

Heart rate increases by 25% in pregnancy, making sinus tachycardia the most common benign arrhythmia, especially in the third trimester. Furthermore, ectopic beats and non-sustained arrhythmia are encountered in more than 50% of pregnant women [19]. Sustained supraventricular tachycardia is the most common serious arrhythmia diagnosed in pregnancy. Interestingly, obese women (BMI >30) have a fourfold increased risk of experiencing a serious rhythm disturbance during gestation, and women with a prior history of arrhythmia have an eightfold increased risk [17].

Echocardiography

Transthoracic echocardiography can be used to evaluate ventricular function, valvular abnormalities, and pericardial disease. It uses high-frequency sound waves to image cardiac structures. Ultrasound waves are harmless to the tissues at the intensities used in diagnostic imaging. Echocardiography should be obtained in pregnant women who complain of chest pain, syncope, shortness of breath out of proportion to pregnancy, and palpitations. Furthermore, an echocardiogram should be performed on women with documented arrhythmia during pregnancy and those with known heart disease, stroke, or prior history of chemotherapy or radiation [20]. Serial echocardiography may be indicated during pregnancy based on the underlying cardiac disease.

It is important to note that significant cardiovascular hemodynamic changes occur during pregnancy, making clinical diagnosis of heart disease challenging. Normal pregnancy is associated with increased blood volume and cardiac output that lead to increases in left and right ventricular chamber size, an increase in left atrial size, and increase in left ventricular wall thickness; however, no change in left ventricular ejection fraction is seen. Other normal cardiac structural changes that can be seen in pregnancy include an increase in aortic root, increase in mitral and tricuspid annular size, and increase in stroke volume (see Table 7.3) [21,24]. In addition, asymptomatic pericardial effusions during the third trimester occur in approximately 40% of pregnant women [22].

TABLE 7.3

Normal Echocardiographic Changes in Pregnancy

Cardiac Chamber Dimensions	Change in Pregnancy
LV dimension and volume	Increases
LA dimension	Increases
LV wall and mass	Increase
RV dimension and volume	Increase
RA dimension	Increases mid to late third trimester
LV Systolic Function	**Change in Pregnancy**
Stroke volume	Increases
Cardiac output	Increases
LV ejection fraction	Unchanged
Doppler Parameters	**Change in Pregnancy**
Mitral E velocity	Slight increase
Mitral A velocity	Significant increase
E/A ratio	Decreases
Deceleration Time	Increases
Peak pulmonary artery pressure	Unchanged
Other	**Change in Pregnancy**
Aortic root diameter	Increases
Mitral/tricuspid annular size	Increases

Source: Adapted from Adeyeye VO et al. *Clin Med Insights Cardiol.* 2016;10:157–62.

Abbreviations: LV, left ventricle; RV, right ventricle; LA, left atrium; RA, right atrium.

Due to physiologic and structural changes in pregnancy, echocardiographic imaging can be technically difficult (i.e., limited subcostal views due to gravid uterus). *The use of echocardiographic contrast agents (ECA) to help discriminate between the blood pool and the endocardium has been used in the United States in at least 10%–15% of patients. To date there are no data about the safety of ECA use in pregnancy, and use of these agents in pregnancy should be limited unless clearly needed [23].*

Exercise Stress Test

In stable women with symptoms of coronary disease but no acute features, it is reasonable to perform exercise stress testing. Studies have shown that exercise stressing in pregnancy is safe. Stress testing can be either ECG-only, or if imaging is needed, exercise echocardiography can be performed. Studies have shown that exercise stress testing in inactive, regularly active, and vigorously active healthy women between 28 and 32 weeks of gestation showed no abnormal fetal bradycardic responses and there were no adverse neonatal outcomes [25,26]. In women who are not able to exercise, pharmacological stress testing using dobutamine would be an alternative. Animal studies to date have shown no evidence of fetotoxicity related to the use of dobutamine, and the FDA has classified it as pregnancy category B (although since 2014 obstetricians no longer classify drugs by categories; rather, each case is assessed individually and ultimately if the benefits outweigh the risks of the drug, it is advised to pursue its use) [5]. Nevertheless, dobutamine stress should only be performed if the benefits of the study outweigh the risks to the fetus and there is no other safer alternative.

Nuclear Perfusion Studies

Cardiovascular nuclear perfusion scans are performed via tagging a chemical agent with a radioisotope. Nuclear studies that may be performed during pregnancy include pulmonary ventilation-perfusion scans that evaluate for PE, and myocardial perfusion images used to assess coronary artery disease (CAD) and ventricular function. The two common nuclear imaging techniques used along with the gamma scintigraphic imaging are positron emission tomography (PET) and single photon-emission computed tomography (SPECT). The most commonly used compound for PET imaging is fluoro-2-deoxyglucose ([18]FDG) [3].

In cardiovascular perfusion scans, technetium 99 m, one of the most commonly used isotopes, may be combined with other compounds that localize to active myocardial cells allowing for identification of ischemic areas in the heart. The half-life of technetium 99 m is 6 hours and it releases a mono-energetic gamma photon of 140 keV [8].

Not all radioisotopes are safe in pregnancy. Radioactive iodine can easily cross the placenta, has a half-life of 8 days, and can lead to fetal thyroid abnormalities, especially after 10 weeks of gestation, given the timing the fetal thyroid commences function. Nuclear T_3 receptors can be identified in the brain of 10-week old fetuses, and they increase tenfold by 16 weeks' gestation before the fetal thyroid becomes fully functional. Myocardial perfusion studies using technetium 99 m result in embryonic

or fetal exposure of ≤17 mGy [27,46]. If cardiac stress testing is indicated in pregnancy, we favor using stress echocardiography over myocardial perfusion imaging to limit fetal exposure to radiation. However, if there is a real clinical indication for the study, such imaging can be performed, and the risk to the mother and fetus is minimal. Counseling pregnant women on the risks of radiation exposure to the fetus is an important duty for the physician. The risk for spontaneous abortions, major malformations, mental retardation, and childhood malignancy is approximately 286/1000 deliveries in the general population [3]; exposing the fetus to 50 mGy of radiation increases that risk by only 0.17% [28].

Cardiac Magnetic Resonance Imaging

Cardiac MRI is indicated when echocardiography cannot provide adequate diagnostic information and better imaging is required to optimize management. Cardiac MRI enables noninvasive evaluation of cardiac chambers, great arteries, and veins, and provides excellent evaluation of both the left and right ventricle, including ventricular size, thickness, wall motion, and ejection fraction. Cardiac MRI can be most helpful in the assessment of complex congenital heart disease and aortic pathology.

Cardiac MRI has been used safely in pregnancy for over 25 years, especially in the second and third trimester. There are no precautions or contraindications specific to the pregnant woman. MRI is free of ionizing radiation and provides high spatial and temporal resolution [8]. Cardiac MRI is reasonable as a diagnostic modality to assess myocardial function, congenital cardiovascular abnormalities, and disease of the aorta [27]. The main safety concerns include potential teratogenicity during the first trimester and acoustic damage to the fetus. A retrospective cohort study of 1737 women in their first trimester found that maternal exposure to MRI was not associated with a higher risk of stillbirth, neonatal death, congenital anomalies, neoplasm, or hearing loss [29].

The diagnostic accuracy of MRI can be improved with gadolinium, an intravenous contrast medium. Gadolinium is used in cardiac MRI for the detection of myocardial scar using late gadolinium enhancement (LGE) methods and detection of myocardial ischemia using stress/rest perfusion techniques [30]. LGE can be useful in identifying myocardial fibrosis and scarring (i.e., to distinguish between coronary disease and infiltrative diseases such as amyloidosis, sarcoidosis, or hemochromatosis) as well as to diagnose pericardial disease. Gadolinium-based contrast agents readily cross the placenta, and massive doses in experimental animals cause post-implantation fetal loss, delayed development, and skeletal and visceral abnormalities [31]. *The administration of gadolinium in pregnancy is discouraged due to the possibility of teratogenicity during organogenesis in the first trimester. In one study, gadolinium MRI used at any time during pregnancy was associated with increased risk of rheumatologic, inflammatory, and infiltrative skin disorders; stillbirth; and neonatal death [29]. Thus, current recommendations are to avoid use of gadolinium-enhanced MRI at any stage of pregnancy unless absolutely essential. The FDA classified all gadolinium-based contrast agents as pregnancy category C.* This category system is frequently misunderstood by health care providers and patients; in 2014 the FDA introduced a new system referred to as the "Pregnancy and Lactation Labeling Rule" that removes the letter ratings from all labels and replaces them with structured narrative summaries of potential risks [5].

Lower Extremity Ultrasound

Lower extremity ultrasound is a noninvasive test that is used in the diagnosis of deep venous thrombosis (DVT). The prevalence of venous thrombi in pregnancy is estimated to range from 0.06% to 8% with a reported predisposition for DVT of the left lower extremity (75%–96% of the cases) [32]. In pregnant women, iliofemoral thrombi involving the pelvic vein are more common than calf vein thrombi, and scanning strategies need to be adapted to take these factors into account [33]. Up to one-quarter of pregnant patients with untreated DVT may develop PE, which is the leading cause of maternal mortality in the developed world [34].

Ventilation-Perfusion Scintigraphy

Diagnostic imaging plays an important role for diagnosis of PE in pregnancy. Ventilation-perfusion (V/Q) scintigraphy and pulmonary CT angiography (CTA) have both been used to diagnose PE in pregnant women. The available literature on fetal radiation remains conflicted, with some authors asserting that both studies confer the same amount of radiation [35], whereas others have shown that pulmonary CTA provides a substantially lower dose [36]. The fetal radiation dose from both studies is approximately 0.1–0.4 mGy. V/Q scan delivers an effective breast dose of 0.22–0.28 mGy, significantly lower than pulmonary CTA (see below) [34]. Thus, one major advantage to V/Q scanning is the lower radiation exposure to the maternal breast tissue, with the major disadvantage being inability to provide an alternative diagnosis in the absence of PE [32]. The accuracy of V/Q scan has been reported to be as high as 96%, although the study can be inconclusive in up to 25% of pregnant patients [37].

In order to avoid nondiagnostic results, it is reasonable to reserve V/Q scanning in women with normal chest radiographic findings and no history of asthma or chronic lung disease. To limit fetal radiation exposure, low-dose perfusion-only scans (LDQ) are used commonly in pregnant women. Dose reduction can be readily achieved by eliminating the ventilation portion and decreasing the dose of the perfusion component by 50%. A retrospective study of 225 pregnant women who underwent LDQ found this imaging modality performed comparably to pulmonary CTA, with indistinguishable negative predictive values (100% and 97.5%, respectively) [32,38].

Pulmonary Computed Tomographic Angiography

Pulmonary CTA is the imaging of choice in the diagnoses of PE due to its high sensitivity and specificity. Disadvantages

include maternal breast radiation exposure of up to 10–70 mGy, fetal radiation exposure, and risks related to iodinated contrast material [32,34]. The most common side effects associated with iodinated contrast media include nausea, vomiting, flushing, and anaphylactoid reaction. Iodine contrast media can readily cross the placenta; however, animal studies have not shown any teratogenic or mutagenic effects with its use [8]. The current recommendation is that contrast may be used when needed and when benefits outweigh the risks.

In a pregnant patient requiring the study, reduced-dose pulmonary CTA is recommended. In addition, other dose reduction methods such as thin-layered bismuth breast shield and abdominal lead shielding for the fetus should always be used [32]. A potential disadvantage to the study is the possibility of reduced image quality due to less pulmonary artery enhancement in pregnancy because a higher percentage of maternal cardiac output is shifted to the fetus [39]. While it remains the imaging choice for PE, in a small retrospective study, pulmonary CTA was diagnostically inadequate in 35.7% of pregnant patients compared with 2.1% in nonpregnant patients [40]. A meta-analysis supported the overall better performance of pulmonary CTA to V/Q scan in the general population [41], whereas an additional study looking at pregnant patients found both imaging modalities to be equivalent [42]. Thus, the choice of study should be based on other considerations, such as radiation concern, radiographic results, and need for an alternative diagnosis.

Coronary Computed Tomographic Angiography

CCTA is used for diagnosis of CAD in patients with chest pain and no prior history of CAD. It uses advanced CT technology along with intravenous contrast material to obtain high-resolution 3D images. CCTA can accurately quantify the presence, extent, angiographic severity, and composition of coronary atherosclerosis with a reported sensitivity of 91% and specificity of 92% [43]. CCTA is noninvasive with potentially less risk and discomfort compared to cardiac catheterization. Although it may provide a safer method to obtain anatomic information, it still carries the risks of fetal radiation and a need to use high doses of a beta-blocker for appropriate heart rate reduction [44].

Left Heart Catheterization

Coronary angiography/left heart catheterization (LHC) is the gold standard diagnostic test in the diagnosis of CAD and management of acute myocardial infarction (AMI). AMI complicating pregnancy is relatively uncommon; it is more likely to occur in older women and has a mortality rate of 7.3%–20% [20,44]. A study of 150 cases of AMI occurring during pregnancy or the postpartum period found that two-thirds of the patients had an anterior wall MI. Coronary artery dissection, a rare cause of AMI in the nonpregnant population, was the most common cause, documented in >40% of the pregnant patients in this study. AMI secondary to coronary artery dissection occurred mostly in late pregnancy or the early postpartum period and involved mostly the left main and left anterior descending artery

TABLE 7.4

Common Diagnostic Tests

Diagnostic Test	Indications	Risks	Safe in Pregnancy
Chest radiograph	Cardiac and pulmonary disease	Estimated fetal exposure to radiation is <0.0001 mGy	Yes
Electrocardiogram	ACS, PE, arrhythmias	Safe	Yes
Echocardiogram	Evaluate cardiac structures and function	Safe	Yes
Rhythm monitors	Palpitations, near-syncope, syncope	Safe	Yes
Exercise stress test	Chest pain, dyspnea	Safe	Yes
Myocardial nuclear perfusion studies	Assess coronary artery disease and ventricular function	Radioactive iodine is teratogenic and should not be used in pregnancy Fetal radiation exposure with technetium is ≤17 mGy	Avoid if possible Use stress echocardiography as first line
Cardiac MRI	Cardiac chambers, great arteries and veins, ventricular size, thickness, wall motion, and ejection fraction	No reported risks in pregnancy without gadolinium Gadolinium readily crosses placenta and may be teratogenic in the first trimester May cause hematologic, inflammatory, infiltrative skin disorders; stillbirth; and neonatal death	Avoid gadolinium
Lower extremity ultrasound	DVT	Safe	Yes
Ventilation-perfusion scintigraphy	PE	Maternal breast radiation 0.22–0.28 mGy Fetal radiation exposure approximately 0.1–0.4 mGy	Yes (weigh risk vs. benefit)
Pulmonary computed tomographic angiography	Imaging of choice for PE	Maternal breast radiation exposure 10–70 mGy Fetal radiation exposure Iodinated contrast exposure	Yes Reduced dose CTPA recommended in pregnancy
Coronary computed tomographic angiography	Used in patients with chest pain but no known coronary disease	Fetal radiation exposure of 1–3 mGy	Use as second line if exercise stress testing and echocardiogram are nondiagnostic
Left heart catheterization	Gold standard for diagnosis of CAD and management of acute MI	Maternal radiation exposure 7 mGy Fetal radiation exposure 1.5 mGy	Weigh risk vs. benefit. Test of choice in STEMI and high-risk NSTEMI

[45]. Clinical presentation of AMI is the same as in the nonpregnant population.

The effects of ionizing radiation should not prevent primary percutaneous coronary intervention (PCI) when there is an indication for revascularization in AMI. The estimated radiation exposure from an LHC to the fetus is approximately 1.5 mGy, and to the mother is about 7 mGy. When PCI or radiofrequency catheter ablation is needed, that exposure increases to 3 mGy for the fetus and 15 mGy for the mother [20]. In stable, low-risk NSTEMI, a noninvasive approach should be considered.

There is little information regarding recommended drug therapy in AMI. Low-dose aspirin appears to be safe in pregnancy. There is little information regarding P2Y$_{12}$ inhibitors, and the most recent recommendations by the European Society of Cardiology suggest using clopidogrel only when strictly needed and for the shortest duration. In the absence of data, they recommend refraining from the use of glycoprotein IIb/IIIa inhibitors, bivalirudin, prasugrel, and ticagrelor. Beta-blockade may be beneficial in reducing shear stress and can be used in pregnancy [44,45]. See Table 7.4.

Conclusion

Physiologic changes in pregnancy may alter results of common diagnostic modalities. A detailed history and physical examination in pregnant patients presenting with cardiac symptoms will help triage and utilize the appropriate test at a given gestational age. Most diagnostic tests and imaging modalities for cardiovascular evaluation are considered safe in pregnancy.

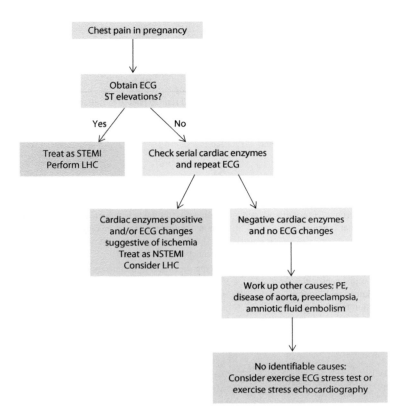

FIGURE 7.1   Chest pain algorithm.

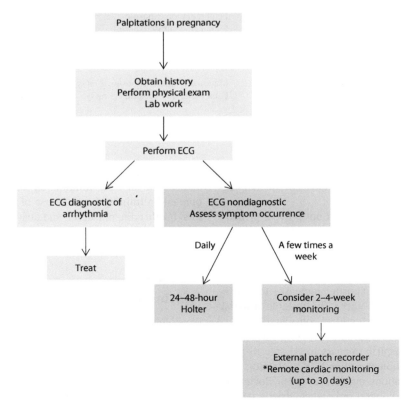

FIGURE 7.2   Palpitations in pregnancy algorithm. *Consider on high-risk patients; ECG-electrocardiogram.

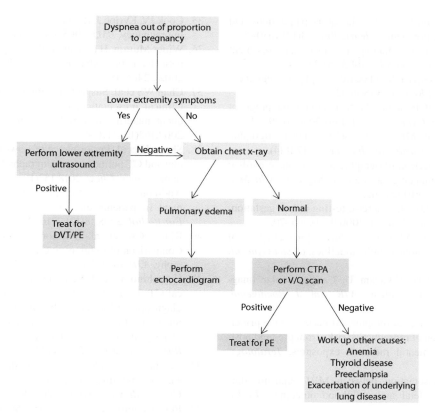

FIGURE 7.3 Shortness of breath algorithm.

REFERENCES

1. Silversides CK et al. Pregnancy outcomes in women with heart disease: The CARPREG II study. *J Am Coll Cardiol.* 2018;71(21):2419–30.
2. Wolfe DS et al. Addressing maternal mortality: The pregnant cardiac patient. *Am J Obstet Gynecol.* 2019;220(2):167 e1–167 e8.
3. Ntusi NA et al. Diagnosing cardiac disease during pregnancy: Imaging modalities. *Cardiovasc J Afr.* 2016;27(2):95–103.
4. Wang PI et al. Imaging of pregnant and lactating patients: Part 1, evidence-based review and recommendations. *AJR Am J Roentgenol.* 2012;198(4):778–84.
5. Chambers C, Friedman JM. Teratogenesis and environmental exposure. In: Resnick R, Lockwood CJ, Moore TR et al., editors. *Creasy & Resnick's Maternal-Fetal Medicine,* 8th ed. Philadelphia: Elsevier; 2019, pp. 539–48.
6. Schwartz DB, Schamroth L. The effect of pregnancy on the frontal plane QRS axis. *J Electrocardiol.* 1979;12(3):279–81.
7. Patel SJ et al. Imaging the pregnant patient for nonobstetric conditions: Algorithms and radiation dose considerations. *Radiographics.* 2007;27(6):1705–22.
8. Jain C. ACOG committee opinion No. 723: Guidelines for diagnostic imaging during pregnancy and lactation. *Obstet Gynecol.* 2019;133(1):186.
9. Troughton R, Michael Felker G, Januzzi JL Jr, Natriuretic peptide-guided heart failure management. *Eur Heart J.* 2014;35(1):16–24.
10. Balaceanu A. B-type natriuretic peptides in pregnant women with normal heart or cardiac disorders. *Med Hypotheses.* 2018;121:149–51.
11. Fryearson J, Adamson DL. Heart disease in pregnancy: Ischaemic heart disease. *Best Pract Res Clin Obstet Gynaecol.* 2014;28(4):551–62.
12. Perrier A et al. D-dimer testing for suspected pulmonary embolism in outpatients. *Am J Respir Crit Care Med.* 1997;156(2 Pt 1):492–6.
13. Borhart J, Palmer J. Cardiovascular emergencies in pregnancy. *Emerg Med Clin North Am.* 2019;37(2):339–350.
14. Ain DL, Narula J, Sengupta PP. Cardiovascular imaging and diagnostic procedures in pregnancy. *Cardiol Clin.* 2012;30(3):331–41.
15. Turner AF, The chest radiograph in pregnancy. *Clin Obstet Gynecol.* 1975;18(3):65–74.
16. Oram S, Holt M. Innocent depression of the S-T segment and flattening of the T-wave during pregnancy. *J Obstet Gynaecol Br Emp.* 1961;68:765–70.
17. Cruz MO et al. Ambulatory arrhythmia monitoring in pregnant patients with palpitations. *Am J Perinatol.* 2013;30(1):53–8.
18. Writing Committee Members et al. 2017 ACC/AHA/HRS guideline for the evaluation and management of patients with syncope: A report of the American College of Cardiology/American Heart Association Task Force on Clinical Practice Guidelines and the Heart Rhythm Society. *Heart Rhythm.* 2017;14(8):e155–e217.

19. Adamson DL, Nelson-Piercy C. Managing palpitations and arrhythmias during pregnancy. *Heart.* 2007;93(12):1630–6.

20. Waksmonski CA. Cardiac imaging and functional assessment in pregnancy. *Semin Perinatol.* 2014;38(5):240–4.

21. Liu S, Elkayam U, Naqvi TZ. Echocardiography in Pregnancy: Part 1. *Curr Cardiol Rep.* 2016;18(9):92.

22. Abduljabbar HS et al. Pericardial effusion in normal pregnant women. *Acta Obstet Gynecol Scand.* 1991;70(4–5):291–4.

23. Muskula PR, Main ML. Safety with echocardiographic contrast agents. *Circ Cardiovasc Imaging.* 2017;10(4).

24. Adeyeye VO et al. Echocardiographic assessment of cardiac changes during normal pregnancy among Nigerians. *Clin Med Insights Cardiol.* 2016;10:157–62.

25. MacPhail A et al. Maximal exercise testing in late gestation: Fetal responses. *Obstet Gynecol.* 2000;96(4):565–70.

26. Szymanski LM, Satin AJ. Exercise during pregnancy: Fetal responses to current public health guidelines. *Obstet Gynecol.* 2012;119(3):603–10.

27. Colletti PM, Lee KH, Elkayam U. Cardiovascular imaging of the pregnant patient. *AJR Am J Roentgenol.* 2013;200(3):515–21.

28. Brent RL. Utilization of developmental basic science principles in the evaluation of reproductive risks from pre- and post-conception environmental radiation exposures. *Teratology.* 1999(59):182–204.

29. Ray JG et al. Association between MRI exposure during pregnancy and fetal and childhood outcomes. *JAMA.* 2016;316(9):952–61.

30. Nacif MS et al. Gadolinium-enhanced cardiovascular magnetic resonance: Administered dose in relationship to United States Food and Drug Administration (FDA) guidelines. *J Cardiovasc Magn Reson.* 2012;14:18.

31. Widmark JM. Imaging-related medications: A class overview. *Proc (Bayl Univ Med Cent).* 2007;20(4):408–17.

32. Pahade JK et al. Quality initiatives: Imaging pregnant patients with suspected pulmonary embolism: What the radiologist needs to know. *Radiographics.* 2009;29(3):639–54.

33. Bennett A, Chunilal S. Diagnosis and management of deep vein thrombosis and pulmonary embolism in pregnancy. *Semin Thromb Hemost.* 2016;42(7):760–773.

34. Wang PI et al. Imaging of pregnant and lactating patients: Part 2, evidence-based review and recommendations. *AJR Am J Roentgenol.* 2012;198(4):785–92.

35. Cook JV, Kyriou J. Radiation from CT and perfusion scanning in pregnancy. *BMJ.* 2005;331(7512):350.

36. Winer-Muram HT et al. Pulmonary embolism in pregnant patients: Fetal radiation dose with helical CT. *Radiology.* 2002;224(2):487–92.

37. Chan WS et al. Suspected pulmonary embolism in pregnancy: Clinical presentation, results of lung scanning, and subsequent maternal and pediatric outcomes. *Arch Intern Med.* 2002;162(10):1170–5.

38. Sheen JJ et al. Performance of Low-dose perfusion scintigraphy and CT pulmonary angiography for pulmonary embolism in pregnancy. *Chest.* 2018;153(1):152–160.

39. Andreou AK et al. Does pregnancy affect vascular enhancement in patients undergoing CT pulmonary angiography? *Eur Radiol.* 2008;18(12):2716–22.

40. Ridge CA et al. Pulmonary embolism in pregnancy: Comparison of pulmonary CT angiography and lung scintigraphy. *AJR Am J Roentgenol.* 2009;193(5):1223–7.

41. Hayashino Y et al. Ventilation-perfusion scanning and helical CT in suspected pulmonary embolism: Meta-analysis of diagnostic performance. *Radiology.* 2005;234(3):740–8.

42. Shahir K et al. Pulmonary embolism in pregnancy: CT pulmonary angiography versus perfusion scanning. *AJR Am J Roentgenol.* 2010;195(3):W214–20.

43. Neglia D et al. Detection of significant coronary artery disease by noninvasive anatomical and functional imaging. *Circ Cardiovasc Imaging.* 2015;8(3).

44. Regitz-Zagrosek V et al. 2018 ESC Guidelines for the management of cardiovascular diseases during pregnancy. *Eur Heart J.* 2018;39(34):3165–3241.

45. Elkayam U et al. Pregnancy-associated acute myocardial infarction: A review of contemporary experience in 150 cases between 2006 and 2011. *Circulation.* 2014;129(16):1695–702.

46. Creasy RK et al. Thyroid disease and pregnancy. In: Charles J Lockwood, Thomas R Moore, and Michael F Greene, editors. *Creasy and Resnik's Maternal-Fetal Medicine: Principles and Practice,* 7th ed. Philadelphia: Elsevier; 2014, p. 1024.

8

Anesthesia and Analgesia in the Pregnant Cardiac Patient

Katherine W. Arendt

KEY POINTS

- The majority of maternal deaths from cardiovascular disease are from acquired heart disease
- The pregnancy heart team is a multidisciplinary team consisting of obstetrician, maternal-fetal medicine, anesthesiologist, and cardiologist working together to optimize outcome of pregnant cardiac patient

- Women with high-risk maternal cardiovascular disease should deliver at a Level 4 Regional Perinatal Health Center
- Neuraxial labor analgesia is an important component of labor management in patients with moderate to severe cardiovascular disease
- In certain circumstances general anesthesia is a safer option than a neuraxial technique for surgical anesthesia

Introduction

Over the past 20 years, cardiovascular disease has gradually become the leading cause of maternal mortality in the United States [1]. Increased survival of congenital heart disease (CHD) patients has resulted in more women reaching childbearing age and presenting to labor and delivery units [2–4]. Factors such as increased maternal age and increased incidence of obesity, chronic hypertension, and diabetes has likely led to expansion of acquired heart disease seen among the childbearing population. *Currently, acquired heart disease comprises the majority of maternal cardiac deaths* [5,6].

Both the European Society of Cardiology and the American College of Obstetricians and Gynecologists (ACOG) guidelines for pregnancy and heart disease recommend that a pregnancy heart team care for pregnant patients with complex cardiovascular disease [7,8]. Such a team involves cardiologists, obstetricians, perinatologists, and anesthesiologists working together to achieve the best outcome for the pregnant patient with complex heart disease. The focus of this chapter is on the role of the anesthesiologist as a member of the pregnancy heart team. Specifically, this chapter will focus on anesthetic risk stratification, the physiologic changes of pregnancy, labor and delivery, hemodynamic goals for patients as they present for delivery, and appropriate anesthetic techniques to achieve those goals.

Anesthetic Risk Stratification

Stratification of the overall risk of pregnancy for women with cardiac disease is discussed elsewhere in this text (see Chapter 4). Tables 8.1 through 8.3 review tools used for risk-stratifying women with cardiac disease who are pregnant [9–11].

Risk stratification is important to the anesthesiologist because anesthesiologists are an integral part of the multidisciplinary team who help identify pregnancies at high risk for maternal harm during childbirth and triage these women to deliver at appropriate hospitals. To do this, anesthesia teams should have the ability to see high-risk pregnant patients in advance of delivery in a clinical setting to obtain an anesthetic, obstetric, and cardiac history; perform a physical exam; and review cardiac testing. The most important aspects of this consultation are reviewed in Box 8.1.

Anesthesiologists often prefer to think in physiologic systems when risk-stratifying patients for surgery or delivery. Understanding the hemodynamic changes of pregnancy and combining these changes with the physiologic vulnerabilities of various cardiac lesions allows the anesthesiologist to understand which lesions will perform poorly during pregnancy, under anesthesia, or under the physiologic stressors of labor, emergency surgery, or obstetric hemorrhage. The physiologic changes of pregnancy are reviewed in Table 8.4. How these changes affect the hemodynamics of a woman with specific cardiac lesions are reviewed in Table 8.5.

The ACOG and the Society for Maternal Fetal Medicine have published a consensus statement that has been endorsed by multiple societies, including the Society for Obstetric Anesthesia and Perinatology [12]. These levels of care are reviewed in Table 8.6. An anesthesiologist should stratify the patient according to their risk of morbidity and mortality in pregnancy and combine that with the level maternal care of the hospital, and then provide recommendations to facilitate triaging patients to the appropriate delivery setting. For example, if an anesthesiologist who works at a Level 2 hospital sees a pregnant patient who has a lesion that is categorized as a modified World Health Organization (WHO) class IV, then the anesthesiologist should recommend and facilitate transfer to their class IV Regional Perinatal Center if it is

TABLE 8.1

CARPREG II Risk Score

Risk Factors	Points
Prior cardiac event or arrhythmia	3
NYHA class >II or cyanosis	3
Mechanical valve	3
Ventricular dysfunction	2
High-risk left-sided valve disease/ LVOT obstruction	2
Pulmonary hypertension	2
Coronary artery disease	2
High-risk aortopathy	2
No prior cardiac intervention	1
Late pregnancy assessment	1

Total Score	Risk of Cardiac Complications
0–1 points	5%
2 points	10%
3 points	15%
4 points	22%
>4 points	41%

Source: Adapted from Silversides CK et al. *J Am Coll Cardiol.* 2018;71(21):2419–30.
Abbreviations: NYHA, New York Heart Association; LVOT, left ventricular outflow tract.

safe and possible to do so at that time. Overall, women with moderate risk maternal cardiovascular disease (e.g., WHO class III) should deliver at a minimum of a Level 3 Subspecialty Care Hospital and women with high-risk maternal cardiovascular disease should deliver at a Level 4 Regional Perinatal Health Center.

TABLE 8.2

ZAHARA Risk Score

Risk Factors	Points
Mechanical valve prosthesis	4.25
Left heart obstruction	2.5
History of arrhythmia	1.5
Cardiac medication prior to pregnancy	1.5
Cyanotic heart disease (corrected or uncorrected)	1.0
NYHA class ≥II	0.75
Systemic atrioventricular valve regurgitation > Mild	0.75
Pulmonic atrioventricular valve regurgitation > Mild	0.75

Total Score	Risk of Cardiac Complications
0–0.5 points	2.90%
0.51–1.5 points	7.50%
1.51–2.5 points	17.50%
2.51–3.5 points	43.10%
>3.51 points	70%

Source: Adapted from Drenthen W et al. *Eur Heart J.* 2010;31(17): 2124–32.
Abbreviation: NYHA, New York Heart Association.

TABLE 8.3

WHO Classification for Pregnancy

Risk Classification	Cardiac Lesions
Class I No detectable increased risk of maternal mortality and no or minimal increase in maternal morbidity	• Uncomplicated mild pulmonary stenosis • Ventricular septal defect • Patent ductus arteriosus • Mitral valve prolapse with no more than trivial mitral regurgitation • Successfully repaired simple lesions (atrial or ventricular septal defect, patent ductus arteriosus, anomalous pulmonary venous drainage) • Isolated ventricular extrasystoles and atrial ectopic beats
Class II Small increased risk of maternal mortality or moderate increase in morbidity	• Unoperated atrial or ventricular septal defect • Repaired tetralogy of Fallot • Most arrhythmias
Class II–III Depends on patient	• Hypertrophic cardiomyopathy • Native or tissue valvular heart disease not considered WHO I or IV • Repaired coarctation • Marfan syndrome without aortic dilatation • Bicuspid valve with aorta <45 mm • Mild ventricular impairment • Heart transplantation
Class III Significantly increased risk of maternal mortality or severe morbidity, and expert cardiac and obstetric pre-pregnancy, antenatal, and postnatal care are required	• Mechanical valve • Systemic RV • Fontan circulation • Unrepaired cyanotic heart disease • Other complex congenital heart disease • Marfan syndrome with aorta 40–45 mm • Bicuspid aortic valve with aorta 45–50 mm
Class IV Pregnancy is contraindicated	• Pulmonary hypertension • Eisenmenger syndrome • Systemic ventricular EF <30% • Systemic ventricular dysfunction with NYHA class III–IV • Severe mitral stenosis • Severe symptomatic aortic stenosis • Marfan syndrome with aorta >45 mm • Bicuspid aortic valve with aorta >50 mm • Native severe coarctation • Prior peripartum cardiomyopathy with any residual impairment of ventricular function

Source: Adapted from Thorne S et al. *Heart* 2006;92(10):1520–5.
Abbreviations: WHO, World Health Organization; EF, ejection fraction; NYHA, New York Heart Association; RV, right ventricle.

HISTORY

- Anesthetic history
- Obstetric history
- Cardiac history with special attention to:
  - All prior cardiac testing including surgeries, echocardiograms, ECGs, Holter monitors, etc.
  - Prior or current episodes of heart failure
  - Intracardiac shunting and cyanosis
  - Prior arrhythmias
  - Left heart obstructive lesions
  - Left and right heart function
  - Pacemaker or defibrillator management
  - Anticoagulation therapy

PHYSICAL EXAM

- Airway
- Cardiac exam
- Pulmonary exam
- Exam of the back to assess for ease of neuraxial techniques

DISCUSS

- Potential hemodynamic monitoring plans for labor or cesarean delivery
- Potential risks, benefits, and alternatives of neuraxial techniques
- Potential need to manage anticoagulation around the time of delivery to facilitate neuraxial techniques
- Potential post-delivery plans for monitoring

TABLE 8.4

Normal Cardiovascular Changes during Pregnancy

Variable	Direction of Change	Average Change
Blood volume	↑	+35%
Plasma volume	↑	+45%
Red blood cell volume	↑	+20%
Cardiac output	↑	+40%
Stroke volume	↑	+30%
Heart rate	↑	+15%
Femoral venous pressure	↑	+15 mmHg
Total peripheral resistance	↓	−15%
Mean arterial blood pressure	↓	−15 mmHg
Systolic blood pressure	↓	−0 to 15 mmHg
Diastolic blood pressure	↓	−10 to 20 mmHg
Central venous pressure	↔	No change

Source: Modified from Bucklin BA, Fuller AJ. Physiologic changes of pregnancy. In: Suresh MS et al (eds). *Shnider and Levinson's Anesthesia for Obstetrics*, 5th ed. Wolters Kluwer Health, Inc. 2013. Chapter 1, pp. 2.

Principles of Labor Analgesia in Cardiac Disease

Neuraxial labor analgesia is an important component of labor management in patients with moderate to severe cardiovascular disease. The principles of neuraxial labor analgesia in women with cardiac disease are reviewed in Box 8.2. If neuraxial analgesia is not an option for a high-risk cardiac patient, then the pregnancy heart team may need to reconsider vaginal delivery. Although patient-controlled analgesia (PCA) via intravascular opioid infusion with remifentanil or fentanyl is provided to some laboring patients, this is not be a good alternative for the moderate- to high-risk cardiac patient. Pain control is typically suboptimal with intravenous opioid analgesia, leading to increased catecholamine release. Furthermore, to achieve even mildly effective analgesia, the dose of opioid required could suppress ventilation. The resultant carbon dioxide retention can cause respiratory acidosis, further catecholamine release, and increased pulmonary hypertension leading to arrhythmias, ischemia, or heart failure in the high-risk cardiac patient.

The most common reasons that a neuraxial technique may not be possible include conditions that increase the risks of the technique causing bleeding, infection, or nerve damage in the patient's spine. In cardiac disease patients, anticoagulation therapy may preclude the ability to perform any neuraxial anesthetic techniques. Although the incidence of epidural hematoma is rare, the consequences can be devastating. Therefore, anesthesiologists are guided by the American Society of Regional Anesthesia and the Society for Obstetric Anesthesia and Perinatology consensus statements in their management of anticoagulation and neuraxial techniques [13,14]. These guidelines are summarized in Figures 8.1 and 8.2. If a patient does not meet the criteria for safe placement, anesthesiologists will not perform a labor analgesic or surgical anesthetic neuraxial technique.

Neuraxial labor analgesia reduces the catecholamine surges from labor pain that can result in tachycardia, arrhythmias, hypertension, increases in cardiac output, and ventricular stress. Maintaining a dense, functional epidural not only decreases such cardiac stress but it also decreases the degree of hemodynamic alteration should an urgent cesarean delivery be required and the epidural need to be converted to a surgical block quickly.

The specific neuraxial catheter technique chosen by the anesthesiologist is less important than simply obtaining an epidural catheter that works well. Epidurals, combined spinal epidurals (CSE), and dural puncture epidurals (DPE) are all reasonable techniques. Some anesthesiologists recommend a loss of resistance with saline technique in patients with intracardiac shunts to minimize the chance of paradoxical air embolism in the event of intravascular needle placement. Others recommend a CSE with opioid-only intrathecal drug administration to minimize the effects of a sympathectomy from neuraxial local anesthetic administration. Still others recommend a DPE technique for greater reassurance that the loss of resistance is, in fact, the epidural space and to facilitate coverage of the sacral nerve roots, and others recommend avoiding epinephrine-containing test doses in patients with a history of arrhythmias. This author believes that all of these recommendations are reasonable, but not critical. What is most important is a catheter safely placed into the epidural space that completely blocks the pain of contractions throughout the entirety of labor.

TABLE 8.5

The Hemodynamic Effects of Pregnancy in Specific Cardiovascular Diseases

Lesion	Hemodynamic Effects of Pregnancy and Delivery
Coronary artery disease	(−) The decreased SVR of pregnancy can result in lesser coronary perfusion to the myocardium (−) The increase in HR during pregnancy can result in decreased coronary filling time (−) Cardiac work can increase significantly during labor, especially painful labor
Severe LV dysfunction (e.g., dilated or peripartum cardiomyopathy)	(−) The increase in cardiac output and blood volume during pregnancy can result in heart failure/pulmonary edema (−) The decrease in oncotic pressure during pregnancy can result in greater risk for pulmonary edema (−) Angiotensive converting enzyme inhibitors must be stopped during pregnancy secondary to teratogenicity (−) Patients with a prior episode of peripartum cardiomyopathy are at risk for further deterioration in LV function with subsequent pregnancies
Pulmonary hypertension	(−) The increased cardiac output of pregnancy may not be accommodated by the fixed pulmonary vasculature resulting in right heart failure and death (−) The decreased SVR of pregnancy can decrease coronary filling to a dilating and failing right ventricle (−) The hypercoagulable state of pregnancy can result in pulmonary emboli which are especially lethal in patients with pulmonary hypertension
Unstable arrhythmia history	(−) Pregnancy, labor, and delivery can trigger tachyarrhythmias
Aortopathy (e.g., Marfan syndrome)	(−) Pregnancy, labor, and delivery may increase dilation of aortic root (−) Pregnancy, labor, and delivery increase the risk of aortic rupture in women with Marfan syndrome
Valvular lesions	
Mechanical prosthetic valve	(−) Hypercoagulable state of pregnancy increases risk of valve thrombosis (−) Vitamin K antagonists (most effective way to prevent valvular clot formation) are teratogenic; often suboptimal anticoagulation regimens are used during pregnancy
Mitral stenosis	(−) Because of relatively fixed preload to the LV, the heart may not be able to generate increased cardiac output and pulmonary edema will develop (−) Decreased oncotic pressure further increases risk of pulmonary edema (−) The increase in blood volume and heart rate in pregnancy increases left atrial pressure and may lead to atrial fibrillation and pulmonary edema
Aortic stenosis	(−) The decreased SVR of pregnancy can result in lesser coronary perfusion pressure to the thickened LV myocardium (−) Because of LV diastolic dysfunction, excess volume can lead to pulmonary edema
Mitral/aortic insufficiency	(+) The decreased SVR results in a lesser regurgitant volume (−) Pregnancy can worsen ventricular dilation
Shunt lesions	
R-to-L shunt (e.g., TOF, Eisenmenger's)	(−) The decrease in SVR increases right-to-left shunting and possible cyanosis (+) In unrepaired TOF and normal RV function, the increase in blood volume is beneficial because adequate RV preload is necessary to eject blood past the outflow obstruction and increase pulmonary blood flow[a]
L-to-R shunt (e.g., VSD or ASD)	(+) The decrease in SVR decreases the left-to-right shunting (−) The increase in blood volume can precipitate failure because the patient is in a state of compensatory hypervolemia

Source: Modified from Arendt KW, Lindley KJ. *Int J Obstet Anesth.* 2019;37:73–85.

Abbreviations: SVR, systemic vascular resistance; HR, heart rate; CD, cesarean delivery; LV, left ventricle; RV, right ventricle; PEEP, positive end expiratory pressure; AICD, automatic implantable cardioverter defibrillator; CCHD, cyanotic congenital heart disease; TOF, tetralogy of Fallot; ASD, atrial septal defect; VSD, ventricular septal defect.

[a] CCHD, Eisenmenger's, and all pulmonary vascular hypertensive diseases carry a high mortality rate in pregnancy, labor, delivery, and the postpartum period; full pregnancy implications and anesthetic management are beyond the scope of this table

The increases in cardiac output during labor are mainly a result of pain and catecholamine release. Therefore, as soon as the pain of labor begins, so do the swings in cardiac output [15]. As labor progresses and becomes more painful, these cardiac output swings increase in amplitude. Therefore, in a patient with cardiac disease, the epidural should be placed upon the onset of labor discomfort and readily replaced if it begins providing suboptimal analgesia. Of note, the greatest cardiac output is immediately after delivery as a result of decompression of the vena

cava and involution of the evacuated uterus contracting and driving blood back into the venous system.

Neuraxial analgesia and anesthesia cause a sympathectomy and, thereby, a decrease in systemic vascular resistance, an increase in heart rate, and a decrease in mean arterial pressure [16]. Overall, the heart experiences a decrease in both preload and afterload. These hemodynamic changes during the onset of neuraxial labor analgesia in patients with cardiovascular disease need to be managed appropriately. To understand how to manage a sympathectomy, it

TABLE 8.6

Maternal Levels of Care

Level	Title	Patients	Examples	Capabilities
Birth Center	Birth Center	Low risk	Low risk, singleton, vertex	
Level 1	Basic Care	Low to moderate risk	TOLAC Uncomplicated twins Uncomplicated CS	Limited OB US Blood bank
Level 2	Specialty Care	Moderate to high risk	*Hypertension* Anticipated complicated CS Placenta previa Maternal pregestational DM	CT/MRI scan Maternal echo Non-obstetric US
Level 3	Subspecialty Care	More complex maternal, obstetric, and fetal conditions	*Moderate Maternal CVD* Suspected accreta Acute fatty liver of pregnancy	Interventional radiology In-house capability of all blood components
Level 4	Regional Perinatal Health Center	Most complex maternal conditions	*Severe Maternal CVD* Severe pulmonary HTN Neurosurgery, cardiovascular surgery, or transplant capabilities	ICU care with MFM co-management

Source: Adapted from American Association of Birth Centers et al. *Am J Obstet Gynecol.* 2019.

Abbreviations: TOLAC, trial of labor after cesarean; US, ultrasound; CVD, cardiovascular disease; HTN, hypertension; ICU, intensive care unit; MFM, maternal-fetal medicine; OB, obstetrics; CS, cesarean delivery; DM, diabetes mellitus.

BOX 8.2   PRINCIPLES OF NEURAXIAL LABOR ANALGESIA IN CARDIAC DISEASE

- Place epidural early in labor
- Do not use a routine pre-epidural fluid bolus patients at risk for pulmonary edema
- Use the epidural technique that the anesthesia provider finds most reliable and consistent in their hands
- If a CSE is utilized, consider an opioid-only technique (e.g., 15 μg fentanyl) in early labor
- Readily replace a suboptimal catheter
- Load epidural catheter slowly with labor epidural solution
- Monitor closely (see Table 8.7) during epidural onset for hypotension and treat with goal-directed fluids and vasopressors (e.g., phenylephrine and ephedrine) to maintain normotension
- Keep epidural block dense enough throughout labor such that it eliminates pain and catecholamine release, and can quickly be converted to a surgical block in the event of an obstetric emergency

is important to understand the physiology. Local anesthetic agents placed in the epidural or intrathecal space ("spinal anesthesia") block motor, sensory, and autonomic nerve fibers. Small, myelinated, easily blocked sympathetic nerve fibers exit the spinal cord from T1 to L2, while parasympathetic nerve fibers exit sacrally and cranially with the vagus nerve. When local anesthetic is placed in the intrathecal space, it spreads through the CSF and rapidly blocks nerves. Likewise, when local anesthetic is spread through the epidural space, it blocks nerve roots as they exit the dura.

As thoracic level sympathetic nerves are blocked with the intrathecal or epidural local anesthetic agent, organs and dermatomes supplied by these nerve roots experience unopposed parasympathetic innervation because the vagus nerve is still supplying parasympathetic innervation at these dermatomal levels. Both the venous and arterial system dilates resulting in a decrease in preload to the heart and a decrease in systemic vascular resistance. Overall, this results in a decrease in mean arterial pressure. This typically happens within 5 minutes following a spinal block but occurs more slowly with an epidural block. Loading an epidural catheter slowly allows the body and the anesthesiologist time to compensate.

To counteract the hemodynamic effects of a sympathectomy, fluids may be given to compensate for the venodilation. In cardiac patients, this may be suboptimal if the patient is in heart failure or is at high risk for pulmonary edema. There is no evidence that a routine preload of intravenous crystalloid prevents hypotension after epidural labor analgesia initiation. Therefore, for cardiovascular patients at high risk for pulmonary edema, it is reasonable for the anesthesiologist to avoid a fluid bolus prior to the epidural placement. For cardiovascular patients not at risk for pulmonary edema who may be dehydrated, it is reasonable for the anesthesiologist to administer a small fluid bolus to counteract the venodilation. Vasopressor medications such as phenylephrine and ephedrine should be immediately available. In women with cardiovascular disease, close monitoring of heart rate and blood pressure during the initiation of neuraxial labor analgesia with rapid treatment of hypotension is paramount. Vasopressors are used to maintain a blood pressure of within 20% of the patient's baseline and a heart rate between 60 and 100 beats per minute. Small doses of intravenous phenylephrine (e.g., 50–100 μg) are used for hypotension with higher heart rates, and small doses of intravenous ephedrine (e.g., 5–10 mg) are used to treat hypotension with lower heart rates.

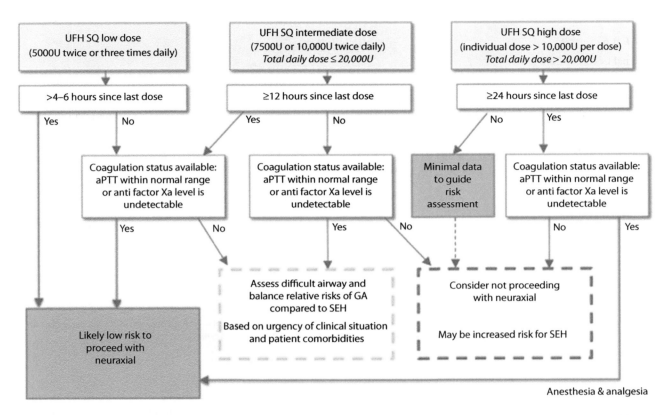

FIGURE 8.1 Neuraxial anesthesia decision aid for pregnant patients receiving unfractionated heparin. Assume normal renal function, body weight >40 kg, and no other contraindications to neuraxial anesthesia. *Abbreviations:* aPTT, activated partial thromboplastin time; GA, general anesthesia; SEH, spinal epidural hematoma; SQ, subcutaneous; UFH, unfractionated heparin. (Adapted from Leffert L et al. *Anesth Analg.* 2018;126(3):928–44 with permission.)

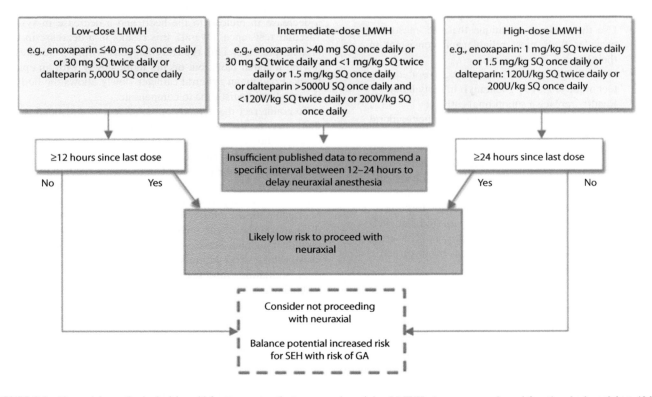

FIGURE 8.2 Neuraxial anesthesia decision aid for pregnant patients managed receiving LMWH. Assume normal renal function, body weight >40 kg, and no other contraindications to neuraxial anesthesia. *Abbreviations:* GA, general anesthesia; LMWH, low molecular weight heparin; SEH, spinal epidural hematoma; SQ, subcutaneous. (Adapted from Leffert L et al. *Anesth Analg.* 2018;126(3):928–44 with permission.)

TABLE 8.7

Cardiovascular Monitoring during Labor

	Low Risk for Cardiac Compromise	**Moderate Risk for Cardiac Compromise**	**High Risk for Cardiac Compromise**
Pulse oximetry	Pulse oximetry without wave form attached to tocodynamometer	1. Pulse oximetry without wave form attached to tocodynamometer along with 2. Pulse oximetry with visible waveform attached to cardiac monitor	
ECG	None	5-lead continuous ECG	
Blood pressure	Noninvasive blood pressure cuff	Noninvasive blood pressure cuff with q 15-minute cycling throughout labor	Intra-arterial blood beat-to-beat pressure monitoring
Central venous pressure	Rarely indicated in labor for monitoring purposes		
Pulmonary artery pressure	Rarely indicated in labor for monitoring purposes		

Because of the hemodynamic effects of labor pain, neuraxial analgesia, the Valsalva maneuver during pushing, potential bleeding, and the hemodynamic effects of obstetric medications, women with cardiovascular disease should be appropriately monitored during labor. In general, typical labor monitoring for women with moderate to severe cardiac disease is inadequate. Appropriate labor monitoring is reviewed in Table 8.7.

Pulse oximetry in laboring women is often incorporated in the tocodynamometer machine and provides neither a visible waveform nor audible tones. The purpose of this pulse oximeter monitor is to assess for concurrency between the maternal and the fetal heart rate indicating that the mother, not the fetus, is being monitored. Laboring women with heart disease should have a pulse oximeter with a visible waveform and audible alarms dedicated to alarm for maternal bradycardia, tachycardia, or hypoxemia. If a patient has a history of a tachyarrhythmia, ischemic heart disease, aortic stenosis, hypertrophic cardiomyopathy, or is otherwise at risk for ischemia or arrhythmia, then it is important that five-lead ECG telemetry is employed during labor and delivery [17]. Specialized nursing may need to be arranged in labor and delivery to interpret electrocardiogram monitoring.

For particular high-risk cardiac patients, an arterial line should be placed for hemodynamic monitoring during labor. This can be critically important in patients at risk for rapid hemodynamic decompensation with hypotension such as severe aortic stenosis, severe left ventricular dysfunction, or pulmonary hypertension with right ventricular dysfunction. This is also important for cardiac patients at risk for proceeding rapidly to cesarean delivery because the beat-to-beat blood pressure measurements of an arterial line can help guide the anesthesiologist though the hemodynamic fluctuations of a rapid induction of regional or general anesthesia. Rarely is a central line or pulmonary artery catheter necessary during labor. With an awake, laboring patient, the central venous pressure tends to be unreliable.

Principles of Cesarean Anesthesia in Cardiac Disease

Anesthesia for cesarean delivery requires complete insensitivity to the pain of a surgical stimulation. The anesthesiologist can provide general or neuraxial anesthesia for cesarean delivery.

Overall, neuraxial anesthesia is the technique of choice for cesarean delivery because it avoids manipulation of the maternal airway, avoids the uterine relaxation effects of volatile anesthetics, and avoids exposure of the fetus to general anesthesia drugs and agents. If neuraxial anesthesia is chosen, then the anesthesiologist must decide between a single-shot spinal, an epidural, a combined spinal-epidural (CSE), or a continuous spinal technique.

The sympathectomy with neuraxial labor analgesia discussed previously is far more pronounced in neuraxial techniques for cesarean delivery because at least a T6 regional anesthetic level is necessary, and the block must be dense enough to block surgical stimulation [18]. The higher and denser a neuraxial block, the greater the sympathectomy. Further, the cardiac acceleration fibers exit the spinal cord at the levels of T1–T5. Blockade of these can result in the rapid onset of bradycardia. When bradycardia occurs in the setting of a sympathectomy (decreased preload and decreased afterload), the cardiac output plummets, compromising blood flow to the mother's organs and the fetus. Therefore, the anesthesiologist employs intense vigilance from the time of spinal block placement to the time of the block establishment. The use of vasoactive medications during this time in cesarean delivery is nearly universal. Prophylactic phenylephrine is the primary drug of choice unless the heart rate drops below 60 beats per minute, at which time bolus doses of ephedrine are added [19,20].

The hemodynamic changes from the rapid onset of a spinal anesthetic for cesarean are far more sudden and pronounced than an epidural [18]. This may carry additional risk in some cardiac lesions (e.g., severe mitral stenosis, severe aortic stenosis, aortic coarctation, or patients at risk for right-to-left shunting). Nonetheless, whenever possible, anesthesiologists typically prefer spinal anesthesia to epidural anesthesia for cesarean delivery because of the simplicity of the spinal technique and the decreased risk of block failure. While epidural anesthesia can provide a more gradual onset of block and far greater hemodynamic stability, the local anesthetic is not traveling in the free-flowing CSF and needs to spread through the epidural space to each of the nerve roots supplying the surgical field. Therefore, epidural anesthesia is far less reliable than spinal anesthesia for cesarean delivery. In fact, it is not uncommon to convert an epidural anesthetic to a general anesthetic during a cesarean delivery as a result of maternal discomfort. Therefore, an arterial

TABLE 8.8

Uterotonic Use in Patients with Cardiac Disease

Drug	Cardiopulmonary Effects	Notes
Oxytocin	↓ MAP Slight ↑ PAP	• Most effective uterotonic agent • Administer cautiously and slowly (via pump) in patients intolerant of ↓ MAP • Consider counteracting ↓ MAP with phenylephrine infusion • Do not administer in bolus IV form in patients with cardiac disease
Methergine	Can cause sudden and profound ↑ SVR, ↑ PVR, and coronary vasospasm	• Generally avoided in cardiac patients
Carboprost (Prostaglandin F2 alpha)	↑↑↑ PAP Bronchospasm can cause ventilation/perfusion mismatch	• Do not use in patients who cannot tolerate increased PA pressure
Misoprostol	Uncommon cardiovascular events reported [23]	• The least effective uterotonic agent • Can be used prophylactically

Abbreviations: MAP, mean arterial pressure; PAP, pulmonary artery pressure; SVR, systemic vascular resistance; PVR, pulmonary vascular resistance; PAP, pulmonary arterial pressure; HTN, hypertension.

line placed prior to the spinal anesthetic with a carefully titrated phenylephrine infusion initiated at the time of the spinal anesthetic may provide adequate hemodynamic stability with a reliable anesthetic block.

An alternative to a single-shot spinal or epidural technique is a low-dose CSE technique that has been reported successful in high-risk cardiac patients [21]. A low-dose CSE technique is performed with an intrathecal dose of 4–5 mg of bupivacaine along with 15 µg fentanyl and long-acting opioid. This is followed by slow loading of the epidural local anesthetic (e.g., 2% lidocaine) to achieve a T4–T6 surgical level. The benefits of the low-dose CSE technique include slow onset of the neuraxial block, which allows the anesthesiologist to maintain preload and afterload during the onset while still achieving the greater block reliability of intrathecal local anesthetic administration.

There are circumstances in which general anesthesia is a safer option than a neuraxial technique for surgical anesthesia. Examples include patients on recently dosed anticoagulation therapy (see Figures 8.1 and 8.2), patients requiring the rapid provision of surgical conditions because of catastrophic maternal or fetal compromise, in the setting of extreme cardiopulmonary compromise such that the patient cannot lie flat, or in the setting of a potential cardiovascular catastrophe during delivery. If a general anesthetic is planned and there is time for the placement of an arterial line, this should be performed prior to induction. This minimizes the time from induction to delivery, thereby minimizing the fetal anesthetic exposure. More importantly, intra-arterial blood pressure monitoring allows for beat-to-beat blood pressure measurements which can guide the anesthesiologist in titrating the induction agent and the vasoactive medications used to counteract the effects of the induction agent.

Obstetric Emergencies

The early recognition and rapid treatment of obstetric hemorrhage in women with cardiac disease is paramount. Further, it is important for the anesthesiologist to understand the cardiovascular effects of the uterotonic agents that can be used to treat uterine atony, the most common cause of postpartum hemorrhage. These are summarized in Table 8.8. *Overall, oxytocin administered via an intravenous pump is the first-line treatment for uterine atony and will cause a decrease in systemic vascular resistance which may need to be counteracted with phenylephrine in the setting of hemorrhage.* For cardiac disease patients, misoprostol per rectum is a second-line therapy, although it is important to note that there have been rare reports of cardiac events and coronary vasospasm with its use [22,23]. Because of the significant cardiovascular effects of methergine and carboprost, which include hypertension, coronary vasospasm, and significant increases in pulmonary artery pressures, these agents are typically avoided in cardiac patients.

Tocolytic therapy may also be administered by the obstetric team in the event of fetal compromise and uterine tetany. Drugs such as ritodrine or terbutaline are beta agonists that cause profound uterine relaxation. They can also cause significant elevation in heart rate and decrease in systemic vascular resistance. Patients with hypertrophic obstructive cardiomyopathy could have infundibular spasm and/or worsen their outflow gradient as a result of beta agonism. Likewise, patients who would not tolerate tachycardia or patients with a history of tachyarrhythmias should not receive beta agonist drugs in labor.

Cardiovascular Emergencies

Maternal arrhythmias with hemodynamic compromise should be treated rapidly in pregnancy. Fetal intolerance of an arrhythmia is an indication for rapid cardioversion. Maternal cardioversion can be performed in pregnancy.

If the patient has a fetal scalp electrode, this should be removed prior to the cardioversion. Automatic implantable cardioverters defibrillators should be left "on" in labor as these provide the most rapid response to a tachyarrhythmia. A magnet should be

BOX 8.3 MODIFICATIONS TO BASIC LIFE SUPPORT AND ADVANCED CARDIAC LIFE SUPPORT IN PREGNANCY

- Perform manual left uterine displacement and focus on excellent chest compressions
- Do not use mechanical chest compression devices
- Place hands on the sternum the same as in the nonpregnant state
- Avoid excessive ventilation
- Place intravenous line above diaphragm
- Immediately begin preparations for cesarean at the time of arrest
- Have a maternal cardiac arrest team which includes the resuscitation team, an obstetric team, an anesthesia team, and a neonatology team
- Use a smaller endotracheal tube (6.0–7.0) and move quickly to a laryngeal mask airway if necessary
- Consider magnesium toxicity and treat with calcium
- Use epinephrine, and generally avoid vasopressin
- Initiate perimortem cesarean delivery within 4 minutes of arrest at the site of arrest

immediately available to use in the event of an emergent cesarean delivery requiring unipolar cautery. In the event of cardiac arrest, the American Heart Association recommends modifications to basic life support and advanced cardiac life support in pregnancy [24]. These are summarized in Box 8.3.

Conclusion

The anesthetic management of labor and delivery in women with cardiac disease requires an understanding of the physiologic changes of labor and delivery, the physiologic vulnerabilities of the woman's cardiovascular disease, and the hemodynamic implications of the various anesthetic techniques employed. For vaginal delivery in moderate- to high-risk cardiac disease, neuraxial labor analgesia is preferred to reduce the hemodynamic consequences of painful labor. For cesarean delivery, neuraxial anesthesia is typically recommended but general anesthesia is sometimes required because of maternal anticoagulation, the emergent nature of the procedure, or the severity of cardiac disease. Women with moderate- to high-risk cardiac disease require additional monitoring for both labor and cesarean delivery. Early recognition and rapid treatment of obstetric, cardiac, or anesthetic complications is paramount. The cardiovascular implications of obstetric medications such as uterotonic or tocolytic medications should be taken into consideration by the entire delivery team.

REFERENCES

1. Creanga AA, Syverson C, Seed K, Callaghan WM. Pregnancy-related mortality in the United States, 2011–2013. *Obstet Gynecol.* 2017;130(2):366–73.

2. Marelli AJ, Ionescu-Ittu R, Mackie AS, Guo L, Dendukuri N, Kaouache M. Lifetime prevalence of congenital heart disease in the general population from 2000 to 2010. *Circulation* 2014;130(9):749–56.

3. Thompson JL, Kuklina EV, Bateman BT, Callaghan WM, James AH, Grotegut CA. Medical and obstetric outcomes among pregnant women with congenital heart disease. *Obstet Gynecol.* 2015;126(2):346–54.

4. Roos-Hesselink JW et al. Outcome of pregnancy in patients with structural or ischaemic heart disease: Results of a registry of the European Society of Cardiology. *Eur Heart J.* 2013;34(9):657–65.

5. Briller J, Koch AR, Geller SE. Maternal cardiovascular mortality in Illinois, 2002–2011. *Obstet Gynecol.* 2017;129(5):819–26.

6. Hameed AB et al. Pregnancy-related cardiovascular deaths in California: Beyond peripartum cardiomyopathy. *Am J Obstet Gynecol.* 2015;213(3):379 e1–10.

7. Regitz-Zagrosek V et al. 2018 ESC Guidelines for the management of cardiovascular diseases during pregnancy. *Eur Heart J.* 2018;39(34):3165–241.

8. ACOG practice bulletin No. 212: Pregnancy and heart disease. *Obstet Gynecol.* 2019;133(5):e320–e56.

9. Silversides CK et al. pregnancy outcomes in women with heart disease: The CARPREG II study. *J Am Coll Cardiol.* 2018;71(21):2419–30.

10. Drenthen W et al. Predictors of pregnancy complications in women with congenital heart disease. *Eur Heart J.* 2010;31(17):2124–32.

11. Thorne S, MacGregor A, Nelson-Piercy C. Risks of contraception and pregnancy in heart disease. *Heart* 2006;92(10):1520–5.

12. American Association of Birth Centers et al. Obstetric Care Consensus #9: Levels of Maternal Care: (Replaces Obstetric Care Consensus Number 2, February 2015). *Am J Obstet Gynecol.* 2019;221(6):B19–30.

13. Horlocker TT, Vandermeuelen E, Kopp SL, Gogarten W, Leffert LR, Benzon HT. Regional Anesthesia in the Patient Receiving Antithrombotic or Thrombolytic Therapy: American Society of Regional Anesthesia and Pain Medicine Evidence-Based Guidelines (Fourth Edition). *Reg Anesth Pain Med.* 2018;43(3):263–309.

14. Leffert L et al. The Society for Obstetric Anesthesia and Perinatology Consensus Statement on the Anesthetic Management of Pregnant and Postpartum Women Receiving Thromboprophylaxis or Higher Dose Anticoagulants. *Anesth Analg.* 2018;126(3):928–44.

15. Robson SC, Dunlop W, Boys RJ, Hunter S. Cardiac output during labour. *Br Med J (Clin Res Ed).* 1987;295(6607):1169–72.

16. Pham LH, Camann WR, Smith MP, Datta S, Bader AM. Hemodynamic effects of intrathecal sufentanil compared with epidural bupivacaine in laboring parturients. *J Clin Anesth.* 1996;8(6):497–501; discussion 2–3.

17. Silversides CK, Harris L, Haberer K, Sermer M, Colman JM, Siu SC. Recurrence rates of arrhythmias during pregnancy in women with previous tachyarrhythmia and impact on fetal and neonatal outcomes. *Am J Cardiol.* 2006;97(8):1206–12.

18. Arendt KW MJ, Tsen LT. Cardiovascular alterations in the parturient undergoing cesarean delivery with neuraxial anesthesia. *Exp Rev Obstet Gynecol.* 2014;7(1).

19. Ngan Kee W, Khaw K, Ng F. Comparison of phenylephrine infusion regimens for maintaining maternal blood pressure during spinal anaesthesia for caesarean section. *Br J Anaesth.* 2004;92(4)469–74.

20. Ngan Kee WD, Lee A, Khaw KS, Ng FF, Karmakar MK, Gin T. A randomized double-blinded comparison of phenylephrine and ephedrine infusion combinations to maintain blood pressure during spinal anesthesia for cesarean delivery: The effects on fetal acid-base status and hemodynamic control. *Anesth Analg.* 2008;107(4):1295.

21. Hamlyn EL, Douglass CA, Plaat F, Crowhurst JA, Stocks GM. Low-dose sequential combined spinal-epidural: An anaesthetic technique for caesarean section in patients with significant cardiac disease. *Int J Obstet Anesth.* 2005;14(4):355–61.

22. Matthesen T, Olsen RH, Bosselmann HS, Lidegaard O. Cardiac arrest induced by vasospastic angina pectoris after vaginally administered misoprostol. *Ugeskr Laeger.* 2017;179(26).

23. Misoprostol: Serious cardiovascular events, even after a single dose. *Prescrire Int.* 2015;24(162):183–4.

24. Jeejeebhoy FM et al. Cardiac arrest in pregnancy: A scientific statement from the American Heart Association. *Circulation.* 2015;132(18):1747–73.

9

Anticoagulation in Pregnancy

Rachel A. Newman, Ather Mehboob, and Judith H. Chung

KEY POINTS

- Venous thromboembolism occurs in 1–4 per 1000 pregnancies, representing a fivefold increase in the risk of VTE as compared to the nonpregnant state
- The highest risk maternal cardiac condition requiring anticoagulation in pregnancy is the presence of a mechanical heart valve
- The highest risk thrombophilias include factor V Leiden homozygosity and prothrombin gene G20210A mutation homozygosity

- Low molecular weight heparin is the anticoagulant of choice in pregnancy; however, it is primarily excreted by the kidney and therefore is relatively contraindicated in significant renal impairment
- The primary advantage for choosing low-dose unfractionated heparin is it the least likely to preclude neuraxial anesthesia

Introduction

Pregnancy is a hypercoagulable state resulting from low-level activation of intravascular coagulation. This physiologic adaptation helps in prevention of hemorrhage at the time of implantation, maintenance of the utero-placental interface, and hemostasis in the third stage of labor. However, hypercoagulability of pregnancy coupled with stasis related to the gravid state leads to an increased risk of venous thromboembolism (VTE) as compared to the nonpregnant state.

Physiologic Changes in Pregnancy

VTE occurs in 1–4 per 1000 pregnancies, representing a fivefold increase in the risk of VTE as compared to the nonpregnant state [1–8]. This increased risk is due to the fact that the three components of Virchow's triad—hypercoagulability, stasis, and endothelial damage—are effected by the physiologic and hormonal changes of pregnancy. Hormonal factors increase the quantity of coagulation factors while decreasing levels of some natural inhibitors of coagulation [9]. These changes are summarized in Table 9.1.

Markers of platelet activation and low levels of fibrin degradation products have been documented in maternal circulation [9], consistent with pregnancy being a state of low level of intravascular coagulation [9,11,12]. These changes occur at the beginning of pregnancy, thus accounting for the increase in VTE occurrence as early as the first trimester [1,13]. Stasis is a result of compression of inferior vena cava and pelvic vessels by the growing uterus and hormone-mediated venous dilation [14]. Furthermore, vascular injury may occur during labor due to fetal descent into the pelvis and possible need for an operative delivery, either vaginal or cesarean, which coincides with the increased risk of VTE in the postpartum period [15–17].

Maternal Cardiac Lesions That May Require Anticoagulation during Pregnancy

Cardiac lesions in which anticoagulation may be considered are summarized in Table 9.2 [18]. They range from valve prosthesis and structural cardiac defects to arrhythmias. The highest risk maternal cardiac condition requiring anticoagulation in pregnancy is the presence of a mechanical heart valve, as there is elevated risk for valve thrombosis, systemic embolism, and even death [19]. In the nonpregnant state, vitamin K antagonists (VKAs) are the preferred agents for anticoagulation. Use of VKA during pregnancy has also been shown to have the lowest risk of valve thrombosis/systemic embolism at a rate of 3.9% [20,21]; however, due to their teratogenic potential, alternate treatment regimens are utilized in pregnancy [22].

Other Considerations for Anticoagulation in Pregnancy

Inherited Thrombophilias

Inherited thrombophilias are a group of genetic disorders that result in an increased risk of venous thromboembolism [23].

TABLE 9.1

Changes in Coagulation Factors during Pregnancy [9,10]

Coagulation Factors	Effect	Change in Pregnancy
I (fibrinogen), VII, VIII, IX, X	Procoagulant	Increased
II, V, and XII	Procoagulant	Unchanged or mildly increased
Protein S, plasminogen activator	Anticoagulant	Decreased
Protein S, antithrombin III	Anticoagulant	Unchanged

The most common and well-studied include factor V Leiden mutation, prothrombin G20210A mutation, protein C deficiency, protein S deficiency, and antithrombin deficiency [23]. Among these, the highest risk thrombophilias include factor V Leiden homozygosity and prothrombin gene G20210A mutation homozygosity. In women with these conditions, the risk of pregnancy-related VTE is approximately 4% [22]. Compound heterozygosity for factor V Leiden and prothrombin gene mutation, in addition to antithrombin deficiency, are also considered to be high risk for VTE [23]. Other less important thrombophilias are methylenetetrahydrofolate reductase (MTHFR) and elevated homocysteine levels. Currently, routine testing is not recommended due to insufficient evidence. In addition, while elevated homocysteine levels, possibly caused by mutations in MTHFR are thought to be a weak risk factor for VTE, MTHFR mutations themselves do not appear to be associated with an increased risk of VTE [23].

Anticoagulation during pregnancy and postpartum women with inherited thrombophilia depends on the underlying diagnosis plus personal or family history of prior thromboembolism. Recommendations vary between the American College of Obstetrics and Gynecology (ACOG) and the American College of Chest Physicians (ACCP) CHEST guidelines summarized in Table 9.3.

Antiphospholipid Syndrome

In contrast to inherited thrombophilias, antiphospholipid syndrome (APS) is an acquired thrombophilia with an increased risk of VTE along with pregnancy complications. It is an autoimmune disorder characterized by the presence of at least one circulating antiphospholipid antibody (present on two or more occasions at least 12 weeks apart) in conjunction with at least one clinical criterion [24,78]. The requirements for the diagnosis of APS is summarized in Table 9.4.

Due to the elevated risk of vascular thrombosis and pregnancy complications, it is imperative that women meeting the criteria for APS should receive treatment before, during, and after pregnancy. Indications for APS testing include a history of venous or arterial thrombosis or a history of pregnancy loss, either three or more unexplained losses prior to 10 weeks' gestation, or one unexplained death after 10 weeks' gestation. While clinical criteria for APS also includes early-onset preeclampsia or growth restriction requiring delivery prior to 34 weeks, expert opinion

TABLE 9.2

Cardiac Lesions in Which Anticoagulation during Pregnancy May Be Considered

Cardiac Lesion	Anticoagulation Indicated	Treatment
Native valve disease	Only in the presence of Atrial fibrillation *or* Atrial flutter *or* Left atrial thrombosis *or* Prior embolism	Therapeutic anticoagulation in combination or without VKA UFH LMWH
Prosthetic heart valve	Yes	Therapeutic anticoagulation VKA UFH LMWH
Cardiomyopathies— Systolic dysfunction	Only in the presence of Intracardiac thrombus *or* Atrial fibrillation *or* Treatment with bromocriptine	Therapeutic anticoagulation in combination or without in Intracardiac thrombus *or* atrial fibrillation VKA UFH LMWH Prophylactic anticoagulation in patients on bromocriptine UFH LMWH
Implantable cardioverter defibrillator (ICD)	No	N/A
Pulmonary hypertension	Yes, in patients with chronic thromboembolic pulmonary hypertension	Therapeutic anticoagulation with UFH *or* LMWH
Congenitally corrected transposition of the great arteries	Yes, anticoagulation should be considered	Therapeutic anticoagulation with UFH *or* LMWH

Note: See further reference [18].

Abbreviations: VKA, vitamin K antagonist; UFH, unfractionated heparin; LMWH, low molecular weight heparin.

does not uniformly recommend screening for APS in women with this history as there is not enough evidence to suggest that diagnosis and treatment of APS in these scenarios improves the outcome of subsequent pregnancies [25]. Other conditions often associated with APS include hemolytic anemia, autoimmune thrombocytopenia, amaurosis fugax, livedo reticularis, systemic lupus erythematosus, and false positive rapid plasma regain test [25]. However, as these are not among the clinical criteria for a diagnosis of APS, the ACOG does not recommend APS testing in these patients for the purposes of pregnancy management. Recommendations for anticoagulation in pregnancy with APS are summarized in Table 9.5.

TABLE 9.3

Anticoagulation Guidelines as a Function of Thrombophilia Status, Prior History, and Time during Pregnancy

Thrombophilia Status	Prior History	American College of Obstetrics and Gynecology (ACOG) Guidelines[a]		American College of Chest Physicians (CHEST) Guidelines	
		Antepartum Anticoagulation	Postpartum Anticoagulation	Antepartum Anticoagulation	Postpartum Anticoagulation
Negative	1 episode of VTE due to transient risk factor that is no longer present	None	• None • Prophylactic dose or • VKA with target INR of 2.0–3.0	None	• Prophylactic dose • Intermediate dose • VKA targeted at INR 2.0–3.0
Negative	1 episode of unprovoked, pregnancy- or estrogen-related VTE and not receiving long-term anticoagulation	None Prophylactic dose	Prophylactic dose or VKA with target INR of 2.0–3.0	• Prophylactic dose • Intermediate dose	• Prophylactic • Intermediate dose • VKA targeted at INR 2.0–3.0
Low risk[b]	No VTE	None	• None • If other risk factors (first degree relative with history of thrombotic event prior to 50 years old, obesity, prolonged immobility), consider prophylactic anticoagulation or VKA with target INR of 2.0–3.0	None	• Prophylactic dose • Intermediate dose • VKA targeted at INR 2.0–3.0 can be considered in women without protein C or S deficiency
Low risk[b]	1 episode of VTE and not receiving long term anticoagulation	Prophylactic Intermediate dose No anticoagulation can also be considered	• Prophylactic or VKA with target INR of 2.0–3.0 • Intermediate dose	No specific recommendations	No specific recommendations
High risk[c]	No VTE	Prophylactic dose	Prophylactic dose or VKA with target INR of 2.0–3.0	• No family history of VTE, no anticoagulation • Positive family history, Prophylactic or Intermediate dose	• Prophylactic • Intermediate dose
High risk[c]	1 episode of VTE and not receiving long term anticoagulation	• Prophylactic • Intermediate • Adjusted dose	• Prophylactic or VKA with target INR of 2.0–3.0 • Intermediate • Adjusted dose	No specific recommendations	No specific recommendations
Thrombophilia or no thrombophilia	Acute VTE during pregnancy	Therapeutic dose	No recommendations given	Adjusted dose for a minimum duration of 3 months followed by Prophylactic or Intermediate dose	• Prophylactic • Intermediate dose • Therapeutic dose if minimum duration of treatment was not achieved prior to delivery
Thrombophilia or no thrombophilia	≥2 episodes of VTE and not receiving long term anticoagulation	• Prophylactic • Therapeutic dose	• Prophylactic or VKA with target INR of 2.0–3.0 • Therapeutic dose	No specific recommendations	No specific recommendations

(Continued)

TABLE 9.3 (Continued)

Anticoagulation Guidelines as a Function of Thrombophilia Status, Prior History, and Time during Pregnancy

Thrombophilia Status	Prior History	American College of Obstetrics and Gynecology (ACOG) Guidelines		American College of Chest Physicians (CHEST) Guidelines	
		Antepartum Anticoagulation	Postpartum Anticoagulation[a]	Antepartum Anticoagulation	Postpartum Anticoagulation
Thrombophilia or no thrombophilia	≥2 episodes of VTE and receiving long term anticoagulation	Therapeutic dose	Resumption of long-term anticoagulation regimen	No specific recommendations	No specific recommendations
Thrombophilia or no thrombophilia	Mechanical heart valve	Therapeutic dose	Therapeutic dose	Therapeutic dose plus low-dose aspirin Options include • Therapeutic LMWH or UFH throughout pregnancy • UFH or LMWH until 13 weeks with transition to VKA until delivery when UFH or LMWH is resumed • VKA through the entirety of the pregnancy with transition to UFH or LMWH at delivery	Therapeutic dose

Abbreviations: LMWH, low molecular weight heparin; UHF, unfractionated heparin; VTE, venous thromboembolism; VKA, vitamin K antagonist; INR, international normalized ratio.

a Postpartum treatment level should minimally be at the level of antepartum coagulation.

b Low-risk thrombophilias include factor V Leiden heterozygote, prothrombin G20210A mutation heterozygote, protein C deficiency, or protein S deficiency.

c High-risk thrombophilias include antithrombin III deficiency, double heterozygote for prothrombin G20210A mutation and factor V Leiden, factor V Leiden homozygote, or prothrombin G20210A mutation homozygote.

TABLE 9.4

Required Laboratory and Clinical Criteria for the Diagnosis of Antiphospholipid Antibody Syndrome (APS)[a]

Laboratory Criteria[b]	Clinical Criteria
1. Circulating lupus anticoagulant	1. Vascular thrombosis
	• History of one or more episodes of arterial, venous, or small vessel thrombosis
	2. Pregnancy morbidity
2. Medium to high titers of anticardiolipin antibodies (IgM and/or IgG)	• Prior pregnancy morbidity including three or more unexplained spontaneous pregnancy losses prior to 10 weeks' gestation with other causes excluded
3. Medium to high titers of anti-B2 glycoprotein I antibodies (IgM and/or IgG)	• One or more unexplained fetal death after 10 weeks' gestation with other causes excluded
	• One or more preterm births prior to 34 weeks' gestation due to eclampsia, preeclampsia with severe features, or evidence of placental insufficiency

[a] For the diagnosis of APS, the patient must have at least one circulating antibody in conjunction with at least one clinical criterion.

[b] Laboratory criteria require at least one circulating antiphospholipid antibody on two more occasions and at least 12 weeks apart [24].

What Are the Options for Anticoagulation in Pregnancy?

There is limited high-quality data regarding specific thromboprophylaxis guidelines in pregnancy [26]. However, multiple guidelines prefer low molecular weight heparin (LMWH) over unfractionated heparin (UFH) in the antepartum outpatient setting [22,27,29]. When choosing a treatment plan, maternal and fetal safety must be balanced. Considerations include altered pharmacokinetics of the drug, concern for teratogenicity to the fetus, and management of anticoagulation around the time of delivery.

There are two categories of anticoagulation dosing: prophylactic and therapeutic. Prophylactic dosing reduces the risk of VTE while minimizing bleeding complications [30]. Therapeutic anticoagulation is utilized for treatment of active thromboembolic disease, or when there is a concern that prophylactic dosing will be inadequate for a patient at high risk of developing a thromboembolism. If required, both prophylactic and therapeutic prophylaxis should be initiated as soon as an intrauterine gestation is confirmed [27,31]. Both ACOG and ACCP have published guidelines to assist in determining whether a patient requires prophylactic versus therapeutic prophylaxis [10,27,32].

Patients with a low-risk thrombophilia (factor V Leiden or prothrombin gene mutation heterozygosity, protein C or S deficiency), low-risk thrombophilia with a family history of VTE, or a prior provoked VTE (associated with a temporary risk factor such as surgery, indwelling catheter, prolonged immobilization) are considered low risk and do not require antepartum prophylactic or therapeutic anticoagulation. The medium-risk category includes:

1. Prior idiopathic VTE
2. Prior VTE with pregnancy or estrogen-containing oral contraception
3. Prior VTE with low-risk thrombophilia
4. Family history of VTE with high-risk thrombophilia
5. High-risk thrombophilia or antiphospholipid syndrome

High-risk thrombophilias include antithrombin III deficiency, factor V Leiden or prothrombin gene mutation homozygosity, or compound heterozygosity. Patients who fall into this category should receive prophylactic LMWH or UFH throughout their pregnancies. Those at high risk of developing a VTE in pregnancy include patients with:

1. Current VTE or multiple prior VTEs
2. Prior VTE with a high-risk thrombophilia
3. Prior VTE with antiphospholipid syndrome

These patients should be started on therapeutic dose LMWH or UFH as soon as a pregnancy is confirmed. If a patient has another medical condition requiring anticoagulation (e.g., mechanical heart valve), she should continue on therapeutic

TABLE 9.5

Anticoagulation Guidelines in Patients with Antiphospholipid Antibody Syndrome (APS)

	American College of Obstetrics and Gynecology (ACOG) Guidelines		American College of Chest Physicians CHEST Guidelines	
Prior History of Thromboembolism	Antepartum Anticoagulation	Postpartum Anticoagulation[a]	Antepartum Anticoagulation	Postpartum Anticoagulation
None	None or prophylactic dose	Prophylactic dose	No specific recommendations	No specific recommendations
Recurrent pregnancy loss	Prophylactic dose and low-dose aspirin	Prophylactic anticoagulation and low-dose aspirin	Prophylactic and low-dose aspirin Intermediate dose and low-dose aspirin	No specific recommendations
History of arterial, venous, or small vessel thrombosis	Prophylactic dose ± low-dose aspirin	Prophylactic anticoagulation		

[a] Postpartum treatment level should minimally be at the level of antepartum coagulation.

thromboprophylaxis throughout her pregnancy. It is recommended that women on therapeutic anticoagulation be co-managed with maternal-fetal medicine and hematology [27].

What Are the Different Options for Anticoagulation Therapy?

Low Molecular Weight Heparin

Heparins (LMWH and UFH) are considered safe in pregnancy as they do not cross the placenta and have not been found to be teratogenic [27]. LMWH is more often recommended as it has a more predictable anticoagulant response and does not require as intensive monitoring as in in the case of UFH [33,34].

LMWH is administered subcutaneously, either once or twice daily, depending on whether therapeutic or prophylactic dosing is needed. There are several formulations of LMWH. As enoxaparin is most widely used in the United States, it will be the basis for the following discussion. For prophylactic dosing, typically enoxaparin 40 mg every 24 hours is used. As a patient's weight increases during pregnancy, dosing can be increased to 1 mg/kg daily [30]. Therapeutic dosing is based on patient's weight (in kilograms) and anti-factor Xa levels. Therapeutic LMWH is often administered as enoxaparin 1 mg/kg every 12 hours. Therapeutic dosing can also be achieved with enoxaparin 1.5 mg/kg daily. This regimen creates greater fluctuation in heparin levels and is avoided in pregnancy [10].

LMWH is metabolized by the liver and is exclusively excreted by the kidney. A baseline platelet and creatinine are drawn prior to starting prophylactic LMWH. Therapeutic LMWH requires regular monitoring. The mechanism of action for LMWH is inhibition of activated factor X (Xa). To assess anticoagulation, an anti-Xa assay is drawn after the third dose, measuring the inactivation of the coagulation factor. In general, anti-Xa 0.6–1.0 IU/mL 4–6 hours after receiving a dose of enoxaparin is considered therapeutic. Of note, anti-Xa levels have not been validated in pregnancy [22,29]. After a therapeutic dose is achieved, routine anti-Xa monitoring is not recommended due to cost and lack of high-quality evidence [22,29].

In addition, for patients on therapeutic LMWH, obtain a baseline platelet count. It should be drawn at regular intervals to monitor for development of heparin-induced thrombocytopenia (HIT), a rare, potentially life-threatening complication of heparin use [22,35]. As the risk of HIT is 14-fold higher with use of UFH compared to LWMH, it will be discussed further under UFH [27]. In heparin-naïve patients, the onset of HIT is typically 5–10 days after initiation; platelets should be watched most closely the first 2 weeks of starting any heparin therapy [36].

Limitations and Benefits of LMWH

- LMWH has a longer half-life than UFH, however it cannot be fully reversed with protamine sulfate.
- Regarding delivery planning, the Society for Obstetric Anesthesia and Perinatology and the American Society of Regional Anesthesia and Pain Medicine (ASRA) state that a patient on LMWH cannot receive neuraxial anesthesia if she has received a prophylactic dose

within the last 12 hours or a therapeutic dose within the last 24 hours [27,37,38]. To avoid this inconvenience, the provider can schedule an induction, or if indicated for obstetric reasons, a cesarean section, and instruct the patient to take the last dose 12 or 24 hours prior to procedure, depending on the dosing.

- LMWH is primarily excreted by the kidney and is relatively contraindicated in significant renal impairment. If a patient shows signs of renal damage, she may need to be switched to UFH, which is cleared by both the kidneys and the liver.

Despite these limitations, LMWH is the preferred anticoagulant for the majority of patients [21,29,41,42]. It is widely available and cost effective. It has greater bioavailability than UFH and does not cross the placenta, minimizing the risk of teratogenicity and fetal anticoagulation. As mentioned, there is a stronger association between dose and anticoagulant response, so it does not have to be monitored too frequently. In addition, HIT is significantly less likely to occur in women using LMWH.

Unfractionated Heparin

UFH has a shorter half-life than LWMH. The majority of women are switched to UFH at 36–37 weeks' gestation, or earlier if there is a concern for preterm labor, to increase the likelihood that a patient will be able to receive neuraxial anesthesia for delivery [10,27,31]. The general exception to this is women at a very high risk for VTE (e.g., mechanical heart valves, atrial fibrillation with thrombus) and time without anticoagulation should be avoided. Separate guidelines exist for managing anticoagulation and delivery planning in these women.

UFH is available as a subcutaneous injection or an intravenous drip. Prophylactic dosing of UFH is often started at 5000–7500 units twice daily and may be titrated up to 10,000 units subcutaneously twice a day in the third trimester.

Therapeutic dosing is titrated based on activated partial thromboplastin time. Therapeutic range is generally 1.5–2.5 times a patient's baseline aPTT but can change based on why the anticoagulation is indicated. Blood sample for aPTT is collected 6 hours after an injection. Activated partial thromboplastin time is measured daily until a therapeutic dose is achieved, and every 1–2 weeks subsequently.

Limitations and Benefits of UFH

- The incidence of HIT is higher in women on UFH due to an autoantibody to the platelet factor 4 heparin complex, which then paradoxically causes thrombosis [27]. To diagnose HIT, a patient must display at least one of the following: 50% decrease in platelet count after administration of heparin, necrosis at the heparin injection site, general skin necrosis, or heparin-dependent platelet-activating IgG antibodies. Obstetric practitioners must consult hematology if there is a concern for HIT [27]. In patients who have received any type of heparin in the preceding 100 days and are restarting UFH or LMWH, HIT can occur in up to 0.8% of patients [36]. A baseline platelet count is drawn within

24 hours of restarting therapy [27,36,44,45]. If a heparin has been used recently, HIT will manifest within the first 24 hours rather than the typical 5–10 days post-heparin initiation [36].

- Studies are inconclusive, though some suggest that prolonged use of UFH can lead to decreased bone mineral density [46,47].

UFH is preferred in the peripartum period as it is less likely to limit a patient's ability to have neuraxial anesthesia. Variation in expert opinion exists regarding time interval between low-dose UFH and spinal and/or epidural administration; a discussion regarding timing should be held between the anesthesia and obstetric teams and the patient [48]. The effects of UFH can be reversed with protamine sulfate. As UFH is primarily cleared by the reticuloendothelial system, it is a preferred agent in renal failure patients with creatinine clearance <30 mL/min.

Heparin Drip

In patients who have been on therapeutic LMWH during pregnancy and require anticoagulation in labor, on admission to the hospital an intravenous heparin drip is often started. Intravenous drip allows for rapid dose adjustments and quicker initiation/termination of therapy, should emergent circumstances arise.

When a patient requiring therapeutic anticoagulation arrives on Labor and Delivery, at minimum, a baseline CBC, PT with international normalized ratio (INR), and aPTT should be obtained. At many institutions, dosing a heparin drip is done by pharmacy. There is a paucity of conclusive evidence regarding the optimal initial dosing of a heparin drip [49]. The 2012 ACCP recommend either a fixed regimen of an initial 5000 unit bolus followed by 1300 units/hr or a weight based regimen (Raschke regimen) [32,49,50]. One has not been shown to be superior to the other regarding VTE prevention in the nonpregnant population [51]. This can be extrapolated to the obstetric patient.

Once a heparin drip has been started, obtain an anti-factor Xa level 6 hours after initiating the treatment. Target therapeutic heparin level is 0.3–0.7 unit/mL [52]. Continue monitoring anti-factor Xa every 4–8 hours while the infusion is running, even if therapeutic levels have been achieved. The heparin infusion is typically stopped six hours prior to expected delivery [27].

It is also crucial to monitor platelets for signs of HIT (platelet drop >50% or decrease <150,000 k/μL).

Limitations and Benefits of UFH Drip

The primary challenge with unfractionated heparin use is the nonlinear dose-response relationship [49]. Nevertheless, UFH drips are preferred in labor as they allow patients to have the option of neuraxial anesthesia more readily than those on LMWH.

- Guidelines recommend that the unfractionated heparin drip should be stopped 4–6 hours prior to placing an epidural [53,54]. A normal aPTT should be verified. After the epidural is placed, only 1 hour needs to elapse prior to restarting therapy [38,50,54].

- Should delivery be required emergently, unfractionated heparin can be fully reversed with protamine sulfate.

Thus, a heparin drip allows for greater flexibility in balancing anticoagulation with comfort and control in labor.

Warfarin

Warfarin, an oral vitamin K antagonist, is generally avoided in pregnancy as it can cross the placenta and cause fetal anticoagulation as well as multiple birth defects [55,56]. Exception to this is women with mechanical heart valves and risk factors such as atrial fibrillation, previous thromboembolic complications, or multiple mechanical valves. It is recommended that warfarin be continued through 36 weeks of gestation. This places highest importance on reducing maternal risk of a thrombotic event. If reduction of fetal risk is prioritized, patients should be counseled that warfarin has been associated with poor development of bone and cartilage, leading to nasal and limb bone hypoplasia and epiphyseal stipping [57]. It may also be associated with early miscarriage and late fetal loss [3,56,58,59]. Studies are not conclusive as to whether this is due to the warfarin itself or the underlying conditions for which it is used.

If warfarin is continued, doses <5 mg/day appear to be the safest, though teratogenic effects have been reported [58,60,61]. At any dose, risk of fetal complication is highest between the 6th and 12th weeks of gestation [57]. If a patient's pre-pregnancy daily dose is >5 mg/day, it is recommended a patient switch to therapeutic LMWH for the first trimester [62].

Warfarin is only used for therapeutic purposes. Prior to initiating treatment, a CBC, basic metabolic panel, and coagulation panel (PT, aPTT, INR) are obtained to assess for baseline abnormalities with platelets, creatinine, liver function, and coagulation. A Cochrane review of randomized trials comparing initial doses of 5 or 10 mg did not demonstrate improved outcomes [63]. In addition, the 10 mg dose was more likely to result in a supra therapeutic INR, increasing the risk of bleeding [64,65]. A starting dose of <5 mg is recommended.

The full anticoagulation effect of warfarin does not occur until 2 or 3 days after first administration. The first lab value to reflect this is PT/INR, as factor VII is quickly depleted [66]. Other vitamin K–dependent factors take longer to deplete, i.e., another 2–3 days. The goal INR may vary based on the clinical setting, but the recommended range is typically 2.0–3.0 times normal. A patient on warfarin must have her INR monitored 3–4 days after the first dose and then serially through the pregnancy. Intervals may vary depending on the dose and indication as determined by the hematology and/or maternal-fetal medicine specialist. Once therapeutic level is achieved, warfarin should be continued until 36 weeks' gestation, at which time the patient is transitioned to therapeutic LMWH or UFH. If a patient is at high risk for early delivery, the timing of this transition may vary.

Limitations and Benefits of Warfarin

Warfarin use is less frequent in pregnancy. As mentioned, the primary drawback is its ability to cross the placenta, resulting in known fetal teratogenicity and increased risk of hemorrhage. It is also challenging because of the narrow therapeutic window and frequent monitoring. As it is a vitamin K antagonist, patients need to comply to avoid food rich in vitamin K (leafy green vegetables, broccoli, liver, etc.).

Despite its limitations, warfarin has distinct advantages. Warfarin is inexpensive and widely available. It is possible to reverse its anticoagulant effect with vitamin K, fresh frozen plasma, or prothrombin complex concentrates. More importantly, it is taken by mouth, which may appeal to patients with a fear of needles.

Other Anticoagulants

There are a multitude of new oral anticoagulants. These include direct thrombin inhibitors, such as dabigatran and argatroban, as well as direct factor Xa inhibitors, such as rivaroxaban and apixaban. In general, they should not be used in pregnancy as little is known about efficacy and fetal safety [21]. If a woman is on one of these medications and becomes pregnant, she should switch to LMWH immediately.

Aspirin

Aspirin (acetylsalicylic acid) is not an anticoagulant but is often used in pregnancy as part of a thromboprophylaxis regimen. The mechanism of action is to prevent platelet aggregation through irreversible inhibition of cyclooxygenase-1 and 2 (COX-1 and 2) enzymes [67].

Studies have shown the efficacy of using aspirin in conjunction with thromboprophylaxis in women with mechanical heart valves as well as those with recent strokes or at high risk for developing an ischemic event [21].

Low-dose aspirin has also been used in pregnancy to help prevent preeclampsia [68]. The etiology of preeclampsia is multifactorial. There is some evidence suggesting that an imbalance of prostacyclin and TXA_2 may result in preeclampsia [69]. At doses <150 mg/day, aspirin may help by preferentially inhibiting TXA_2 [70,71]. Initially, use of low dose aspirin for preeclampsia prevention was based on results of several small trials. More recently, larger randomized controlled trials and multiple meta-analyses have confirmed these findings [70,72–76]. Treatment is generally initiated between 12 and 28 weeks of pregnancy, but a recent meta-analysis demonstrated that maximal efficacy only occurs when started prior to 16 weeks [73]. While no consensus exists on timing or dosage of treatment, multiple guidelines, including the World Health Organization (WHO), ACOG, and U.S. Preventative Task Force recommend use of low-dose aspirin for preeclampsia prevention as there is clear benefit and few maternal or fetal adverse effects.

Low-dose aspirin has also been used to treat women with APS. There are three antiphospholipid proteins assessed as part of the diagnosis for APS: lupus anticoagulant, anticardiolipin, and anti-β_2 glycoprotein. β_2 glycoprotein is primarily clinically relevant as it may have a regulatory role in coagulation and fibrinolysis [77]. In women with APS who have had a thrombotic event, prophylactic anticoagulation is recommended throughout pregnancy and 6 weeks postpartum [22,25]. Low-dose aspirin is also added, though the evidence remains inconclusive about the benefit of this treatment [25].

The optimal treatment for women with APS without a preceding thrombotic event is not well studied. Expert consensus recommends either clinical surveillance or prophylactic heparin in addition to 6 weeks of postpartum anticoagulation [22,25]. A recent meta-analysis found that in women with recurrent pregnancy loss and antiphospholipid antibodies, prophylactic heparin and low-dose aspirin can reduce pregnancy loss by 50% [79]. This combination is superior to low-dose aspirin or prednisone alone [79].

To date, there is insufficient evidence to recommend use of low-dose aspirin for prevention of stillbirth, fetal growth restriction, or preterm birth [69].

Preconception Period

The majority of women will not require thromboprophylaxis during the antenatal period. Women who are already on anticoagulation or have a high-risk condition that will necessitate thromboprophylaxis in pregnancy require preconception counseling. Patients at high risk can be identified by existing ACOG and ACCP guidelines. See Chapter 4 on preconception counseling for further information.

Delivery Planning

Delivery is a time at which women are at increased risk of hemorrhage. Therefore, careful multidisciplinary planning must be done for patients on thromboprophylaxis. LMWH is the preferred anticoagulant during pregnancy; however, the duration of its half-life can limit a patient's ability to receive neuraxial anesthesia and theoretically increase her risk of postpartum hemorrhage. For this reason, after 36 weeks' gestation, or earlier if preterm labor is suspected, alternative anticoagulation plans are made [27,80]. A patient may choose to continue LMWH (either prophylactic or therapeutic), transition to low-dose UFH twice daily (5000 units), or transition to high-dose UFH twice daily (10,000 units, ACOG recommended).

If a patient chooses to continue LWMH, the main advantage is the close correlation between dose and anticoagulant effect. In addition, monitoring requirements are limited. The primary disadvantage is the prolonged length of time between the last dose of LMWH and the possibility of neuraxial anesthesia.

The primary advantage for choosing low-dose UFH is that it the least likely to preclude neuraxial anesthesia. The potential disadvantages include twice-daily dosing, increased dose requirements in the third trimester, and significant variation in guidelines between timing of last dose and neuraxial anesthesia.

High-dose UFH may be advantageous over low-dose UFH for providing more effective thromboprophylaxis, but there is no high-quality research to substantiate this [10]. Similar to low-dose UFH, the primary disadvantages include variable dose-response relationship, frequent lab monitoring, and twice-daily dosing.

There is no established gestational age for delivery; it depends on indication for anticoagulation. Patients are instructed to take the last dose 12–24 hours prior to a planned induction of labor or scheduled cesarean delivery [38,48].

Induction of Labor

For an induction, patients who have been on therapeutic anticoagulation are started on an unfractionated heparin drip. Close monitoring of the therapeutic level is monitored with aPTT. When a patient desires neuraxial anesthesia, preliminary ASRA guidelines recommend 4–6 hours between administration of a therapeutic dose and neuraxial blockade [27,48]. Prior to placement, aPTT should have normalized. If it has not, aPTT is rechecked in 1 hour, and repeated until the value has normalized before placing the catheter for neuraxial anesthesia.

After the epidural catheter or spinal is placed, the 2018 ASRA guidelines recommend that 4 hours elapse prior to restarting the UFH drip [53]. If the placement of neuraxial anesthesia is complicated, the obstetric and anesthesia teams must work together to balance the need for maternal anticoagulation with the rare but serious risk of a spinal hematoma. If a UFH drip has been restarted and the patient continues to labor, the clinical expertise of the provider is used to determine at what cervical dilation it should be stopped. This is often between 6–8 cm dilation. See the below section for a discussion of when thromboprophylaxis should be restarted in the postpartum period.

Spontaneous Labor

If a patient presents in spontaneous labor, recent anticoagulation use often makes her ineligible for an immediate epidural. LMWH effect cannot be reliably reversed with protamine sulfate and therefore is not used for reversal purposes in these patients. Instead, the patient's primary pain control in labor will be intravenous medication. If, in the course of her labor, anesthesia determines that it is safe to place an epidural catheter, it is at the discretion of their team. If the patient has been receiving UFH for her anticoagulant, it can be reversed with protamine sulfate and has a shorter half-life. These patients may be candidates for neuraxial anesthesia.

Emergency Cesarean Section

Should a patient who has been fully anticoagulated require an emergency cesarean section, protamine sulfate is given regardless of whether she has been on LWMH or UFH. All members of the team should be aware of the type of anticoagulant the patient has been on and have a contingency plan outlined accordingly in conjunction with anesthesia and hematology. In the event of postpartum- or surgery-related hemorrhage, blood products should be made available immediately.

Risk of Postpartum Hemorrhage

Use of anticoagulation in pregnancy increasing the risk of postpartum hemorrhage (PPH) has not been borne out in the literature. A small retrospective cohort study on the effects of LWMH on bleeding at the time of vaginal delivery found that the risk of PPH was significantly higher in the cohort of women on therapeutic LMWH [39]. However, the risk of severe PPH (>1000 cc estimated blood loss) was comparable between the two groups [39]. There was no significant difference in PPH for patients who delivered by cesarean section, including emergent deliveries [39]. Overall, the PPH risk was not increased in women who delivered within 24 hours after the last dose of LMWH versus those who delivered more than 24 hours after the last dose [39].

Another retrospective cohort study (n = 77) found that antepartum anticoagulation had a greater incidence of wound complications, but there were no differences in the mean estimated blood loss or women receiving blood products [81]. Although these studies are small, the findings have been replicated [40].

Postpartum

There is an absence of high-quality evidence regarding the best postpartum prophylactic anticoagulation regimen. For patients who have been on UFH prophylaxis, the first dose may be administered 1 hour after the spinal needle was placed or the epidural catheter has been removed [31,82]. If LMWH has been used for prophylaxis, the CMQCC Maternal VTE Task Force and ASRA recommends that a minimum of 12 hours elapse between removal of the epidural catheter or spinal needle placement and administration of LWMH.

For patients who have been on therapeutic anticoagulation during pregnancy, ACOG and ASRA recommend waiting at least 24 hours after delivery (vaginal or cesarean) prior to initiating therapeutic LMWH (e.g., enoxaparin 1 mg/kg every 12 hours) [10,27,48]. The most recent preliminary ASRA guidelines also support waiting an hour after neuraxial block or epidural catheter removal prior to administration of therapeutic UFH (>10,000 units per day) [38,48]. ACOG recommends that the dose of therapeutic anticoagulation be equal or greater to that required in pregnancy [10].

For women at a high risk of postpartum VTE, anticoagulation should continue for 6 weeks postpartum [10,27]. This includes women with a high-risk thrombophilia, personal history of VTE, or a low-risk thrombophilia with a family history of VTE. Women at very high risk of postpartum VTE (antithrombin III deficiency, mechanical heart valves, recent VTE) will also require 6 weeks of postpartum anticoagulation.

If a patient has had a single prior provoked pulmonary embolism or a low-risk thrombophilia, she does not require antepartum coagulation. As the risk for a VTE increases in the postpartum period, the National Partnership for Maternal Safety, ACCP, and Royal College of Obstetricians and Gynecologists recommend postpartum prophylaxis for 6 weeks [15,28,44]. ACOG allows for 4 weeks of postpartum treatment [10].

Bridging Anticoagulation

If a patient will not require anticoagulation greater than 6 weeks postpartum, she will often choose to remain on LMWH rather than bridge to warfarin. For patients on warfarin prior to pregnancy or who will require anticoagulation longer than 6 weeks, a bridge to warfarin is recommended [15,27,31]. There are varying opinions on when to (re)start warfarin postpartum. It is not uncommon to see warfarin restarted 24–48 hours after delivery. However, the CMQCC Maternal VTE Task Force does not recommend bridging sooner than 2 weeks postpartum [27]. While bridging, a patient typically requires simultaneous warfarin and heparin. This increases a patient's bleeding risk. Frequent monitoring is required until the INR is in therapeutic range. The patient should be closely followed by an anticoagulation specialist and/or hematologist during this period of transition.

Breastfeeding

Neither heparin nor warfarin is contraindicated in breastfeeding. Should a patient desire to transition to one of the newer oral anticoagulants, there is insufficient data to support safety of use while breastfeeding.

Contraception

Contraception options depend on the indication for thromboprophylaxis in pregnancy. In general, the risk of a VTE is increased during pregnancy and in the postpartum period. The risk is most pronounced in the first 3 weeks after delivery, declining to baseline levels by 42 days postpartum [15,16,28]. Please refer to the chapter on contraception for further information.

Conclusion

Pregnancy affords unique challenges in women with an underlying risk of venous and/or arterial thrombosis. Pregnancy itself may increase the inherent risk of thrombosis in such women due to the hypercoagulable changes that occur as the result of the pregnant state. Pregnancy may also require individualization of therapy in women on VKA given the potential fetal risks. The management of labor and delivery can be particularly complex for women requiring anticoagulation given the innate risk of hemorrhage during this process. The role of multidisciplinary planning with the anesthesiologist and hematologist cannot be overemphasized.

REFERENCES

1. Jacobsen AF, Skjeldestad FE, Sandset PM. Incidence and risk patterns of venous thromboembolism in pregnancy and puerperium-a register-based case-control study. *Am J Obstet Gynecol*. 2008. doi:10.1016/j.ajog.2007.08.041
2. James AH, Jamison MG, Brancazio LR, Myers ER. Venous thromboembolism during pregnancy and the postpartum period: Incidence, risk factors, and mortality. *Am J Obstet Gynecol*. 2006. doi:10.1016/j.ajog.2005.11.008
3. Chan WS, Anand S, Ginsberg JS. Anticoagulation of pregnant women with mechanical heart valves: A systematic review of the literature. *Arch Intern Med*. 2000.
4. Bourjeily G, Khalil H, Rodger M. Pulmonary embolism in pregnancy—Authors' reply. *Lancet*. 2010. doi:10.1016/S0140-6736(10)60800-8
5. Marik PE, Plante LA. Venous thromboembolic disease and pregnancy. *N Engl J Med*. 2008. doi:10.1056/NEJMra0707993
6. Kujovich JL. Hormones and pregnancy: Thromboembolic risks for women. *Br J Haematol*. 2004. doi:10.1111/j.1365-2141.2004.05041.x
7. Heit J et al. Trends in the incidence of venous thromboembolism during pregnancy or postpartum: A 30-year population-based study. *Ann Intern Med*. 2005. doi:10.7326/0003-4819-143-10-200511150-00006
8. Simpson EL, Lawrenson RA, Nightingale AL, Farmer RDT. Venous thromboembolism in pregnancy and the puerperium: Incidence and additional risk factors from a London perinatal database. *Br J Obstet Gynaecol*. 2001. doi:10.1016/S0306-5456(00)00004-8
9. Gabbe SG et al. Obstetrics: Normal and Problem Pregnancies. 2012. doi:10.1017/CBO9781107415324.004
10. Barbour LA. ACOG practice bulletin: Thromboembolism in pregnancy. *Int J Gynecol Obstet*. 2001. doi:10.1016/S0020-7292(01)00535-5
11. Lockwood CJ, Krikun G, Rahman M, Caze R, Buchwalder L, Schatz F. The role of decidualization in regulating endometrial hemostasis during the menstrual cycle, gestation, and in pathological states. *Semin Thromb Hemost*. 2007. doi:10.1055/s-2006-958469
12. Lockwood CJ, Krikun G, Schatz F. The decidua regulates hemostasis in human endometrium. *Semin Reprod Endocrinol*. 1999. doi:10.1055/s-2007-1016211
13. Clark P, Brennand J, Conkie JA, McCall F, Greer IA, Walker ID. Activated protein C sensitivity, protein C, protein S and coagulation in normal pregnancy. *Thromb Haemost*. 1998.
14. Macklon NS, Greer IA, Bowman AW. An ultrasound study of gestational and postural changes in the deep venous system of the leg in pregnancy. *BJOG An Int J Obstet Gynaecol*. 1997. doi:10.1111/j.1471-0528.1997.tb11043.x
15. Jackson E, Curtis KM, Gaffield ME. Risk of venous thromboembolism during the postpartum period: A systematic review. *Obstet Gynecol*. 2011. doi:10.1097/AOG.0b013e31820ce2db
16. Kamel H, Navi BB, Sriram N, Hovsepian DA, Devereux RB, Elkind MSV. Risk of a thrombotic event after the 6-week postpartum period. *N Engl J Med*. 2014. doi:10.1056/NEJMoa1311485
17. Sultan AA, West J, Tata LJ, Fleming KM, Nelson-Piercy C, Grainge MJ. Risk of first venous thromboembolism in and around pregnancy: A population-based cohort study. *Br J Haematol*. 2012. doi:10.1111/j.1365-2141.2011.08956.x
18. Regitz-Zagrosek V et al. ESC Guidelines on the management of cardiovascular diseases during pregnancy. *Eur Heart J*. 2011. doi:10.1093/eurheartj/ehr218
19. Whitlock RP, Sun JC, Fremes SE, Rubens FD, Teoh KH. Antithrombotic and thrombolytic therapy for valvular disease: Antithrombotic therapy and prevention of thrombosis, 9th ed: American College of Chest Physicians evidence-based clinical practice guidelines. *Chest*. 2012. doi:10.1378/chest.11-2305
20. Hall JG, Pauli RM, Wilson KM. Maternal and fetal sequelae of anticoagulation during pregnancy. *Am J Med*. 1980. doi:10.1016/0002-9343(80)90181-3
21. Guyatt GH, Akl EA, Crowther M, Gutterman DD, Schünemann HJ. Executive summary: Antithrombotic therapy and prevention of thrombosis, 9th ed: American College of Chest Physicians evidence-based clinical practice guidelines. *Chest*. 2012. doi:10.1378/chest.1412S3
22. Bates SM, Greer IA, Middeldorp S, Veenstra PharmD DL, Prabulos A-M, Olav Vandvik P VTE, thrombophilia, antithrombotic therapy, and pregnancy. *Chest*. 2012;141:e691S–736S. doi:10.1378/chest.11-2300

23. Silverman NS. ACOG Practice Bulletin No. 197: Inherited thrombophilias in pregnancy. *Obstet Gynecol.* 2018. doi:10.1097/AOG.0000000000002703

24. APA Syndrome-ACOG Pr Bulletin No 132.

25. ACOG. Practice Bulletin No. 132: Antiphospholipid syndrome. *ObstetGynecol.*2012.doi:10.1097/01.AOG.0000423816.39542.0f

26. Cantwell R et al. Saving mothers' lives: Reviewing maternal deaths to make motherhood safer: 2006–2008. The Eighth Report of the Confidential Enquiries into Maternal Deaths in the United Kingdom. *Bjog.* 2011. doi:10.1111/j.1471-0528.2010.02847.x

27. Hameed AB. Improving Health Care Response to Maternal VTE: A California Quality Improvement Toolkit. 2018.

28. Petersen JF, Bergholt T, Nielsen AK, Paidas MJ, Lokkegaard ECL. Combined hormonal contraception and risk of venous thromboembolism within the first year following pregnancy. Danish nationwide historical cohort 1995–2009. *Thromb Haemost.* 2014. doi:10.1160/TH13-09-0797

29. Bates SM, Middeldorp S, Rodger M, James AH, Greer I. Guidance for the treatment and prevention of obstetric-associated venous thromboembolism. *J Thromb Thrombolysis.* 2016. doi:10.1007/s11239-015-1309-0

30. Hunt BJ et al. Thromboprophylaxis with low molecular weight heparin (Fragmin) in high risk pregnancies. *Thromb Haemost.* 1997.

31. D'Alton ME et al. National Partnership for Maternal Safety: Consensus bundle on venous thromboembolism. *Obstet Gynecol.* 2016;128(4):688–98.

32. Geerts WH et al. Prevention of venous thromboembolism: American College of Chest Physicians evidence-based clinical practice guidelines (8th edition). *Chest.* 2008. doi:10.1378/chest.08-0656

33. Weitz JI. Low-molecular-weight heparins. *N Engl J Med.* 1997. doi:10.1056/NEJM199709043371007

34. Litin SC, Gastineau DA. Current concepts in anticoagulant therapy. *Mayo Clin Proc.* 1995. doi:10.1016/S0025-6196(11)64947-1

35. Greer IA, Nelson-Piercy C. Low-molecular-weight heparins for thromboprophylaxis and treatment of venous thromboembolism in pregnancy: A systematic review of safety and efficacy. *Blood.* 2005. doi:10.1182/blood-2005-02-0626

36. Warkentin TE, Kelton JG. Temporal aspects of heparin-induced thrombocytopenia. *N Engl J Med.* 2001. doi:10.1056/NEJM200104263441704

37. Leffert L et al. The society for obstetric anesthesia and perinatology consensus statement on the anesthetic management of pregnant and postpartum women receiving thromboprophylaxis or higher dose anticoagulants. *Anesth Analg.* 2017. doi:10.1213/ANE.0000000000002530

38. Horlocker TT et al. Regional anesthesia in the patient receiving antithrombotic or thrombolytic therapy: American Society of Regional Anesthesia and Pain Medicine Evidence-Based Guidelines (Third Edition). *Reg Anesth Pain Med.* 2010. doi:10.1097/Aap.0b013e3181c15c70

39. Knol HM, Schultinge L, Veeger NJGM, Kluin-Nelemans HC, Erwich JJHM, Meijer K. The risk of postpartum hemorrhage in women using high dose of low-molecular-weight heparins during pregnancy. *Thromb Res.* 2012;130(3):334–8. doi:10.1016/j.thromres.2012.03.007

40. Kominiarek MA, Angelopoulos SM, Shapiro NL, Studee L, Nutescu EA, Hibbard JU. Low-molecular-weight heparin in pregnancy: Peripartum bleeding complications. *J Perinatol.* 2007;27(6):329–34. doi:10.1038/sj.jp.7211745

41. Chan WS et al. Venous thromboembolism and antithrombotic therapy in pregnancy. *J Obstet Gynaecol Can.* 2014. doi:10.1016/S1701-2163(15)30569-7

42. Gyamfi C, Cohen R, Desancho MT, Gaddipati S. Prophylactic dosing adjustment in pregnancy based upon measurements of anti-factor Xa levels. *J Matern Neonatal Med.* 2005. doi:10.1080/14767050500275796

43. Brancazio LR, Roperti KA, Stierer R, Laifer SA. Pharmacokinetics and pharmacodynamics of subcutaneous heparin during the early third trimester of pregnancy. *Am J Obstet Gynecol.* 1995. doi:10.1016/0002-9378(95)91362-9

44. Royal College Obstetricians and Gynaecologists. *Reducing the Risk of Venous Thromboembolism during Pregnancy and the Puerperium Green-top Guideline No. 37a.* RCOG Press; 2015.

45. Linkins L-A et al. Treatment and prevention of heparin-induced thrombocytopenia. *Chest.* 2012. doi:10.1378/chest.11-2303

46. Snijder CA, Cornette JMW, Hop WCJ, Kruip MJHA, Duvekot JJ. Thrombophylaxis and bleeding complications after cesarean section. *Acta Obstet Gynecol Scand.* 2012. doi:10.1111/j.1600-0412.2012.01351.x

47. Osterman MJK, Martin JA. Epidural and spinal anesthesia use during labor: 27-state reporting area, 2008. *Natl Vital Stat Rep.* 2011;133(6 Suppl):381S–453S.

48. Leffert LR, Dubois HM, Butwick AJ, Carvalho B, Houle TT, Landau R. Neuraxial anesthesia in obstetric patients receiving thromboprophylaxis with unfractionated or low-molecular-weight heparin: A systematic review of spinal epidural hematoma. *Anesth Analg.* 2017. doi:10.1213/ANE.0000000000002173

49. Smythe MA, Priziola J, Dobesh PP, Wirth D, Cuker A, Wittkowsky AK. Guidance for the practical management of the heparin anticoagulants in the treatment of venous thromboembolism. *J Thromb Thrombolysis.* 2016;41(1):165–86. doi:10.1007/s11239-015-1315-2

50. Douketis JD et al. Perioperative management of antithrombotic therapy. Antithrombotic therapy and prevention of thrombosis, 9th ed: American College of Chest Physicians evidence-based clinical practice guidelines. *Chest.* 2012. doi:10.1378/chest.11-2298

51. Garcia DA, Baglin TP, Weitz JI, Samama MM. Parenteral anticoagulants—Antithrombotic therapy and prevention of thrombosis, 9th ed: American College of Chest Physicians evidence-based clinical practice guidelines. *Chest.* 2012. doi:10.1378/chest.11-2291

52. Spruill WJ, Wade WE, Huckaby WG, Leslie RB. Achievement of anticoagulation by using a weight-based heparin dosing protocol for obese and nonobese patients. *Am J Heal Pharm.* 2001.

53. Horlocker TT, Vandermeuelen E, Kopp SL, Gogarten W, Leffert LR, Benzon HT. Regional anesthesia in the patient receiving antithrombotic or thrombolytic therapy: American Society of Regional Anesthesia and Pain Medicine Evidence-Based Guidelines (Fourth Edition). *Reg Anesth Pain Med.* 2018. doi:10.1097/AAP.0000000000000763

54. Gogarten W, Vandermeulen E, Van Aken H, Kozek S, Llau JV, Samama CM. Regional anaesthesia and antithrombotic agents: Recommendations of the European Society of Anaesthesiology. *Eur J Anaesthesiol.* 2010. doi:10.1097/EJA.0b013e32833f6f6f

55. Pauli RM, Lian JB, Mosher DF, Suttie JW. Association of congenital deficiency of multiple vitamin K-dependent coagulation factors and the phenotype of the warfarin embryopathy: Clues to the mechanism of teratogenicity of coumarin derivatives. *Am J Hum Genet.* 1987.

56. Schaefer C et al. Vitamin K antagonists and pregnancy outcome. A multi-centre prospective study. *Thromb Haemost.* 2006. doi:10.1160/TH06-02-0108

57. Barbour LA. Current concepts of anticoagulant therapy in pregnancy. *Obstet Gynecol Clin North Am.* 1997. doi:10.1016/S0889-8545(05)70319-3

58. Cotrufo M et al. Risk of warfarin during pregnancy with mechanical valve prostheses. *Obstet Gynecol.* 2002. doi:10.1016/S0029-7844(01)01658-1

59. D'Souza R et al. Anticoagulation for pregnant women with mechanical heart valves: A systematic review andmeta-Analysis. *Eur Heart J.* 2017. doi:10.1093/eurheartj/ehx032

60. Vitale N, De Feo M, De Santo LS, Pollice A, Tedesco N, Cotrufo M. Dose-dependent fetal complications of warfarin in pregnant women with mechanical heart valves. *J Am Coll Cardiol.* 1999. doi:10.1016/S0735-1097(99)00044-3

61. Basu S, Aggarwal P, Kakani N, Kumar A. Low-dose maternal warfarin intake resulting in fetal warfarin syndrome: In search for a safe anticoagulant regimen during pregnancy. *Birth Defects Res Part A - Clin Mol Teratol.* 2016. doi:10.1002/bdra.23435

62. Goland S, Schwartzenberg S, Fan J, Kozak N, Khatri N, Elkayam U. Monitoring of anti-xa in pregnant patients with mechanical prosthetic valves receiving low-molecular-weight heparin: Peak or trough levels? *J Cardiovasc Pharmacol Ther.* 2014. doi:10.1177/1074248414524302

63. Garcia P, Ruiz W, Loza Munárriz C. Warfarin initiation nomograms of 5 mg and 10 mg for venous thromboembolism. *Cochrane Database Syst Rev.* 2013. doi:10.1002/14651858.CD007699.pub3. http://www.cochranelibrary.com

64. Kovacs MJ et al. Comparison of 10-mg and 5-mg Warfarin initiation nomograms together with low-molecular-weight heparin for outpatient treatment of acute venous thromboembolism: A randomized, double-blind, controlled trial. *Ann Intern Med.* 2003. doi:10.7326/0003-4819-138-9-200305060-00007

65. Crowther MA et al. A randomized trial comparing 5-mg and 10-mg warfarin loading doses. *Arch Intern Med.* 1999. doi:10.1001/archinte.159.1.46

66. Becker DM, Humphries JE, Walker IV FB, DeMong LK, Bopp JS, Acker MN. Standardizing the prothrombin time: Calibrating coagulation instruments as well as thromboplastin. *Arch Pathol Lab Med.* 1993.

67. Paez Espinosa EV, Murad JP, Khasawneh FT. Aspirin: Pharmacology and clinical applications. *Thrombosis.* 2012. doi:10.1155/2012/173124

68. Roberts JM et al. *ACOG Guidelines: Hypertension in Pregnancy*; 2012. doi:10.1097/01.AOG.0000437382.03963.88

69. ACOG. ACOG Committee opinion No. 743: Low-dose aspirin use during pregnancy. *Obstet Gynecol.* 2018. doi:10.1097/AOG.0000000000002708

70. Schiff E et al. The use of aspirin to prevent pregnancy-induced hypertension and lower the ratio of thromboxane A2to prostacyclin in relatively high risk pregnancies. *Obstet Gynecol Surv.* 1990. doi:10.1097/00006254-199003000-00008

71. Benigni A et al. Effect of low-dose aspirin on fetal and maternal generation of thromboxane by platelets in women at risk for pregnancy-induced hypertension. *N Engl J Med.* 1989. doi:10.1056/NEJM198908103210604

72. Caritis S et al. Low-dose aspirin to prevent preeclampsia in women at high risk. National Institute of Child Health and Human Development Network of Maternal-Fetal Medicine Units. *N Engl J Med.* 1998. doi:10.1056/NEJM199803123381101

73. Rolnik DL et al. ASPRE trial: Performance of screening for preterm pre-eclampsia. *Ultrasound Obstet Gynecol.* 2017. doi:10.1002/uog.18816

74. Roberge S, Nicolaides KH, Demers S, Villa P, Bujold E. Prevention of perinatal death and adverse perinatal outcome using low-dose aspirin: A meta-analysis. *Ultrasound Obstet Gynecol.* 2013. doi:10.1002/uog.12421

75. Bujold E, Morency A-M, Roberge S, Lacasse Y, Forest J-C, Giguère Y. Acetylsalicylic acid for the prevention of pre-eclampsia and intra-uterine growth restriction in women with abnormal uterine artery Doppler: A systematic review and meta-analysis. *J Obstet Gynaecol Can.* 2009. doi:10.1016/S1701-2163(16)34300-6

76. Roberge S, Nicolaides K, Demers S, Hyett J, Chaillet N, Bujold E. The role of aspirin dose on the prevention of pre-eclampsia and fetal growth restriction: Systematic review and meta-analysis. *Am J Obstet Gynecol.* 2017. doi:10.1016/j.ajog.2016.09.076

77. De Laat B, Derksen RHWM, Urbanus RT, De Groot PG. IgG antibodies that recognize epitope Gly40-Arg43 in domain I of β_2-glycoprotein I cause LAC, and their presence correlates strongly with thrombosis. *Blood.* 2005. doi:10.1182/blood-2004-09-3387

78. Levine JS, Branch DW, Rauch J. The antiphospholipid syndrome. *N Engl J Med.* 2002. doi:10.1056/NEJMra002974

79. Empson M, Lassere M, Craig JC, Scott JR. Recurrent pregnancy loss with antiphospholipid antibody: A systematic review of therapeutic trials. *Obstet Gynecol.* 2002. doi:10.1016/S0029-7844(01)01646-5

80. Pacheco LD, Saade GR, Costantine MM, Vadhera R, Hankins GD V. Reconsidering the switch from low-molecular-weight heparin to unfractionated heparin during pregnancy. *Am J Perinatol.* 2014. doi:10.1055/s-0033-1359719

81. Limmer JS, Grotegut CA, Thames E, Dotters-Katz SK, Brancazio LR, James AH. Postpartum wound and bleeding complications in women who received peripartum anticoagulation. *Thromb Res.* 2013;132(1):e19–23. doi:10.1016/j.thromres.2013.04.034

82. Sultan AA et al. Development and validation of risk prediction model for venous thromboembolism in postpartum women: Multinational cohort study. *BMJ.* 2016. doi:10.1136/BMJ.I6253

10

Congenital Heart Disease in Pregnancy

Jeannette P. Lin

KEY POINTS

- Congenital heart disease (CHD) is the most common congenital defect, affecting approximately 0.8% of live births
- Over 80% of patients born with congenital heart disease will survive to adulthood
- Aside from bicuspid aortic valves, atrial septal defects (ASDs) are the most common type of congenital heart defect, accounting for 10%–20% of congenital heart defects

- A delivery plan readily accessible to all care providers should be outlined for patients who are at moderate or high risk for maternal cardiac complications
- Patients with Eisenmenger syndrome are at high risk for maternal morbidity and mortality and therefore pregnancy is contraindicated

Introduction

Congenital heart disease (CHD) refers to structural malformations of the heart and/or great vessels that result from abnormal cardiac development in utero or persistence of embryologic structure(s) beyond the first weeks of life (e.g., patent ductus arteriosus). CHD is the most common congenital defect, affecting approximately 0.8% of live births. With improvements in diagnostic tools and advances in surgical and transcatheter techniques, over 80% of patients born with CHD will survive to adulthood. As more women with CHD reach childbearing age, care of these patients requires a multidisciplinary approach with specialists in maternal-fetal medicine, adult CHD, and obstetric anesthesia with expertise in care of this patient population.

When caring for the pregnant patient with CHD, the first step is to identify the patient's congenital cardiac diagnoses. While some patients have received cardiac care since childhood for their conditions and are well-versed in their diagnoses, others may be unfamiliar with the terminology and unable to name or describe their cardiac condition to their providers. In the latter case, review of imaging and knowledge of CHD may help clarify their diagnoses. While the majority of patients with CHD are diagnosed in childhood, 30% of patients with CHD do not receive their diagnoses of CHD until adulthood. For some, the hemodynamic changes of pregnancy unmask symptoms or murmurs, leading to their congenital cardiac diagnosis.

The second step in caring for the pregnant patient with CHD is to understand their prior congenital cardiac interventions. As Dr. Perloff, one of the founders of the field of adult CHD, eloquently wrote in 1983, nearly all patients with CHD will have either *residua* or *sequelae* that warrant lifelong cardiac care [1]. *Residua* refers to "physiologically unimportant uncorrected defects," such as

bicuspid aortic valve in a patient with coarctation. *Sequelae* refers to the undesired (but often unavoidable) consequence of a surgical intervention, such as heart block after subaortic stenosis resection. Knowledge of patients' surgical or procedural history guide surveillance for such *residua* and *sequelae*. For example, patients who underwent surgical closure of an atrial septal defect are more likely to have atrial arrhythmias than patients who underwent transcatheter closure of an atrial septal defect due to the presence of atriotomy scars. Finally, providers should seek to understand the patient's current physiology to guide surveillance and management throughout pregnancy. Although many patients with CHD carry the belief that they were "cured" of their CHD with their childhood surgeries, nearly all patients require lifelong cardiac care [2].

In this chapter, we will review common CHD diagnoses and common *residua* and *sequelae* of each defect, and then review the hemodynamic issues often seen in patients with CHD and strategies for management in pregnancy. Table 10.1 outlines a basic checklist for a cardiology or obstetric visit in the pregnant patient with CHD.

Care of the patient with CHD requires an understanding of the hemodynamic burden of their repaired or unrepaired defect. Hemodynamic burdens can be understood as one or a combination of the following: volume loading, pressure loading, or low cardiac output states (Table 10.2). An overview of common congenital defects and pregnancy management is summarized in Table 10.3.

Shunts

Atrial Septal Defects

Aside from bicuspid aortic valves, atrial septal defects (ASDs) are the most common type of congenital heart defect, accounting for 10%–20% of congenital heart defects [3]. *Ostium secundum*

TABLE 10.1

Checklist for CHD Visit in Pregnancy

Past cardiac history	Congenital cardiac diagnosis
	Prior surgeries and/or catheter-based interventions
	Prior arrhythmias and/or electrophysiology study/ablation
	Implantable cardiac device (pacemaker, implantable cardioverter-defibrillator, loop recorder) and device settings
	Antiplatelet/anticoagulation, and indication
Current status	Last cardiology visit
	Last echocardiogram
	Last EKG
	Current NHYA functional class
Risk assessment	mWHO class
	ZAHARA
	CARPREG2
	Physiologic stage
Pregnancy management	Add/hold antiplatelet medications or anticoagulation
	Echocardiogram frequency
	BNP frequency
	EKG frequency
	CXR frequency
	Additional testing
	Additional consultations: Maternal-fetal medicine, adult congenital heart disease specialists
Fetal surveillance	Risk for anomalies
	Fetal anatomy, including fetal echo
	Serial growth
	Antepartum fetal heart rate testing

ASDs and primum ASDs are the most common, accounting for 75% and 20% of ASDs, respectively. Sinus venous defects and unroofed coronary sinus defects are, strictly defined, not ASDs as they do not involve the primum or secundum septum, but nonetheless are included here as the result in the same physiology

as ASDs [4]. Sinus venosus defects occur at the juncture of the superior vena cava (SVC) or inferior vena cava (IVC) and the right atrium, and account for 15% of ASDs. Unroofed coronary sinus defects result from a fenestration in the roof of the coronary sinus as it passes posterior to the left atrium in the atrioventricular groove, allowing oxygenated blood to shunt from the left atrium into the coronary sinus, which then drains into the right atrium [5]. Unroofed coronary sinus defects are rare, estimated to account for 1% of atrial level shunts.

Atrial level shunts result in volume loading of the right atrium and right ventricle, which in turn dilate over time. Symptoms of exertional dyspnea and palpitations may develop at any stage of life, even late in adulthood, as the degree of shunting across the defect increases as the left ventricle stiffens with age.

If an ASD is suspected but not clearly seen on transthoracic echocardiogram (TTE), a "bubble study" can aid in diagnosis of an atrial level shunt. In a bubble study, agitated saline is injected into a peripheral IV while an echocardiogram is being performed. In patients without shunts, the bubbles are visualized on the echocardiogram filling the right atrium and ventricle, and are then filtered out in the lungs, with no bubbles appearing in the left atrium or ventricle. Appearance of bubbles in the left atrium or ventricle suggests right-to-left intracardiac (or intrapulmonary) shunting. Notably, a negative agitated saline contrast study does not definitively exclude an atrial level communication, as patients who are shunting predominantly from the left to right atrium may have a negative agitated saline contrast study.

Patients with unrepaired atrial level shunts typically shunt blood from the left atrium to the right atrium, as left atrial pressure is typically higher than right atrial pressures due to greater right ventricular compliance. However, transient increases in right atrial pressure or volume can cause transient right to left atrial shunting. The risk of paradoxical embolism across the atrial septal defect is increased in pregnancy due to the increased volume and hypercoagulable state of pregnancy. Labor and delivery is a particularly high-risk period due to the increase in venous return with release

TABLE 10.2

Hemodynamic Burdens of Congenital Heart Defects

Hemodynamic Burden	Example(s)	Pregnancy Symptoms	Management Strategies	Comments
Right heart volume loading	Atrial level shunts	Exertional dyspnea, increased lower extremity edema, atrial arrhythmias	Diuretics	Generally well tolerated in pregnancy but may require diuretic therapy
Right heart pressure loading	Pulmonary valve/artery stenosis, double chambered right ventricle	Exertional dyspnea, increased lower extremity edema, ventricular arrhythmias	Diuretics, beta-blockers	Consider transcatheter interventions (balloon angioplasty or valvuloplasty) if refractory symptoms
Left heart volume loading	Mitral or aortic regurgitation	Exertional dyspnea, orthopnea, paroxysmal nocturnal dyspnea, atrial arrhythmias. Ventricular arrhythmias, especially if LV dysfunction	Diuretics, beta-blockers	Generally well tolerated in pregnancy but may require diuretic therapy
Left heart pressure loading	Coarctation of the aorta, aortic stenosis	Exertional dyspnea, orthopnea, paroxysmal nocturnal dyspnea, atrial arrhythmias. Ventricular arrhythmias, especially if LV dysfunction	Diuretics, beta-blockers	Consider transcatheter interventions (balloon angioplasty or valvuloplasty) if refractory symptoms

TABLE 10.3

An Overview of Common Congenital Defects and Pregnancy Management

Congenital Heart Defect	Hemodynamics	Physical Exam Findings	Findings on Testing	Modified WHO Risk Class	Pregnancy Concerns	Management Recommendation
Unrepaired atrial level shunts (secundum or primum ASDs, sinus venosus defects, unroofed coronary sinus)	• Left to right interatrial shunt causes volume loading of the right heart • Right ventricular dysfunction (variable) • Mild-moderately elevated pulmonary artery pressures, particularly in older patients	• Split second heart sound • Right ventricular heave • Systolic flow murmur at the left upper sternal border	• EKG: incomplete right bundle branch block • Echo: right atrial and right ventricular dilation • Primum or secundum defects usually well visualized by TTE • Sinus venosus defects and unroofed coronary sinus often require TEE, MRI or CT for diagnosis	II	Paradoxical emboli may cause stroke or myocardial infarction	• Consider aspirin 81 mg daily • Consider anticoagulation with low molecular weight heparin if patient has a cardioembolic event • SBE prophylaxis at time of delivery is reasonable given potential for transient right to left shunting • Bubble/particle filters on IVs
Unrepaired ventricular septal defect (all types), unrepaired PDA						
Small VSD or PDA	No significant hemodynamic impact	Small VSD: holosystolic murmur at the left sternal border Small PDA: faint, continuous murmur below the left clavicle	EKG: normal TTE: small VSD or PDA with high-velocity left to right shunt. Normal chamber sizes	II	No significant additional risk	Small VSDs SBE prophylaxis reasonable given small risk of endocarditis
Medium-sized VSD or PDA	Pressure loading of the right ventricle Mild-moderate pulmonary arterial hypertension Volume loading of the left atrium/left ventricle	Moderate sized VSD: softer holosystolic murmur RV lift if pulmonary hypertension Moderate-sized PDA: continuous murmur below the left clavicle	EKG: may demonstrate RV hypertrophy TTE: • VSD with left to right shunt or PDA with aorta-to-pulmonary artery shunt • Right ventricle hypertrophy and hypertension • Left atrium/ventricle dilation	II-III	Risk for heart failure	• Avoid volume loading • Bubble/particle filters on IVs • SBE prophylaxis reasonable given small risk of endocarditis
Left ventricular outflow tract obstruction (subvalvar or supravalvar aortic stenosis)	Pressure loading of the left ventricle	• Harsh systolic crescendo murmur at the right upper sternal border • LV impulse may be enlarged if LV hypertrophy is present	EKG: left ventricular hypertrophy TTE: • Left ventricular hypertrophy • Left atrial dilation if longstanding LVH • Subvalvar aortic stenosis (discrete membrane or tunnel-like) with flow acceleration • Supravalvar aortic stenosis typically at the level of the sinotubular junction	II if moderate stenosis III if severe obstruction and patient is symptomatic	If severe: • Risk for heart failure • Right for ventricular or atrial arrhythmias	• Avoid volume loading • SBE prophylaxis reasonable if aortic valve is thickened

(Continued)

TABLE 10.3 (*Continued*)

An Overview of Common Congenital Defects and Pregnancy Management

Congenital Heart Defect	Hemodynamics	Physical Exam Findings	Findings on Testing	Modified WHO Risk Class	Pregnancy Concerns	Management Recommendation
Aortic coarctation						
Mild native coarctation, or repaired coarctation without significant residual narrowing	No significant hemodynamic impact	• No significant delay between right brachial and femoral pulses • Left upper extremity pulse may be diminished or absent if patient had prior subclavian flap repair	EKG: normal	II	May be prone to hypertension due to aortic stiffness	Avoid checking BP in LUE if prior subclavian flap repair. If unsure whether patient has prior subclavian flap repair, check bilateral upper extremity blood pressures, and follow the higher of the two
Moderate or severe native or residual coarctation	Left ventricular pressure overload	• Femoral pulse delayed and diminished compared with (right) upper extremity pulse • LV impulse may be enlarged if LV hypertrophy is present	EKG: left ventricular hypertrophy	III (severe asymptomatic) IV (severe symptomatic)	• Hypertension in the upper body, with relative hypotension of the lower body due to gradient across the coarctation • Risk for heart failure	• Monitor upper and lower extremity BPs; placental perfusion will correlate best with LE BPs • Titration of anti-hypertensives as tolerated by mother and fetus • Pain control to avoid fluctuations in blood pressure
Ebsteins anomaly	• Right heart volume overload if moderate or severe regurgitation • Right ventricular systolic function often abnormal	Widely split-second heart sound, additional heart sounds common If ASD is also present, patient may have cyanosis	EKG: right bundle branch block, PR prolongation are common. Evaluate for preexcitation (Wolff- Parkinson-White syndrome) TTE: right atrial dilation, displaced septal leaflet of the tricuspid valve with elongation of the anterior leaflet, tricuspid regurgitation. Evaluate right ventricular function and assess for secundum ASD	II-III depending on right/left ventricular function, history of arrhythmias, and presence of cyanosis	• Risk for atrial arrhythmias (SVT with or without preexcitation, PACs) • Risk for ventricular arrhythmia, especially if poor ventricular function • Risk for paradoxical embolus if ASD is present	• Monitor for arrhythmias • Avoid volume loading • Bubble/particle filters if ASD is present • SBE prophylaxis if ASD is present
Pulmonary stenosis, subvalvar pulmonary stenosis, pulmonary artery stenosis	Right heart pressure overload	Systolic crescendo murmur at the left upper sternal border	EKG: right ventricular hypertrophy TTE: stenosis of subvalvar/valvar/ supravalvar region(s); right ventricular hypertrophy; right atrial dilation	• I if mild or moderate • II-III if severe	• Risk for atrial or ventricular arrhythmias, particularly with severe stenosis • Risk for right heart failure if RV function is decreased	• Monitor for arrhythmias • Avoid volume loading • SBE prophylaxis
Tetralogy of Fallot, status post repair	• If chronic severe pulmonary valve regurgitation, right heart volume overload • If pulmonary valve is functional, patient may have relatively normal hemodynamics	• Fixed split-second heart sound • Short diastolic decrescendo murmur if severe PR	EKG: right bundle branch block TTE: repaired VSD Right atrium and right ventricle dilation if chronic severe pulmonary valve regurgitation	II	• Right for atrial or ventricular arrhythmias, particularly if history of prior arrhythmias and/or severe RA/RV dilation • Risk for right heart failure if severe RA/RV dilation or severe RV dysfunction	• Monitor for arrhythmias • Avoid volume loading • SBE prophylaxis

(Continued)

TABLE 10.3 (Continued)

An Overview of Common Congenital Defects and Pregnancy Management

Congenital Heart Defect	Hemodynamics	Physical Exam Findings	Findings on Testing	Modified WHO Risk Class	Pregnancy Concerns	Management Recommendation
Double outlet right ventricle, status post Rastelli repair Truncus arteriosus, status post repair	Variable, depending on presence or absence of residual lesions: • RV-PA conduit stenosis or regurgitation • Aortic regurgitation	• Systolic crescendo murmur (flow through RV-PA conduit) • Diastolic decrescendo murmur at the left upper sternal border (RV-PA conduit regurgitation) or right upper sternal border (aortic regurgitation)	EKG: right bundle branch block TTE: repaired VSD; right atrium and right ventricle size, wall thickness and function dependent on status of the RV-PA conduit	II-III, depending on residual lesions	Variable, depending on residual lesions. If significant RV-PA conduit dysfunction, then increased risk of right heart failure	Avoid volume loading if significant RV-PA conduit dysfunction or severe RV dysfunction
D-Transposition of the great arteries, status post arterial switch	Normal, if no residual lesions Potential late complications include aortic root dilation, aortic regurgitation, and stenosis of the reimplanted coronary arteries	Normal	EKG: normal TTE: abnormal positioning of the aorta and pulmonary artery post-arterial switch. LV function normal in most patients	II if no significant residual lesions	Low risk for complications if no significant residual lesions	Low risk for complications if no significant residual lesions
D-Transposition of the great arteries, status post atrial switch procedure	• Systemic right ventricle, typically with at least mild systolic dysfunction by adulthood • Tricuspid regurgitation is common, with associated RA/RV volume overload	• Right ventricular lift/heave • Holosystolic murmur (tricuspid regurgitation)	EKG: right ventricular hypertrophy TTE: abnormal position of the aorta (anterior and rightward). Systemic right ventricular systolic function is usually abnormal. Tricuspid regurgitation is common	III if normal or mildly decreased systemic right ventricular function; IV if moderate-severe systemic right ventricular dysfunction	• Risk of heart failure • Risk of ventricular and arrhythmias, especially if prior history of arrhythmias	• Monitor for arrhythmias • Avoid volume loading • SBE prophylaxis
Congenitally corrected transposition of the great arteries (ccTGA)	• Systemic right ventricle, typically with at least mild systolic dysfunction by adulthood • Tricuspid regurgitation is common, with associated RA/RV volume overload	Right ventricular lift/heave Holosystolic murmur (tricuspid regurgitation)	EKG: right ventricular hypertrophy; q waves in the right precordial leads V1-V2 TTE: leftward systemic right ventricle; Ebstenoid malformation of the tricuspid valve is associated with ccTGA	• III if normal or mildly decreased systemic right ventricular function • IV if moderate-severe systemic right ventricular dysfunction	• Risk of heart failure • Risk of ventricular and arrhythmias, especially if prior history of arrhythmias	• Monitor for arrhythmias • Avoid volume loading • SBE prophylaxis
Univentricular hearts, status post Fontan operation	• Systemic venous return flows passively to the pulmonary arteries • Decreased LV preload due to slow transit through the pulmonary arteries • Variable single ventricle function, depending on anatomy	Single S1 and S2 Saturations may be as high as low-mid 90s, or may be lower	EKG: variable depending on underlying anatomy Typically ventricular hypertrophy is seen TTE: variable depending on anatomy. Severe right atrial dilation if patient had an atriopulmonary Fontan	III	• Risk of heart failure • Right of thromboembolic complications • Right of atrial arrhythmias	• Monitor for arrhythmias • Avoid volume loading • SBE prophylaxis • Bubble/particle filters on IVs

of Valsalva, and postpartum due to relief of IVC compression and increase in systemic venous return to the right atrium. Bubble/particle filters can decrease the risk of paradoxical embolism and should be utilized in all patients with potential right-to-left cardiac shunts. Providers caring for patients with unrepaired atrial level shunts should be vigilant for neurologic signs or symptoms that suggest a cerebral vascular accident (CVA) or chest pain/pressure or unexplained dyspnea to suggest myocardial infarction due to a coronary artery embolus. Though data are scarce, aspirin is generally recommended to minimize this risk. Anticoagulation with low molecular weight heparin should be recommended in the pregnant patient who experiences an embolic event.

The decision for ASD closure should be made together with an experienced adult congenital cardiology team. Patients with secundum type ASDs are often candidates for transcatheter ASD closure. For the patient at high risk for a recurrent thromboembolic event, closure during pregnancy may be considered but the risks of fetal loss or preterm labor with the administration of general anesthesia must be weighed against the risk for recurrent thromboembolic event. The other types of atrial shunts (primum, sinus venosus, unroofed coronary sinus) require a surgical approach (Figure 10.1) [6].

Ventricular Septal Defects

The incidence of ventricular septal defects (VSDs) varies widely in the literature, as many patients are asymptomatic, and many small defects close spontaneously but are among the most common forms of CHD in childhood. Approximately 10,000–11,000 isolated VSDs are diagnosed in infants in the United States annually [7,8]. Ventricular septal defects are divided into four types, based on their location within the interventricular septum:

1. Perimembranous VSDs account for 80%
2. Muscular VSDs account for 50%–10%
3. Inlet VSDs account for 5%
4. Supracristal VSDs account for 5%–7%

VSDs result in pressure loading of the right ventricle and pulmonary artery due to exposure of the right heart to systemic pressures. VSDs also result in volume loading of the left atrium and left ventricle, as the oxygenated blood shunted from the left ventricle to the right ventricle through the VSD is recirculated through the lungs and back to the left heart. Patients with small VSDs have normal pulmonary artery pressures and normal left atrial and

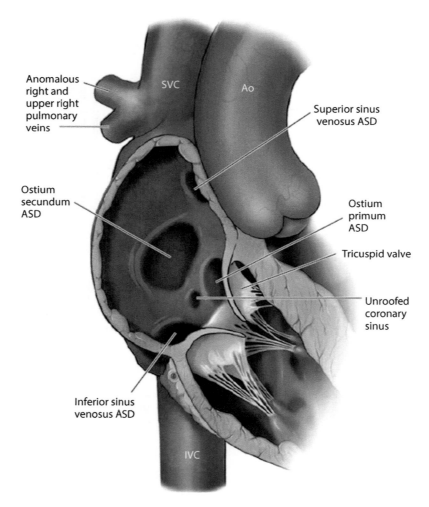

FIGURE 10.1   Locations of atrial level shunts, en face view. RA view of the interatrial septum demonstrating the location of different types of atrial level shunts. ASD, atrial septal defects. (Adapted from Otto CM et al. *Textbook of Clinical Echocardiography*, 6th ed. Philadelphia: Elsevier; 2019, ch. 1. With permission.)

ventricular size. Patients with moderate VSDs will develop moderate pulmonary arterial hypertension and have dilation of the left atrium and ventricle. Patients with large nonrestrictive VSDs will develop heart failure symptoms early in life. If left unrepaired, patients with large VSDs will begin to have progressive pulmonary arterial hypertension by 2–3 years of age and have severe pulmonary hypertension and bidirectional or right to left shunting (Eisenmenger physiology) by the time they reach adulthood.

Patent Ductus Arteriosus

The ductus arteriosus is a vessel between the proximal descending aorta and the main pulmonary artery near the origin of the left pulmonary artery. In fetal life, the ductus arteriosus diverts blood from the pulmonary artery away from the lungs, into the aorta. The ductus arteriosus typically closes after birth; persistence of the ductus arteriosus beyond the first few weeks of life is abnormal and represents a congenital heart defect termed patent ductus arteriosus (PDA). The incidence of PDA is approximately 1 in 2000, accounting for 5%–10% of all congenital heart defects [7].

Similar to VSDs, the PDA may be a small, moderate, or large shunt, and moderate or large PDAs result in pressure loading of the right ventricle and pulmonary arteries, and volume loading of the left heart. Small shunts are typically well-tolerated lifelong and may never require intervention, while large shunts result in heart failure and Eisenmenger syndrome if not addressed early in life. Transcatheter device closure is now preferred over surgical closure, and may be performed in patients of all ages, though may be more difficult in adults with calcification of the PDA. PDA closure is contraindicated in patients with severe pulmonary arterial hypertension and Eisenmenger syndrome.

Left Ventricular Outflow Tract Obstruction

Subvalvar, Valvar, and Supravalvar Aortic Stenosis

Subvalvar aortic stenosis (SAS) accounts for approximately 30% of congenital left ventricular outflow tract obstruction (LVOT) lesions, and can be caused by a spectrum of malformations, from a discrete fibrous membrane to a tunnel-like fibromuscular band encompassing the circumference of the left ventricular outflow tract. It can be progressive and cause a significant pressure load on the left ventricle, with resultant hypertrophy, diastolic dysfunction, and eventual systolic dysfunction if left untreated. Surgical treatment of SAS depends on the type of obstruction and may range from resection of a discrete fibrous membrane to a septomyectomy to enlarge the left ventricular outflow tract in patients with tunnel-like obstruction. Recurrence of SAS is unfortunately common, with recurrence rates of 14%–27% [9–12]. Mild to moderate aortic regurgitation is common, seen in approximately 60% of patients with subaortic stenosis, as the aortic valve leaflets develop fibrous thickening from repeated shear stress of the high velocity SAS flow on the leaflets.

Valvar aortic stenosis is typically due to a bicuspid aortic valve in young adults, but in rare cases may be due to a unicuspid aortic valve. Bicuspid aortic valve (BAV) is the most common congenital heart defect, affecting up to 3% of the population, more often in males than females. Patients may present in the neonatal period with critical congenital aortic stenosis requiring emergent balloon valvotomy; other patients may remain asymptomatic with adequate valve function into advanced age. Approximately 50% of patients with BAV will require valve intervention by their fifth or sixth decade of life.

Supravalvar aortic stenosis (SVAS) is the least common cause of LVOT obstruction, accounting for 8% cases. Approximately 60% of patients with SVAS have Williams syndrome, which is characterized by elfin facies, stellate iris, short stature, and a "cocktail personality." The remaining 40% of SVAS cases may be familiar or sporadic. SVAS is defined by a fixed aortic narrowing at the level of the sinotubular junction and is associated with a generalized arteriopathy which can affect both the aorta and its branches, as well as the pulmonary arterial system. Surgical intervention is recommended for severe SVAS.

Aortic Coarctation

Aortic coarctation (CoA) is a focal narrowing of the aorta, almost always at the junction of the distal aortic arch and descending aorta, just below the origin of the left subclavian artery. It is associated with a generalized arteriopathy and hypertension. CoA accounts for 5%–8% of congenital cardiac disease and is associated with bicuspid aortic valves in approximately 70% of patients, ventricular septal defects, and mitral valve abnormalities. Intracranial aneurysms, typically berry aneurysms of the circle of Willis, are seen in 3%–5% of patients with CoA. Treatment of CoA in childhood in infants and small children is typically surgical; in older children, adolescents, and adults, angioplasty and stent implantation is preferred in patients with suitable anatomy. Residua and sequelae include hypertension due the underlying arteriopathy, residual focal narrowing after stenting or surgical repair, or saccular aneurysms at suture lines after surgical repair.

Right Ventricular Outflow Tract Obstruction

Pulmonary Stenosis

Pulmonary valve stenosis (PS) accounts for 7%–10% of congenital heart defects, and typically occurs in isolation. The pulmonary valve may be fused and have an appearance of "doming" on the TTE or may be dysplastic with thickened leaflets. Pulmonary stenosis results in right ventricular pressure overload. The treatment of choice for pulmonary stenosis is balloon valvuloplasty. Dysplastic valves may require surgical valvotomy if valvuloplasty is unsuccessful. Pulmonary regurgitation is a common sequela of surgical valvotomy and may require reintervention with a pulmonary valve replacement later in life.

Double-Chambered Right Ventricle

Double-chambered right ventricle (DCRV) is an uncommon congenital heart defect which occurs when anomalous or hypertrophied muscle bundles in the mid ventricle or outflow tract cause intraventricular obstruction. The obstructing muscles divide the ventricle into a high-pressure proximal inflow chamber that communicates with the tricuspid valve, and a low-pressure distal outflow chamber that communicates with the pulmonary valve. DCRV accounts for 0.5%–2% of all CHD and is associated with VSDs, pulmonary stenosis, and tetralogy of Fallot. Surgical resection of the anomalous or hypertrophied muscle bundles is an effective cure and is indicated for patients with moderate or greater obstruction.

Other Complex Congenital Heart Disease

Ebstein Anomaly

Ebstein anomaly is a congenital malformation of the tricuspid valve defined by failure of delamination of the septal leaflet from the septum, apical and posterior displacement of the functional tricuspid annulus, and elongation of the anterior leaflet. Part of the anatomic right ventricle is "atrialized," and the right atrioventricular junction (true tricuspid annulus) is dilated. The right ventricular wall is typically thinned and dilated, and Wolf-Parkinson-White is often seen due to disruption of the normal electrical separation between the right atrium and the right ventricle. Patients with more mild forms of Ebstein anomaly may not ever require intervention, whereas those with very severe forms may require transplant consideration as infants due to severe ventricular dysfunction. Adults with a diagnosis of Ebstein anomaly may be unrepaired with chronic tricuspid regurgitation, may have had prior tricuspid valve repair with variable degrees of residual tricuspid regurgitation, or may have had prior tricuspid valve replacement.

Double-Outlet Right Ventricle

Double-outlet right ventricle (DORV) is defined as "a type of ventriculoarterial connection in which both great vessels arise either entirely or predominantly from the right ventricle" [13]. DORV accounts for 1% of all CHD [14] and is often associated with other anomalies such as coarctation, heterotaxy, and chromosomal mutations such as trisomy 13, trisomy 18, and chromosome 22q11 deletion. Surgical approach to DORV, and thus the associated residua and sequelae, depend on the relationship of the VSD to the great arteries, the size of the VSD, the size of the great arteries, size of the ventricles, and the atrioventricular valves. Ventricular-to-pulmonary artery conduits and baffles are typically used in two-ventricle repairs, and are associated with conduit stenosis or regurgitation, and baffle stenoses or leaks. Single-ventricle repairs are discussed below.

Truncus Arteriosus

Truncus arteriosus, also known as persistent truncus arteriosus, is an uncommon cyanotic congenital heart defect, accounting for 1%–4% of cardiac heart defects in a large autopsy series [15] and 0.6–1.4 per 10,000 live births [16]. In truncus arteriosus, the main pulmonary artery or branch pulmonary arteries arise from the aorta, typically the ascending aorta. Patients nearly always have a large nonrestrictive ventricular septal defect. The truncal (aortic) valve has normal trileaflet morphology in 69%, is quadricuspid in 22%, and bicuspid in 9%. The abnormality, as well as the

dilation of the aorta and valve annulus, predisposes patients with truncus arteriosus to aortic regurgitation.

Patients with truncus arteriosus typically present in the neonatal period or early infancy with signs of heart failure from pulmonary overcirculation. Survival into adulthood without surgical repair is rare; those who survive suffer from severe pulmonary arterial hypertension. Surgical repair for truncus arteriosus, known as the Rastelli repair, was first performed in 1967, involving closure of the VSD, separation of the pulmonary artery from the aorta, and placement of a right ventricular to pulmonary artery (RV-PA) conduit to separate the venous and arterial circulation [17]. Unfortunately, due to the small size of the RV-PA conduits, conduit degeneration, and patient growth, patients with truncus arteriosus often require reoperation(s) to replace the RV-PA conduits before they reach adulthood.

Care of the repaired patient with truncus arteriosus requires an understanding of (i) the degree of stenosis or regurgitation across the RV-PA conduit which may impose volume or pressure loading on the right ventricular, respectively; (ii) presence of truncal/aortic valve regurgitation which may impose volume loading on the left ventricular; and (iii) biventricular function which may be normal or abnormal, depending on the severity and degree of both prior and current pressure/volume loading. Physical exam findings and management strategies in pregnancy will vary depending on the presence of the above residua.

D-Transposition of the Great Arteries

In D-transposition of the great arteries (D-TGA), the aorta arises from the right ventricle and the pulmonary artery arises from the left ventricle. This results in two parallel circulations, with the deoxygenated blood traveling via systemic veins to the right atrium, right ventricle, aorta, and back to the systemic veins, and the oxygenated blood traveling via the pulmonary veins to the left atrium, left ventricle, pulmonary artery, back to the pulmonary veins. Mixing of the systemic and venous circulation is necessary for the neonate to be viable, and typically occurs via a ventricular septal defect which is present in 40%–45% of cases, atrial septal defect, or patent ductus arteriosus. If none of these are present, or if they are inadequate, a balloon atrial septostomy early in life will permit greater mixing of the circulation.

The first definitive surgical repairs for D-TGA were the Senning [18] and Mustard [19] atrial switch procedures. The atrial switch procedure is a physiologic correction that uses surgically placed baffles to redirect systemic venous return across the atrial septum to the left atrium, thus allowing deoxygenated blood to flow to the pulmonary artery; the pulmonary venous baffle directs the pulmonary venous return rightward across the atrial septum to the right atrium, thus allowing oxygenated blood to travel to the aorta. In the atrial switch procedure, the right ventricle thus serves as the systemic ventricle, pumping oxygenated blood to the aorta, while the left ventricle is the subpulmonary ventricle, pumping deoxygenated blood to the pulmonary artery. Long-term sequelae of the atrial switch procedures include baffle stenoses which can increase pressures in the systemic or pulmonary veins, baffle leaks which would result in an atrial level shunt, systemic right ventricle systolic and diastolic dysfunction, tricuspid regurgitation, atrial tachyarrhythmias, and sinus node dysfunction.

Due to the late complications of the atrial switch operation, it was eventually developed and first performed successfully in 1975 by Jatene and associates [20]. However, due to early operative complications with coronary ischemia, the arterial switch operation was not performed routinely until the early 1990s. In the arterial switch operation, the aorta and pulmonary artery are transected above the sinuses, and the coronary arteries are disconnected from the native aorta. The great arteries are then re-anastomosed in a "switched" manner, with the aorta now surgically anastomosed to the native pulmonary root (which arises from the left ventricle), and the pulmonary artery now surgically anastomosed anteriorly to the native aortic root (which arises from the right ventricle). The coronary arteries are implanted into the new constructed aortic ("neoaortic") root. Long-term sequelae of the arterial switch operation include ventricular dysfunction and risk for myocardial ischemia, particularly due to the reimplantation of the coronary arteries. Neoaortic dilation and neoaortic valve regurgitation may also occur.

Congenitally Corrected Transposition of the Great Arteries

In congenitally corrected transposition of the great arteries (ccTGA), the positions of the ventricles are reversed, so that the right atrium drains systemic venous return into the right-sided anatomic left ventricle, which then pumps the deoxygenated blood to the pulmonary artery. The pulmonary venous return to the left atrium drains across the tricuspid valve to the left-sided anatomic right ventricle that functions as the systemic ventricle, pumping oxygenated blood to the aorta. Thus, discordance of the atrioventricular (i.e., right atrium to left ventricle, and left atrium to right ventricle) and ventricular arterial (i.e., left ventricle to pulmonary artery, and right ventricle to aorta) results in physiologic connections in spite of abnormal anatomic connections.

A common sequela of these congenital heart defects is heart block, which occurs at a rate of approximately 2% per year. The tricuspid valve may be abnormal, with Ebstein-like malformation and associated regurgitation, or may be initially competent but develop secondary regurgitation due to tricuspid annular dilation. Tricuspid valve replacement should be considered for patients with severe tricuspid regurgitation, though the optimal timing of this surgery is subject to debate. With increasing age, right ventricular dysfunction also becomes more prevalent, and significant systemic ventricular dysfunction leading to heart failure symptoms often presents in the fourth or fifth decade of life.

Single-Ventricle Physiology

Various degrees of ventricular hypoplasia may be seen in many of the congenital heart defects discussed in this chapter. True single-ventricle *anatomy*, in which a second hypoplastic ventricle is not able to be identified, is unusual but can be seen in some cases of double-inlet left ventricle. Single-ventricle *physiology* is more prevalent and refers to a patient who has undergone surgical Fontan palliation.

In the Fontan surgery, the systemic venous return can be redirected to the pulmonary artery by one of several methods. Early Fontan palliations were performed by anastomosing the right atrial appendage to the pulmonary artery, thus allowing SVC

and IVC flow to enter the right atrium and then the main pulmonary artery. This resulted in right atrial hypertension, right atrial dilation, and atrial arrhythmias, so was largely abandoned in the early 1990s in favor of the lateral tunnel and extracardiac Fontans. The lateral tunnel (LT) Fontan uses an intra-atrial baffle to direct IVC flow superiorly through an atrial tunnel, anastomosing to the inferior aspect of the right pulmonary artery. A Glenn shunt is an anastomosis of the SVC to the superior aspect of the (usually right) pulmonary artery, thereby directing SVC flow directly to the pulmonary arteries. An extracardiac (EC) Fontan is similar to the LT Fontan but uses an extracardiac conduit rather than an intra-atrial tunnel to direct blood from the IVC to the pulmonary arteries.

The Fontan palliation has allowed many patients with cyanotic congenital heart defects not amenable to a biventricular repair to survive to adulthood. However, their physiology remains markedly abnormal. Patients with Fontan physiology depend on a pressure gradient, low pulmonary vascular resistance, and negative intrathoracic pressure to promote systemic venous return. Preload, or filling, of the single ventricle depends on transit of blood through the pulmonary vasculature, assisted by diastolic relaxation of the single ventricle drawing blood forward from the pulmonary venous atrium and pulmonary veins. Diastolic dysfunction, atrioventricular valve regurgitation, pulmonary vein stenosis, pulmonary artery stenosis, or pulmonary vascular disease would further impede pulmonary blood flow, ventricular filling, and would result in elevated pressures in the Fontan circuit (IVC, SVC, and right atrium/intra-atrial tunnel/extracardiac conduit). Chronic hepatic congestion is the rule, and patients may develop advanced fibrosis or even cirrhosis due to hepatic congestion. Maternal Fontan physiology is a major predictor for adverse fetal outcomes of prematurity and small-for-gestational age, likely due to multifactorial causes of chronic low cardiac output and, for some patients, variable levels of desaturation from venovenous collaterals.

Eisenmenger Syndrome

Eisenmenger syndrome was first coined by Paul Wood in 1958 and defined as "pulmonary hypertension due to a high pulmonary vascular resistance with reversed or bidirectional shunt at aortopulmonary, ventricular, or atrial level" [21]. The prevalence of Eisenmenger syndrome in developed nations has decreased by an estimated 50% over the past 50 years due to advances in diagnostic and surgical techniques in pediatric cardiology [22] that allow for earlier diagnoses and closure of large shunts before patients develop pulmonary vascular disease. For those who develop Eisenmenger syndrome, survival has improved due to advancements in medical management and the development of pulmonary vasodilators.

Severe pulmonary arterial hypertension in the presence of an intra- or extracardiac shunt results in cyanosis due to right-to-left shunting, right ventricular hypertrophy and diastolic dysfunction, and variable right ventricular systolic dysfunction. However, Eisenmenger syndrome is also a multi-organ disease. Patients have a bleeding diathesis due to low platelets and dysfunction of von Willebrand factor but may also have in situ thrombosis in the pulmonary arteries and are predisposed to thromboembolic events such as strokes due to paradoxical embolism across the shunt. The right-to-left shunt also increases risk for infection, particularly endocarditis and brain abscesses from septic emboli. Renal dysfunction can occur due to a nephrotic syndrome, or due to cardiorenal syndrome.

Patients with Eisenmenger syndrome are modified WHO (mWHO) class IV, and at high risk for maternal morbidity and mortality with pregnancy. All patients of reproductive age should be counseled to avoid pregnancy. If pregnancy occurs, termination should be discussed with the patient. For patients who elect to continue the pregnancy, a multidisciplinary approach with cardiologist experienced in the care of Eisenmenger syndrome, cardiac and obstetric anesthesiologists, and maternal-fetal medicine specialists is strongly recommended.

Preconception and Pregnancy Counseling

The patient should be counseled in detail regarding the following:

1. The risk of maternal and fetal adverse outcomes during pregnancy and postpartum period.
2. The potential for adverse long-term outcomes after pregnancy such as the risk of worsening ventricular function in patients with systemic ventricular dysfunction, and the risk for progressive aortic dilation due to pregnancy.
3. Offspring of parents with congenital defects are at a higher risk for congenital heart defects. For those with de novo mutation, risk of CHD recurrence for most lesions is 3%–5%, though the relative risk is higher in patients with atrioventricular septal defect and left ventricular outflow tract obstructive lesions. The relative risk of recurrence is 80-fold for patients with heterotaxy syndrome [23]. Genetic counseling should be offered to patients with known heritable conditions, such as Marfan syndrome, Holt-Oram, Noonan, Alagille, CHARGE, 22q11.2 microdeletion, and Williams syndrome.

Management of Congenital Heart Disease in Pregnancy, Peripartum, and Postpartum

In addition to the above risk assessment schemes, the 2018 AHA/ACC Guidelines for the Management of adults with CHD outline four physiological classes, A–D, which include consideration of residua and sequela (Table 10.4; ref [2]).

Frequency of cardiology visits should be individualized based on level of risk as assessed by the risk stratification schemes, understanding of the severity of the patient's hemodynamic burden from residual lesions (see Table 10.3), and physiological stage of CHD, which accounts for common residua and sequelae. Those who are at physiological stage A, such as a patient with a bicuspid aortic valve with normal valve function and no aortic dilation, may only require a single cardiology visit in the late second or early third trimester. Those at physiological stage B, such as a patient with a bicuspid aortic valve with normal valve function but mild aortic dilation, may benefit from cardiology visits and surveillance echocardiograms every trimester. Those in physiological stage C, such as a patient with bicuspid aortic valve and moderate aortic stenosis and/or regurgitation may require visits every 1 or 2 months. Those in physiological stage D, such

TABLE 10.4

Physiological Stage of Congenital Heart Disease

A

NYHA functional class I symptoms
No hemodynamic or anatomic sequelae
No arrhythmias
Normal exercise capacity
Normal renal, hepatic, pulmonary function

B

NYHA functional class II symptoms
Mild hemodynamic sequelae (mild aortic enlargement, mild
  ventricular enlargement, mild ventricular dysfunction)
Mild valvular disease
Trivial or small shunt (not hemodynamically significant)
Arrhythmia not requiring treatment
Abnormal, objective cardiac limitation to exercise

C

NYHA functional class III symptoms
Moderate or greater valvular disease; moderate or greater
  ventricular dysfunction (systemic, pulmonic, or both)
Moderate aortic enlargement
Venous or arterial stenosis
Mild or moderate hypoxemia/cyanosis
Hemodynamically significant shunt
Arrhythmias controlled with treatment (ablation or medication)
Pulmonary hypertension (less than severe)
End-organ dysfunction responsive to therapy

D

NYHA functional class IV symptoms
Severe aortic enlargement
Arrhythmias refractory to treatment
Severe hypoxemia (cyanosis)
Severe pulmonary hypertension
Eisenmenger syndrome
Refractory end-organ dysfunction

Source: Stout KK et al. *J Am College Cardiol.* 2019;73(12):1494–
          563. With permission.

as a patient with bicuspid aortic valve and severe aortic enlargement, may require more frequent visits, including the possibility of weekly visits for close monitoring and medication titration.

Similarly, prenatal obstetric care should be individualized to the patient risk. Patients at physiological stage A may be cared for by a maternal-fetal medicine specialist but may also be cared for by a general obstetrician. However, those at physiological stage B, C, or D should be managed by an obstetrician trained in maternal-fetal medicine or experienced in the care of pregnant patients with CHD. For patients in physiologic stage C or D, a multidisciplinary meeting including the obstetric, cardiology, and anesthesia teams should be convened once the fetus reaches viability at 23–24 weeks.

The rate of fetal loss in CHD patients is approximately 15%–25%, slightly higher than that of the general population [24,25]. Rate of premature delivery (10%–12%) was more common in patients with CHD compared with the general population, particularly in patients with complex CHD [24]. Neonatal events such as small for gestational age, respiratory distress syndrome, interventricular hemorrhage, and neonatal death also occur at a

TABLE 10.5

Sample Delivery Plan Checklist

Patient risk category
- ☐ *WHO 1* (The risk of maternal morbidity and mortality is not detectably higher than that in the general population)
- ☐ *WHO 2 or 3* (WHO 2 conditions carry a small increased risk of maternal mortality or morbidity. WHO 3 conditions carry a significant increased risk of maternal morbidity or mortality)
  - WHO 2 (if otherwise well and uncomplicated) 6.8% (*Heart 2014*)
  - WHO 2–3 (depending on individual)
  - WHO 3 (*24.5% Heart 2014*)
- ☐ *WHO 4* (WHO 4 conditions carry an extremely high risk of maternal mortality or severe morbidity; pregnancy is contraindicated. If pregnancy occurs, termination should be discussed. If pregnancy continues, care as for WHO 3) (*100% Heart 2014*)

Patient is at risk for
- ☐ Atrial arrhythmias
- ☐ Ventricular arrhythmias
- ☐ Heart failure/volume overload
- ☐ Other

Admission
- ☐ Notify cardiac or adult congenital heart disease (ACHD) team of patient admission
- ☐ No additional monitoring required beyond normal L&D monitoring
- ☐ Continuous telemetry upon admission. Continue telemetry until 24 hours postpartum or per ACHD recommendations
- ☐ Continuous pulse oximetry during active labor and delivery
- ☐ Cardiac or ICU nurse recommended due to risk for maternal cardiac event
- ☐ Invasive hemodynamic monitoring:
  - ☐ CVP line
  - ☐ Arterial line
- ☐ EKG on admission
- ☐ BNP, CMP, magnesium, CBC on admission
- ☐ PT/INR on admission
- ☐ Additional labs on admission

Ob anesthesia
- ☐ No contraindications to epidural placement if desired by the patient
- ☐ Epidural is recommended from cardiac perspective

Inpatient peripartum management
- ☐ Compression socks
- ☐ Sequential compression devices
- ☐ Bubble/particle filters
- ☐ Avoid volume loading. 0.5 mL/kg/hour maintenance fluids if NPO >6 hours. IVF boluses not to exceed 250 mL except if resuscitating for significant blood loss
- ☐ Strict I/Os

Infective endocarditis prophylaxis
- ☐ None indicated
- ☐ Ampicillin 2 g IV OR cefazolin or ceftriaxone 1 g IV, 30–60 minutes prior to anticipated delivery
- ☐ PCN allergy, use alternative: clindamycin 600 mg IV, 30–60 minutes prior to anticipated delivery

Delivery management
- ☐ No cardiac indication for cesarean delivery, but this is acceptable if indicated for obstetric reasons
- ☐ May push during second stage of labor
- ☐ Minimize pushing during second stage of labor
- ☐ Cesarean delivery planned for obstetric reasons
- ☐ Cesarean delivery recommended for cardiac reasons

Recovery/postpartum
- ☐ Routine postpartum recovery and nursing care
- ☐ Transfer to CCU for monitoring postpartum
- ☐ Echocardiogram postpartum, prior to discharge. Please order "congenital transthoracic echo" and specify in comments "ACHD attending to read"
- ☐ BNP postpartum

Discharge planning
- ☐ ACHD team will provide recommendations for f/u testing and visit prior to discharge
- ☐ Contraception management

---

higher frequency of 27.8%. Maternal cyanosis, subaortic ventricular outflow tract obstruction, and low cardiac output are known predictors of adverse perinatal events [24,25].

Due to the increased incidence of CHD in the offspring of patients with CHD, a comprehensive fetal echocardiogram should be performed between 18 and 23 weeks' gestation to evaluate the fetus for congenital heart defects if either biological parent has CHD.

A delivery plan (Table 10.5) should be outlined for patients who are at moderate or high risk for maternal cardiac complications and should be readily accessible to all staff caring for the patient.

Maintenance IV fluids are often administered to patients who are NPO for an extended period of time but should be used judiciously in patients susceptible to heart failure, particularly those requiring diuretics at baseline or during pregnancy. However, fluid resuscitation in the event of extensive blood loss is acceptable and should be administered when clinically necessary.

Medications for cervical ripening are generally considered safe. Use of tocolytic agents is generally safe, except terbutaline, which should be used with caution in patients with a history of arrhythmia. Nitrates should be used in caution in patients with severe obstructive lesions (e.g., aortic stenosis). Hypermagnesemia may result in hypotension and bradycardia and should be used with caution in patients with severe obstructive lesions or at risk for bradyarrhythmias.

Endocarditis prophylaxis is controversial given the scarcity of data to guide recommendations. Current recommendations from the American College of Obstetricians and Gynecologists [26] mirror that of the American Heart Association and American College of Cardiology guidelines [27]. In both documents, antibiotic prophylaxis for vaginal deliveries is recommended only for those at highest risk for endocarditis: those with prosthetic valves or prosthetic material used in valve repair, those with previous infective endocarditis, those with unrepaired cyanotic CHD, those who underwent transcatheter or surgical intervention involving prosthetic material in the first 6 months after the intervention, and those with repaired congenital heart defects with residual shunt at the prosthetic device. However, this does not preclude consideration or usage of antibiotic prophylaxis for other patients who are at risk for endocarditis compared with the general population (e.g., bicuspid aortic valves, restrictive ventricular septal defects). Patients and providers should engage in shared decision about use of antibiotics, given the significant morbidity associated with endocarditis.

Vaginal delivery is preferred for the majority of patients with CHD, with a few exceptions. For patients at high risk for aortic dissection, such as those with bicuspid aortic valve and a significantly dilated ascending aorta, or Marfan syndrome with a dilated aorta, pain control with neuraxial anesthesia, a passive second stage of labor, or cesarean delivery are reasonable to minimize the aortic stress associated with labor and delivery.

Postpartum, "autotransfusion" of blood from the uterus may trigger heart failure in patients susceptible to volume overload. In patients at high risk for heart failure or arrhythmias, management on the cardiac ward or intensive care unit for the first 24–48 hours after delivery should be considered.

Conclusion

As a majority of patients born with CHD will reach adulthood, management of the pregnant patient with CHD will be increasingly important for the obstetrician, cardiologist, and anesthesiologist. An understanding of the congenital heart defect, the sequelae, and residua helps with maternal risk stratification and management. A multidisciplinary approach with a maternal-fetal medicine specialist and a congenital cardiac team is strongly recommended, particularly for the patient with complex CHD.

REFERENCES

1. Perloff JK. Adults with surgically treated congenital heart disease. Sequelae and residua. *JAMA*. 1983;250(15):2033–6.
2. Stout KK et al. 2018 AHA/ACC Guideline for the Management of Adults with Congenital Heart Disease: Executive Summary: A Report of the American College of Cardiology/American Heart Association Task Force on Clinical Practice Guidelines. *J Am Coll Cardiol*. 2019;73(12):1494–563.
3. Campbell M. Natural history of atrial septal defect. *Br Heart J*. 1970;32(6):820–6.
4. Van Praagh S, Carrera ME, Sanders SP, Mayer JE, Van Praagh R. Sinus venosus defects: Unroofing of the right pulmonary veins—Anatomic and echocardiographic findings and surgical treatment. *Am Heart J*. 1994;128(2):365–79.
5. Kirklin JK, Barratt-Boyes B. *Cardiac Surgery*. New York: Wiley; 1986, pp. 463–97.
6. Otto CM. *Textbook of Clinical Echocardiography*, 6 ed. Philadelphia: Elsevier; 2019, ch. 1.
7. Mitchell SC, Korones SB, Berendes HW. Congenital heart disease in 56,109 births. Incidence and natural history. *Circulation*. 1971;43(3):323–32.
8. Hoffman JI. Congenital heart disease: Incidence and inheritance. *Pediatr Clin North Am*. 1990;37(1):25–43.
9. Brauner R, Laks H, Drinkwater DC, Jr., Shvarts O, Eghbali K, Galindo A. Benefits of early surgical repair in fixed subaortic stenosis. *J Am Coll Cardiol*. 1997;30(7):1835–42.
10. Serraf A et al. Surgical treatment of subaortic stenosis: A seventeen-year experience. *J Thorac Cardiovasc Surg*. 1999;117(4):669–78.
11. van Son JA, Schaff HV, Danielson GK, Hagler DJ, Puga FJ. Surgical treatment of discrete and tunnel subaortic stenosis. Late survival and risk of reoperation. *Circulation*. 1993;88(5 Pt 2):II159–69.
12. Geva A, McMahon CJ, Gauvreau K, Mohammed L, del Nido PJ, Geva T. Risk factors for reoperation after repair of discrete subaortic stenosis in children. *J Am Coll Cardiol*. 2007;50(15):1498–504.
13. Walters HL 3rd, Mavroudis C, Tchervenkov CI, Jacobs JP, Lacour-Gayet F, Jacobs ML. Congenital Heart Surgery Nomenclature and Database Project: Double outlet right ventricle. *Ann Thorac Surg*. 2000;69(4 Suppl):S249–63.
14. Sondheimer HM, Freedom RM, Olley PM. Double outlet right ventricle: Clinical spectrum and prognosis. *Am J Cardiol*. 1977;39(5):709–14.
15. Van Praagh R, Van Praagh S. The anatomy of common aorticopulmonary trunk (truncus arteriosus communis) and its embryologic implications. A study of 57 necropsy cases. *Am J Cardiol*. 1965;16(3):406–25.
16. Hoffman JI, Kaplan S. The incidence of congenital heart disease. *J Am Coll Card*. 2002;39(12):1890–900.
17. McGoon DC, Rastelli GC, Ongley PA. An operation for the correction of truncus arteriosus. *JAMA*. 1968;205(2):69–73.
18. Senning A. Surgical correction of transposition of the great vessels. *Surgery*. 1959;45(6):966–80.
19. Mustard WT. Successful two-stage correction of transposition of the great vessels. *Surgery*. 1964;55:469–72.
20. Jatene AD et al. Anatomic correction of transposition of the great vessels. *J Thorac Cardiovasc Surg*. 1976;72(3):364–70.
21. Wood P. The Eisenmenger syndrome or pulmonary hypertension with reversed central shunt. *Br Med J*. 1958;2(5099):755–62.
22. Diller GP, Gatzoulis MA. Pulmonary vascular disease in adults with congenital heart disease. *Circulation*. 2007;115(8):1039–50.
23. Oyen N, Poulsen G, Boyd HA, Wohlfahrt J, Jensen PK, Melbye M. Recurrence of congenital heart defects in families. *Circulation*. 2009;120(4):295–301.
24. Drenthen W et al. Outcome of pregnancy in women with congenital heart disease: A literature review. *J Am Coll Cardiol*. 2007;49(24):2303–11.
25. Khairy P, Ouyang DW, Fernandes SM, Lee-Parritz A, Economy KE, Landzberg MJ. Pregnancy outcomes in women with congenital heart disease. *Circulation*. 2006;113(4):517–24.
26. American College of Obstetricians and Gynecologists et al. ACOG Practice Bulletin No. 120: Use of prophylactic antibiotics in labor and delivery. *Obstet Gynecol*. 2011; 117(6):1472–83.
27. Nishimura RA et al. 2017 AHA/ACC Focused Update of the 2014 AHA/ACC Guideline for the Management of Patients With Valvular Heart Disease: A Report of the American College of Cardiology/American Heart Association Task Force on Clinical Practice Guidelines. *J Am Coll Cardiol*. 2017;70(2):252–89.

11

Valve Disease in Pregnancy

Tanush Gupta, Thomas Boucher, and Anna E. Bortnick

KEY POINTS

- Many patients with significant VHD are not aware of their diagnosis until pregnancy when hemodynamic stress precipitates symptoms
- Stenotic valvular lesions pose a higher risk of maternal and fetal adverse events than regurgitant lesions
- Women with severe, symptomatic aortic stenosis (AS) should be counseled against pregnancy until the lesion is surgically corrected and if pregnant, consider their options including termination of pregnancy

- Manipulating the intensity and duration of anesthesia improves hemodynamic changes on valvular heart disease during labor and delivery
- Hemodynamic changes peak within 24–72 hours after delivery, a vulnerable period when women with valvular heart disease are most likely to manifest symptomatic heart failure

Introduction

Cardiovascular disease complicates ~1%–3% of all pregnancies and is a leading cause of maternal mortality [1–3]. With advances in cardiovascular medical and surgical care over the last few decades, more women with congenital or acquired heart disease are reaching reproductive age [4,5], with a wide spectrum of congenital and acquired valvular heart disease (VHD) seen in pregnant women (Figure 11.1) [6]. Although VHD due to rheumatic heart disease (RHD) has declined in industrialized countries, it continues to be a major cause of global maternal cardiovascular morbidity and mortality [4,6–10]. Despite the improvements in diagnosis and management, VHD remains associated with adverse maternal and fetal events [11,12]. Many patients with significant VHD are not aware of their diagnosis until pregnancy, when hemodynamic stress precipitates symptoms [12].

Hemodynamic Effects of Valvular Heart Disease in Pregnancy

Hemodynamic changes of pregnancy can lead to clinical decompensation of women with VHD due to increases in cardiac output (CO), intravascular volume expansion, and a drop in systemic vascular resistance (SVR) [2,13,14]. Early in pregnancy, there is a 30%–50% increase in CO largely attributable to rises in circulating blood volume and heart rate [14,15]. During the later stages of pregnancy, increases in heart rate contribute more to increased CO. Pregnancy is also accompanied by physiologic anemia with a greater increase in plasma volume than red blood cell volume, resulting in increased flow and increased gradients across preexisting valvular lesions

[16]. In addition, SVR decreases toward the end of the second trimester as placental circulation matures and then slowly rises until term [17]. The gravid uterus may compress the inferior vena cava in the second trimester, decreasing preload to the heart, and increasing afterload by compressing the abdominal aorta. These changes, in turn, modulate CO so that it plateaus between the second and third trimesters [2,12,18].

Clinical Implications: Pregnancy leads to a series of hemostatic changes leading to hypercoagulability and risk of thromboembolism, which is of particular concern in patients with known VHD or prosthetic heart valves (PHVs). Uterine obstruction to vena cava flow may also predispose to increased risk of deep venous thrombosis [19]. Importantly, the pharmacokinetics of cardiac drugs may be altered during pregnancy, necessitating more frequent monitoring and/or dose adjustment in women [20].

During labor and delivery (L&D), maternal hemodynamics are influenced by an array of factors including pain, anxiety, mode of delivery, analgesia, blood loss, and uterine contractions [21]. Abrupt changes can have a significant effect on pregnant women with VHD. CO increases by ~30% in the first stage of labor and by ~80% early postpartum [22]. There are catecholamine-induced increases in stroke volume and heart rate, which in turn increase CO. Each uterine contraction is accompanied by autotransfusion of up to 500 mL of blood from the placental to systemic circulation [23,24]. Systemic blood pressure can increase by ~15–20 mmHg with each contraction. The use of epidural and spinal analgesia can attenuate some of these hemodynamic alterations associated with L&D [25]. Manipulating the intensity and duration of anesthesia for optimal vasodilation, decreasing anxiety/stress to reduce maternal heart rate and afterload, controlled permissive blood loss, and postpartum diuresis are ways to counteract the effects of hemodynamic changes on VHD at the time of L&D.

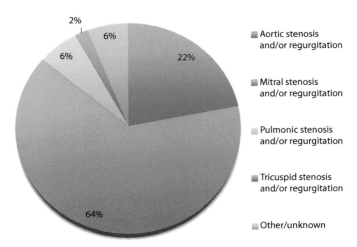

FIGURE 11.1 Frequency of valvular heart disease in pregnancy. (Compiled from references [3,18].)

Cardiac hemodynamics change rapidly in the early postpartum period. Delivery is accompanied by loss of intravascular volume, which can be up to 500 mL with vaginal delivery and up to 1000 mL with cesarean delivery [24]. The relief of caval obstruction by the gravid uterus results in redistribution of blood from the lower limbs and an increase in preload and circulating volume [21]. Also, there is an overall increase in afterload due to loss of the low-resistance placental circulation and mobilization of interstitial fluid. Hemodynamic changes peak within 24–72 hours after delivery, a vulnerable period when women with VHD are most likely to manifest symptomatic heart failure (HF) [10,12].

Stenotic versus Regurgitant Valvular Heart Disease in Pregnancy

In general, stenotic valvular lesions pose a higher risk of maternal and fetal adverse events than regurgitant lesions [26]. With stenotic lesions, the increase in CO associated with pregnancy and labor results in increased transvalvular flows and gradients. Increases in heart rate are poorly tolerated in pregnant women with stenotic valvular lesions such as mitral stenosis (MS), where left ventricular filling is heavily dependent on the duration of the diastolic filling period. The combined effect of increased transvalvular flow and shortened diastolic filling time can result in symptomatic HF, pulmonary edema, and arrhythmias such as atrial fibrillation [27].

Transthoracic echocardiography (TTE) is essential for diagnosis and evaluation of stenotic VHD [28–31]. Tachycardia and increased CO in pregnancy increase transvalvular gradients on TTE but do not affect the calculated valve area by the continuity equation. Direct planimetry is a flow-independent measure of valve area and is likely more accurate than flow-dependent measures such as pressure half time. Despite this, the mean gradient across a valve is likely the best reflection of the hemodynamic significance of valvular stenosis at that particular point in time [27,32].

Left-sided chronic regurgitant lesions (mitral regurgitation [MR] and aortic regurgitation [AR]) are typically well tolerated during pregnancy, as the low-resistance placental circulation decreases SVR, and in turn decreases regurgitant volume [32,33]. However, severe regurgitant lesions in the context of impaired left or right ventricular systolic function or acute valvular regurgitation can result in HF [10]. Table 11.1 provides details on the commonly encountered valvular lesions in pregnant women, their etiology, risk to mother and fetus, management, and preferred mode of delivery.

In general, evaluation of VHD should be performed prior to pregnancy and significant symptomatic VHD should be corrected beforehand, particularly if surgery is required, as bypass increases maternal and fetal risk [34,35]. Treating VHD in the setting of symptomatic HF, arrhythmias, or hemodynamic deterioration is necessary to prevent maternal and fetal adverse events (Table 11.2) [12].

Specific Valvular Heart Disease Lesions

Mitral Stenosis

MS is the most common acquired VHD in pregnant women [2,36]. MS is considered clinically important if the valve area is ≤1.5 cm² (Table 11.3) [18]. The gold standard method of estimating MS severity on TTE is direct planimetry; however, this method can be technically challenging and is dependent on optimal image quality. Doppler-derived pressure half time depends on heart rate, with lower gradients observed at slower heart rates. Estimations of transvalvular mean gradients and pulmonary artery pressures on Doppler echocardiography are informative regarding the hemodynamic effects of MS. The assessment of mitral valve anatomy, specifically, leaflet calcification, thickening, subvalvular apparatus, and concomitant MR, elements captured by the Wilkins score, is important prior to consideration for percutaneous mitral commissurotomy (valvuloplasty) [28,37,38]. For asymptomatic women prior to pregnancy, exercise TTE may be useful in assessing exertional tolerance, changes in Doppler-derived gradients, and prognosis [18]. During pregnancy, clinical and echocardiographic follow-up is recommended monthly or bimonthly with moderate or severe MS [18].

Mild MS is usually well tolerated during pregnancy [32]. HF occurs in up to 1/3 of pregnant women with moderate MS and up to 1/2 with severe MS, even in previously asymptomatic patients, and most often during the second or third trimesters [39]. Sustained AF occurs in up to 10% of pregnant women with moderate/severe MS and can predispose to symptomatic HF and thromboembolism [40]. Maternal mortality from MS is reported to vary from 0%–3% in the West but may be higher in other parts of the world [8,32,39–41]. Fetal morbidity includes intrauterine growth restriction and premature birth, and is directly proportional to the severity of MS, ranging from ~14% in mild MS to ~35% in severe MS. Fetal death has been reported in 1%–5% with significant MS [32,39,40].

Management:

1. Exertion should be restricted in patients with symptomatic MS [2].
2. Beta-1 selective blockers are first-line drugs in management of MS during pregnancy.
3. Diuretics are often used to avoid volume overload.
4. Digoxin may be utilized in those with HF and concomitant AF not rate-controlled with beta-blockers.

TABLE 11.1

Risk Stratification and Management of Specific Valvular Lesions during Pregnancy

Lesion	Most Common Etiology	Risk to Mother	Risk to Fetus	Possible Intervention	Preferred Mode of Delivery
Mitral stenosis	Rheumatic	• Mild MS (area >1.5 cm²)/asymptomatic: low risk • Moderate-to-severe MS (area <1.5 cm², in AF): may develop heart failure; mortality up to 3%	Prematurity 20%–30%, intrauterine growth retardation 5%–20%, still birth 1%–3%. Offspring risk higher in women in NYHA class III/IV	• Nonpregnant: moderate–severe MS should be counseled before pregnancy and may need intervention • In pregnancy: beta-blockers and diuretics; in AF: digoxin • Percutaneous mitral commissurotomy in NYHA III/IV or PAP >50 mmHg on medical therapy	Vaginal delivery in mild MS Cesarean in moderate–severe MS in NYHA III/IV or having severe PH on medical therapy
Aortic stenosis	Congenital bicuspid	• Severe AS and asymptomatic on exercise test: low risk • Severe AS with symptoms or drop in BP on exercise test: heart failure in 10% and arrhythmias in 3%–25%	Fetal complications increased in moderate and severe AS. Preterm birth, intrauterine growth retardation, low birth weight in up to 25%	• Nonpregnant: symptomatic severe AS or asymptomatic AS with LV dysfunction or aortic dilatation >45 mm should be counseled against pregnancy or have an intervention first • In pregnancy: restrict activities and in AF, beta-blocker or a non-dihydropyridine calcium channel blocker for rate control • Percutaneous valvuloplasty in severely symptomatic patient despite bedrest and medical therapy	Non-severe AS: vaginal delivery; in selected cases of severe AS, cesarean delivery can be considered
Mitral regurgitation	Rheumatic, congenital	• Moderate-to-severe MR with good LV function: low risk with good care • Severe MR with LV dysfunction: high risk of heart failure or arrhythmia	No increased risk of fetal complications has been reported	• Nonpregnant: patients with severe regurgitation and symptoms or impaired LV function or dilatation should be referred for pre-pregnancy surgery. • Pregnant: symptoms of fluid overload can be managed with diuretics. Surgery in women with intractable HF	Vaginal delivery is preferable Epidural anesthesia and shortened second stage is advisable
Aortic regurgitation	Rheumatic, congenital, degenerative	• Moderate-to-severe AR with good LV function: low risk with good care • Severe AR with LV dysfunction: high risk of heart failure or arrhythmia	No increased risk of fetal complications has been reported	• Nonpregnant: patients with severe regurgitation and symptoms or impaired LV function or severe dilatation should be referred for pre-pregnancy surgery • Pregnant: symptoms of fluid overload can be managed with diuretics and bedrest. Surgery in women with intractable HF, preferably after delivery	Vaginal delivery is preferable Epidural anesthesia and shortened second stage is advisable
Tricuspid regurgitation	Functional, Ebstein's anomaly, endocarditis	• Moderate-to-severe TR with good RV function: arrhythmias • Moderate-to-severe TR with impaired RV function: heart failure	No increased risk of fetal complications has been reported	• Nonpregnant: patients with severe regurgitation and symptoms or impaired LV and/or RV function or dilatation should be referred for pre-pregnancy TV repair • Pregnant: severe TR can usually be managed medically with diuretics	Vaginal delivery is preferable

Source: Reproduced with permission from Sliwa K et al. *Eur Heart J.* May 7 2015;36(18):1078–89.

Abbreviations: AF, atrial fibrillation; AR, aortic regurgitation; AS, aortic stenosis; BP, blood pressure; LV, left ventricular; MR, mitral regurgitation; MS, mitral stenosis; NYHA, New York Heart Association; RV, right ventricular; TR, tricuspid regurgitation; TV, tricuspid valve; PAP, pulmonary arterial pressure; PH, pulmonary hypertension.

TABLE 11.2

Pharmacologic Management of Symptomatic Valvular Heart Disease during Pregnancy

Drug/Class	Purpose	Comment
Diuretics		
Furosemide	• Avoidance or treatment of volume overload or pulmonary edema • Use of lowest possible dose	• Can result in uteroplacental hypoperfusion • Contraindicated in settings in which uteroplacental hypoperfusion is already reduced (IUGR, preeclampsia)
Antiarrhythmics		
Carvedilol, Labetalol, Metoprolol, Propranolol	• Essential in chronic heart failure • Agents that are beta-1 selective are preferable	• Generally safe and effective in pregnancy • Can cause IUGR • Infants born to mothers on beta-blockers should be observed for at least 72 hours after birth
Digoxin	• Not considered first-line therapy for heart failure in nonpregnant patients • No improvement in mortality • Considered useful in pregnancy given toxicities of other antiarrhythmics	• Generally considered safe • Useful in treatment of persistent symptoms despite beta-blockers
Vasodilators		
Hydralazine	• Commonly used oral antihypertensive agent in pregnancy • Common substitute for ACE inhibitor during pregnancy	• Demonstrated efficacy in hypertension • Risk of hypotension • Pregnancy already reduces SVR • Avoid large or precipitous decreases in blood pressure
ACE inhibitors/ARBs	• Proven benefit in treatment of chronic heart failure in nonpregnant patients	• Contraindicated throughout pregnancy due to teratogenic effects. Associated with oligohydramnios, neonatal death secondary to renal failure, renal agenesis
Amlodipine	• Alternative to ACE inhibitor in pregnancy	• Can be used with hydralazine if needed
Nitrates	• May be used to treat decompensated heart failure	
Aldosterone Antagonists		
Spironolactone, Eplerenone	• Prolongs survival in selected heart failure patients • Not routinely used in pregnancy	• Limited data to support safety in pregnancy

Source: Modified with permission from Stergiopoulos K et al. *J Am Coll Cardiol.* Jul 19 2011;58(4):337–50.
Abbreviations: ACE inhibitor, angiotensin converting enzyme inhibitor; ARB, angiotensin receptor blocker; IUGR, intrauterine growth retardation; SVR, systemic vascular resistance.

TABLE 11.3

Grading Mitral Stenosis (MS) Severity by Transthoracic Echocardiogram

Severity	Mitral Valve Area (cm²)	Diastolic Pressure Half-Time (ms)	Mean Pressure Gradient (mmHg)	Pulmonary Artery Systolic Pressure (mmHg)
Mild	>1.5	<150	<5	<30
Moderate	1.0–1.5	≥150	5–10	>30
Severe	≤1.5, ≤1.0 for very severe	≥150, ≥220 for very severe	>10	>30

Source: Adapted from Nishimura RA et al. *J Am Coll Cardiol.* Jun 10 2014;63(22):2438–88; Zoghbi WA et al. *J Am Soc Echocardiogr.* Apr 2017;30(4):303–71; Baumgartner H et al. *J Am Soc Echocardiogr.* Jan 2009;22(1):1–23. quiz 101–102.
Note: The revised AHA/ACC grading system adds the category of "at risk for MS" and "progressive MS" to describe mild disease, and divides severe MS into Asymptomatic, severe MS, and severe, symptomatic MS.

5. Anticoagulation is recommended for paroxysmal or permanent AF, left atrial thrombus, or history of prior thromboembolism [2,18].

Women with moderate or severe MS should be counseled against pregnancy until the lesion is treated, and intervention should be performed prior to pregnancy, with preference given to percutaneous valvuloplasty if the valve is anatomically favorable for the procedure, and termination may be recommended if currently pregnant [32,37]. During pregnancy, percutaneous mitral valvuloplasty should be considered in women with New York Heart Association (NYHA) class III/IV HF or with estimated

TABLE 11.4

Grading Aortic Stenosis (AS) Severity by Transthoracic Echocardiogram

Severity	Aortic Valve Area (cm²)	Mean Pressure Gradient (mmHg)	Aortic Jet Velocity (m/s)	Indexed AVA (cm²/m²)
Mild	>1.5	<20	2.0–2.9	>0.85
Moderate	1.0–1.5	20–39	3.0–3.9	0.6–0.85
Severe	≤1.0	≥40	≥4.0	≤0.6

Source: Adapted from Nishimura RA et al. *J Am Coll Cardiol.* Jun 10 2014;63(22):2438–88; Zoghbi WA et al. *J Am Soc Echocardiogr.* Apr 2017;30(4):303–71; Baumgartner H et al. *J Am Soc Echocardiogr.* Jan 2009;22(1):1–23. quiz 101–102.

Note: The revised AHA/ACC grading system uses categories of "at risk of AS" and "progressive AS" to describe mild and moderate disease, and divides the category of "severe" into asymptomatic, severe AS, and severe, symptomatic AS.

pulmonary artery systolic pressures of ≥50 mmHg and preferably delayed until after the 20th week of gestation [18,37]. Surgical mitral valve replacement should be considered only in pregnant women with medically refractory symptoms when percutaneous valvuloplasty fails or is not an option, as open heart surgery is highly morbid for both mother and fetus [42].

Vaginal delivery is often preferred in patients with mild MS and in those with moderate or severe MS in the presence of NYHA class I/II symptoms without significant pulmonary hypertension (PH). Cesarean section is often considered for women with NYHA class III/IV symptoms, severe PH, or in whom percutaneous mitral valvuloplasty has failed or is not possible [18].

Aortic Stenosis

The leading causes of aortic stenosis (AS) in pregnant women are bicuspid aortic valve disease, often associated with dilation of the ascending aorta, followed by RHD [43]. Most with mild or moderate AS can tolerate pregnancy (Table 11.4) [44]. HF is infrequent, with an estimated prevalence of <10% in women with moderate AS who were asymptomatic pre-pregnancy. Even in patients with severe AS, maternal mortality is reported to be <1% in presence of close follow-up and treatment [32,33,45,46]. Maternal and fetal adverse events are directly proportional to the severity of AS. Approximately one-third of women with severe AS require hospitalization during pregnancy. Fetal adverse events including growth restriction, low birth weight, and preterm birth have been reported in 20%–25% of babies of mothers with moderate or severe AS [44,46]. TTE is the gold standard for grading severity of AS (Table 11.4) [28,37,38]. Exercise TTE testing can be considered for women with asymptomatic, severe AS prior to pregnancy. Favorable maternal and fetal outcomes were reported for those who remained asymptomatic on exercise testing even in the presence of severe AS. However, surgery should be considered pre-pregnancy for exercise-induced symptoms (like shortness of breath, chest pain, dizziness), drop in blood pressure, or left ventricular dysfunction [18]. In bicuspid aortic valve disease, ascending aortic diameters should be assessed before, during, and after pregnancy to rule out worsened dilation. In pregnant women with severe AS, monthly or bimonthly clinical and echocardiographic follow-up is recommended [18].

Women with severe, symptomatic AS should be counseled against pregnancy until the lesion is surgically corrected and if pregnant, consider termination [28,37]. The American Heart Association/American College of Cardiology (AHA/ACC)

guidelines have further subdivided stages of valvular AS [28]. Included in these stages are asymptomatic, severe or symptomatic, and severe AS with left ventricular dysfunction. Symptoms can be self-reported or elicited during exercise stress test if asymptomatic. Pregnancy was well tolerated in severe AS patients who had a normal prior exercise test, while abnormal results were predictive of adverse pregnancy outcomes [47,48]. All symptomatic and asymptomatic AS patients with impaired left ventricular function should be counseled against pregnancy without pre-pregnancy intervention to the lesion, and termination may be recommended [18,28].

Management:

1. Pregnant women with severe AS should limit exertion.
2. HF should be treated with diuresis and afterload reduction; however, dehydration and nitrates should be avoided due to preload dependence.
3. In patients with medically refractory symptoms during pregnancy, balloon aortic valvuloplasty can be considered [18,49].
4. Surgical aortic valve replacement can be considered in severely symptomatic patients not responding to medical therapy and who are not candidates for valvuloplasty, with careful consideration of maternal and fetal morbidity.
5. Transcatheter aortic valve replacement may be an option in pregnant women but the clinical experience with this approach is extremely limited [18].
6. Women proceeding with pregnancy in the context of severe, symptomatic AS typically undergo cesarean delivery, whereas those with asymptomatic severe AS or mild/moderate AS typically undergo vaginal delivery [5].

Mitral and Aortic Regurgitation

The most common cause of MR in pregnant women in developed countries is mitral valve prolapse, followed by RHD [50]. The causes of aortic regurgitation (AR) include bicuspid aortic valve disease, aortopathies leading to ascending aorta and aortic annular dilatation (i.e., Marfan's), infective endocarditis, and RHD [2,39,51]. Evaluation for MR or AR should be performed prior to pregnancy (Tables 11.5 and 11.6). Exercise testing in those without symptoms but with severe valvular regurgitation is

TABLE 11.5

Grading Mitral Valve Regurgitation (MR) Severity by Transthoracic Echocardiography

Severity	Effective Regurgitant Orifice (cm²)	Regurgitant Volume (ml)	Regurgitant Fraction (%)	Jet Width (% of LA)	Vena Contracta[a] (cm)
Mild	<0.20	<30	NA	<20	<0.3
Moderate	<0.40	<60	<50	20–40	<0.7
Severe	≥0.40	≥60	≥50	>40	≥0.7

Source: Adapted from Nishimura RA et al. *J Am Coll Cardiol.* Jun 10 2014;63(22):2438–88; Zoghbi WA et al. *J Am Soc Echocardiogr.* Apr 2017;30(4):303–71; Baumgartner H et al. *J Am Soc Echocardiogr.* Jan 2009;22(1):1–23. quiz 101–102; Lancellotti P et al. *Eur Heart J Cardiovasc Imaging.* Jul 2013;14(7):611–44.

Note: The revised AHA/ACC grading system uses categories of "at risk" and "progressive MR" to describe mild and moderate disease, and divides the category of "severe" into asymptomatic, severe MR, and symptomatic, severe MR. It also divides criteria according to primary MR (due to intrinsic valvular disease) and secondary MR.

Abbreviations: LA, left atrium; NA, not available.

[a] Vena contracta is the narrowest area of the jet.

TABLE 11.6

Grading Aortic Valve Regurgitation (AR) Severity by Transthoracic Echocardiography

Severity	Effective Regurgitant Orifice (cm²)	Regurgitant Volume (ml/beat)	Regurgitant Fraction (%)	Jet Width (% of LV Outflow Tract)	Vena Contracta (cm)
Mild	<0.10	<30	<30	<25	<0.3
Moderate	0.10–0.29	30–59	30–49	25–64	0.3–0.6
Severe[a]	≥3.0	≥60	≥50	≥65	>0.6

Source: Adapted from Nishimura RA et al. J Am Coll Cardiol. Jun 10 2014;63(22):2438–88; Zoghbi WA et al. *J Am Soc Echocardiogr.* Apr 2017;30(4):303–71; Baumgartner H et al. *J Am Soc Echocardiogr.* Jan 2009;22(1):1–23. quiz 101–102; Lancellotti P et al. *Eur Heart J Cardiovasc Imaging.* Jul 2013;14(7):611–44.

Note: The revised AHA/ACC grading system adds the category of "at risk for AR," "progressive AR" to describe mild/moderate disease, and divides severe AR into the categories of asymptomatic, severe AR, and severe, symptomatic AR.

[a] Severe also requires evidence of LV dilation.

prognostic [33,37]. Women with severe symptomatic regurgitation or associated left ventricular dysfunction were reported to have HF rates of 20%–25% during pregnancy [33,39]. Despite this, the reported rate of fetal adverse events is low [39]. Pregnant women with mild to moderate MR/AR are recommended to get follow-up every trimester with more frequent follow-up for severe regurgitant lesions based on symptoms [18].

Women with severe MR or AR with symptoms or left ventricular compromise should ideally undergo surgery prior to pregnancy, with repair preferred over replacement for MR if the repair is expected to be durable [28,37]. Surgical treatment of severe left-sided regurgitation is rarely indicated during pregnancy [52]. If surgery is necessary, delivery should be attempted before cardiac surgery. Shared decision making for surgery in severe MR and AR should be informed by current guidelines [28,37,53].

In pregnant women with MR, exertional restriction, diuretics, beta-blockers, and vasodilators are recommended (Table 11.2) [28]. In contrast, beta-blockers are considered unfavorable for AR as they can prolong diastole and increase regurgitation. Vaginal delivery with epidural anesthesia and a shortened second stage of labor is considered a preferred approach to MR and AR with diuresis and afterload reduction [18].

Tricuspid Regurgitation

Tricuspid regurgitation (TR) is commonly secondary to annular dilatation due to right ventricular (RV) pressure or volume overload related to left-sided heart disease [12]. Primary TR may be secondary to RHD, endocarditis, or Ebstein's anomaly, a congenital downward displacement of the tricuspid valve resulting in an enlarged right atrium and small right ventricle, associated with atrial septal defect, and predisposing to atrial arrhythmia and right-sided HF [18,54,55]. When surgical repair is performed for left-sided valve lesions prior to pregnancy, concomitant tricuspid repair is also indicated in those with severe TR (Table 11.7). Isolated severe TR without RV dysfunction is often well tolerated during pregnancy and repair is rare prior to pregnancy [18,28,37]. For women with severe, symptomatic TR, or already undergoing left-sided valve surgery having a tricuspid annulus ≥40 mm or evidence of prior right-sided HF, repair is recommended before pregnancy (with replacement an option) [18,28,37]. Those with Ebstein's anomaly and severe TR can develop interatrial right-to-left shunting, right-sided dilatation, and HF intrapartum, which may prompt correction prior to pregnancy [56]. Of the various manifestations of VHD, tricuspid stenosis is least common and not reviewed in this chapter.

TABLE 11.7

Limited Criteria for Grading Tricuspid Valve Regurgitation (TR) Severity by Transthoracic Echocardiography

Severity	Valve Morphology	RA/RV/IVC Size	Hepatic Vein Flow	EROA (cm²)
Mild	Normal, mildly abnormal leaflets	Normal	Normal systolic flow	<0.20
Moderate	Moderately abnormal leaflets	Mild dilation	Flow blunted in systole	
Severe	Severe abnormalities of valve	Dilated	Flow reversed in systole	≥0.40

Source: Adapted from Nishimura RA et al. *J Am Coll Cardiol.* Jun 10 2014;63(22):2438–88; Zoghbi WA et al. *J Am Soc Echocardiogr.* Apr 2017;30(4):303–71; Baumgartner H et al. *J Am Soc Echocardiogr.* Jan 2009;22(1):1–23. quiz 101–102; Lancellotti P et al. *Eur Heart J Cardiovasc Imaging.* Jul 2013;14(7):611–44.

Note: The revised AHA/ACC grading system adds the category of "at risk for TR" and "progressive TR" to describe mild/moderate disease, and divides severe TR into asymptomatic, severe TR, and severe, symptomatic TR.

Abbreviations: EROA, effective regurgitant orifice area; IVC, inferior vena cava; RA, right atrium; RV, right ventricle.

Pulmonic Stenosis and Regurgitation

Pulmonic stenosis (PS) is either congenital or results from homograft degeneration after a prior Ross procedure [12]. PS severity is often defined by TTE (Table 11.8), is generally well-tolerated during pregnancy, and pregnant women with mild or moderate PS are considered at low risk of adverse maternal and fetal events as compared to those with AS or MS [57,28,58,59]. Evaluation of PS should be performed pre-pregnancy with TTE. Those with severe, asymptomatic PS (peak pressure gradient >60 mmHg, mean pressure gradient >40 mmHg) or severe, symptomatic PS (peak pressure gradient >50 mmHg, mean pressure gradient >30 mmHg) should have balloon pulmonary valvuloplasty prior to attempting to become pregnant [28,37,58].

Severe PS is associated with adverse fetal outcomes, such as prematurity in ~20% and fetal mortality of up to 5% [55]. Pregnant women with severe PS should be managed with exertional restriction and diuresis to decrease RV volume. Balloon pulmonic valvuloplasty during pregnancy is typically for medically refractory symptoms [57,60]. Vaginal delivery is considered preferred in pregnant women with mild/moderate PS, severe asymptomatic PS, or in those with NYHA class I/II symptoms without severe PH. Cesarean delivery should be considered in pregnant women with severe PS and NYHA class III/IV symptoms in whom percutaneous valvuloplasty is not feasible or has failed [18].

TABLE 11.8

Grading Pulmonic Stenosis Severity

Severity	Pulmonic Jet Velocity (m/s)	Peak Pressure Gradient (mmHg)
Mild	<3	<36
Moderate	3–4	36–64
Severe	>4	>64

Source: Adapted from Nishimura RA et al. *J Am Coll Cardiol.* Jun 10 2014;63(22):2438–88; Zoghbi WA et al. *J Am Soc Echocardiogr.* Apr 2017;30(4):303–71; Baumgartner H et al. *J Am Soc Echocardiogr.* Jan 2009;22(1):1–23. quiz 101–102.

Note: The revised AHA/ACC grading system eliminates mild/moderate categories.

Severe PR can be a consequence of prior balloon valvuloplasty, a degenerated homograft, or previously repaired tetralogy of Fallot, and is an independent predictor of adverse maternal events [12]. In patients with severe, symptomatic PR and RV dilatation or HF, surgical replacement should be considered pre-pregnancy [54].

Risk Assessment

As discussed previously, pregnancy for women with VHD carries increased risk for adverse maternal and fetal events including HF, thromboembolism, and mortality [11,12,61–63]. The woman's risk for adverse events should be assessed as early as possible by a multidisciplinary team, ideally preconception (Figure 11.2). Representation from cardiology, obstetrics, anesthesia, and maternal-fetal medicine (MFM) is strongly recommended, and additional expertise from other disciplines, including cardiothoracic surgery or adult congenital heart disease, should be individualized to the patient [18,28,64–66]. Scoring tools can help to quantify pre-pregnancy risk of mortality and adverse events and may be useful in preconception discussions for patients with VHD. The CARPREG I model uses four variables: prior cardiac event or arrhythmia, NYHA functional class >II or cyanosis, left heart obstruction (mitral valve area <2 cm², aortic valve area <1.5 cm², or peak left ventricular outflow tract gradient <30 mmHg by TTE), and reduced LVEF <40% [4]. CARPREG II adds general, lesion-specific, and delivery-of-care variables to improve prediction [67]. ZAHARA, builds upon the CARPREG I to include moderate to severe PR or MR, cyanotic heart disease, the previous use of cardiac drugs, and the presence of mechanical valve prosthesis as predictors [55]. The WHO score was developed based on expert consensus and then modified (Modified WHO [mWHO]) [18]. Two multicenter cohort studies evaluated CARPREG I, ZAHARA, and mWHO models and found mWHO to be the most accurate in predicting maternal adverse events [3,26]. However, scoring systems are not an absolute method to ascertain risks for all patients [63].

The risk associated with each pregnancy is derived from the specific underlying cardiac diagnosis and comorbidities, making each patient distinctive. Because of the shortfalls of the current predictive models and the uniqueness of each patient's medical

1. Patient history and maternal risk assessment	2. Patient/doctor education	3. Pregnancy planning
VHD diagnosis: ☐ Specific disease: _____ ☐ Time and context of diagnosis ☐ Current medical treatment ☐ Most recent visit to cardiologist ☐ Current NYHA functional class ☐ Severity of disease according to AHA/ACC guidelines ☐ Recent disease progression? **Past medical history:** ☐ Past cardiac events (i.e., arrhythmia, heart failure, stroke/TIA) ☐ Obstetric history (gravidity and parity, vaginal/cesarean birth, complications, etc.) ☐ Comorbidities (hypertension, diabetes mellitus, history of smoking, etc.) ☐ Surgical history **Risk assessment:** ☐ Multidisciplinary assessment of maternal risk for morbidity and mortality based on past medical history, clinical evaluation, and current valve hemodynamics ☐ CARPREG I and II, ZAHARA, and mWHO models as tools to guide assessment ☐ Use of disease-specific diagnostic tools to assess severity	**Things for the patient to understand:** ☐ Long-term complications and prognosis living with her VHD ☐ Normal hemodynamics of the heart ☐ Effect of her lesion on hemodynamics ☐ Normal hemodynamic changes that occur during pregnancy ☐ How her VHD would affect hemodynamic changes during pregnancy ☐ The risk of maternal morbidity and mortality associated with her VHD ☐ The fetal risks associated with her VHD ☐ Recommendations according to guidelines on whether or not she is contraindicated for pregnancy ☐ Potential long-term effect of pregnancy on her VHD ☐ How her medications would change during pregnancy (see Table 11.2) ☐ The difficulty distinguishing between normal gestational symptoms with signs of progression of her VHD and therefore, the need for consistent follow-up with the pregnancy heart team **Things for the physicians to understand:** ☐ Woman's familial or cultural values ☐ Woman's life plan ☐ Woman's social determinants of health affecting her access to specialized care	**Patient decides to avoid risks of pregnancy:** ☐ Offer access to safe and appropriate contraception ☐ Offer information on the safe termination of undesired pregnancy ☐ Offer information about adoption or surrogate pregnancies **Patient decides to continue with pregnancy:** ☐ Consultation with cardiology, maternal-fetal medicine, and anesthesiology as pregnancy heart team ☐ Determine whether the patient needs preconception intervention based on guidelines ☐ Perform preconception counseling with pregnancy heart team ☐ Adjust medications to avoid teratogenicity ☐ Arrange schedule of follow-up visits with pregnancy heart team ☐ Determine location of care based on specialization needed ☐ Determine location and mode of delivery (see Table 11.1) and need for telemetry or intensive care

FIGURE 11.2 Multidisciplinary care of women with VHD contemplating pregnancy. ACC, American College of Cardiology; AHA, American Heart Association; VHD, valvular heart disease; NYHA, New York Heart Association, CARPREG, Cardiac Disease in Pregnancy score; TIA, transient ischemic attack; ZAHARA, Zwangerschap bij vrouwen met een Aangeboren HARtAfwijking score; mWHO, modified World Health Organization score. (Compiled from references [4,18,28,53,55,64,75].)

history and diagnosis, the estimation of the risk for adverse events should be individualized. A multidisciplinary team of experienced physicians should ascertain the risk using the medical history, general cardiac assessments, and diagnostic tools specific to the lesion. Based on the timing of the diagnosis and the patient's specific lesion, the team will need to tailor the care to best serve the patient's needs and health. For example, for preconception patients with asymptomatic AS or MS, an exercise stress test can be used to better determine symptomatic classification, and thus individual pregnancy risk [18,28].

While there is no all-encompassing predictive model, the care team can use different tools to guide them in determining the level of risk associated with each pregnancy, like NYHA and AHA classes of HF. The NYHA and AHA designate functional classes defined by the severity of heart failure and the presence of symptoms. Moving from NYHA class I–IV and AHA A–C, the symptoms increase in severity and impairment of daily activities. Risk scores and the patient's functional class can be useful in ascertaining and communicating the patient's risk of adverse events during pregnancy and symptomatic progression over time [68,69].

Bioprosthetic versus Mechanical Valves

For patients who must undergo valve replacement prior to pregnancy, preconception counseling may include discussion of bioprosthetic vs. mechanical valves. While mechanical valves are highly durable, they also require consistent therapeutic anticoagulation and pose a higher risk of major cardiac events during pregnancy than bioprosthetic valves [18,70–72]. In contrast, bioprosthetic use at a younger age risks structural valve deterioration during the reproductive years of life. Dysfunctional bioprosthetic valves have comparable risks during pregnancy as native diseased valves [18]. For these reasons, women with VHD should make final decisions after careful consideration of the risks, benefits, and alternatives associated with all of their options and in consultation with the pregnancy heart team.

Preconception Counseling for Women with VHD

Guidelines pertaining to women with VHD support preconception counseling with the goal of forming a detailed reproductive plan based on the desires of the patient and advice from the specialists [18,28]. If possible, this should be a longitudinal conversation beginning early in her reproductive years. For patients with congenital heart disease, it has been shown that by starting conversations in adolescence, girls have a significantly better understanding of their disease, their need for lifelong monitoring, and that they should have their condition evaluated before becoming pregnant [73]. Preconception counseling should include a review of contraception compatible with individual comorbidities, based on individual preferences, efficacy, the risk/benefit of each method, and cost [74]. A patient-centered approach to preconception counseling should include education about the specific VHD, anticipated effect of hemodynamic changes in the setting of VHD, risks associated with the lesion, concerning signs and symptoms, and management options (Table 11.4) [75]. This conversation should be accompanied by a thorough evaluation of the patient's current condition and if pregnancy is considered contraindicated, as in severe, symptomatic AS, MS, or LVEF <40%.

Part of preconception counseling is considering whether to carry out an intervention before the pregnancy, or if the patient can tolerate the hemodynamic changes that occur during pregnancy and peripartum. This conversation should include a list of symptoms that may signify deterioration in their clinical status. This could include dyspnea, dizziness, syncope, palpitations, and others. Oftentimes, these symptoms are very similar to the experience of pregnant patients who do not have VHD. This makes it difficult to distinguish between benign and pathologic symptoms. Therefore, it is important to have routine follow-up with cardiology and MFM, often with serial TTE, in order to determine if evolving symptoms are caused by a change in hemodynamics, arrhythmia, or LVEF [28]. If experiencing pregnancy poses too great a risk, other options may be appropriate to discuss, such as adoption and surrogacy.

Conclusion

Women with VHD, particularly those with moderate to severe disease, VHD in the context of HF, arrhythmia, or lower LVEF, and mechanical valves or degenerated bioprostheses, are at risk of adverse outcomes. A woman's individual risk for pregnancy with her VHD should ideally be addressed with preconception counseling. For those pursuing pregnancy, careful monitoring with serial cardiac examination is recommended, at minimum every trimester, but potentially more often with moderate to severe disease, with repeat TTE to detect changes in LVEF and evaluate gradients, and measurement of BNP for detection of HF. Medical therapy is often directed at avoiding volume overload and arrhythmia. Percutaneous intervention or surgery should be considered when medical therapy is insufficient to avoid HF.

REFERENCES

1. Cantwell R et al. Saving Mothers' Lives: Reviewing maternal deaths to make motherhood safer: 2006–2008. The Eighth Report of the Confidential Enquiries into Maternal Deaths in the United Kingdom. *BJOG*. Mar 2011;118(Suppl 1):1–203.
2. Elkayam U, Goland S, Pieper PG, Silverside CK. High-risk cardiac disease in pregnancy: Part I. *J Am Coll Cardiol*. Jul 26 2016;68(4):396–410.
3. van Hagen IM et al. Global cardiac risk assessment in the Registry of Pregnancy and Cardiac disease: Results of a registry from the European Society of Cardiology. *Eur J Heart Fail*. May 2016;18(5):523–33.
4. Siu SC et al. Prospective multicenter study of pregnancy outcomes in women with heart disease. *Circulation*. Jul 31 2001;104(5):515–21.
5. European Society of G, Association for European Paediatric C, German Society for Gender M. et al. ESC Guidelines on the management of cardiovascular diseases during pregnancy: The Task Force on the Management of Cardiovascular Diseases during Pregnancy of the European Society of Cardiology (ESC). *Eur Heart J*. Dec 2011;32(24):3147–97.
6. Kassebaum NJ et al. Global, regional, and national levels and causes of maternal mortality during 1990–2013: A systematic analysis for the Global Burden of Disease Study 2013. *Lancet*. Sep 13 2014;384(9947):980–1004.
7. Sliwa K et al. Spectrum of cardiac disease in maternity in a low-resource cohort in South Africa. *Heart*. Dec 2014;100(24):1967–74.
8. Diao M et al. Pregnancy in women with heart disease in sub-Saharan Africa. *Arch Cardiovasc Dis*. Jun-Jul 2011; 104(6–7):370–4.
9. Carapetis JR, Steer AC, Mulholland EK, Weber M. The global burden of group A streptococcal diseases. *Lancet Infect Dis*. Nov 2005;5(11):685–94.
10. Sliwa K, Johnson MR, Zilla P, Roos-Hesselink JW. Management of valvular disease in pregnancy: A global perspective. *Eur Heart J*. May 7 2015;36(18):1078–89.
11. Roos-Hesselink JW et al. Outcome of pregnancy in patients with structural or ischaemic heart disease: Results of a registry of the European Society of Cardiology. *Eur Heart J*. Mar 2013;34(9):657–65.
12. Nanna M, Stergiopoulos K. Pregnancy complicated by valvular heart disease: An update. *J Am Heart Assoc*. Jun 5 2014;3(3):e000712.
13. van Oppen AC, van der Tweel I, Alsbach GP, Heethaar RM, Bruinse HW. A longitudinal study of maternal hemodynamics during normal pregnancy. *Obstet Gynecol*. Jul 1996;88(1):40–6.
14. Hunter S, Robson SC. Adaptation of the maternal heart in pregnancy. *Br Heart J*. Dec 1992;68(6):540–3.
15. Robson SC, Hunter S, Boys RJ, Dunlop W. Serial study of factors influencing changes in cardiac output during human pregnancy. *Am J Physiol*. Apr 1989;256(4 Pt 2):H1060–1060–5.
16. James AH. Pregnancy and thrombotic risk. *Crit Care Med*. Feb 2010;38(2 Suppl):S57–63.
17. Cornette J et al. Hemodynamic adaptation to pregnancy in women with structural heart disease. *Int J Cardiol*. Sep 30 2013;168(2):825–31.
18. Regitz-Zagrosek V et al. 2018 ESC Guidelines for the management of cardiovascular diseases during pregnancy. *Eur Heart J*. Sep 7 2018;39(34):3165–241.
19. Rossi A et al. Quantitative cardiovascular magnetic resonance in pregnant women: Cross-sectional analysis of physiological parameters throughout pregnancy and the impact of the supine position. *J Cardiovasc Magn Reson*. Jun 27 2011;13:31.
20. Anderson GD. Pregnancy-induced changes in pharmacokinetics: A mechanistic-based approach. *Clin Pharmacokinet*. 2005;44(10):989–1008.
21. Robson SC, Dunlop W, Boys RJ, Hunter S. Cardiac output during labour. *Br Med J (Clin Res Ed)*. Nov 7 1987;295(6607):1169–72.
22. Robson SC, Dunlop W, Moore M, Hunter S. Combined Doppler and echocardiographic measurement of cardiac output: Theory and application in pregnancy. *Br J Obstet Gynaecol*. Nov 1987;94(11):1014–27.

23. Lee W, Rokey R, Miller J, Cotton DB. Maternal hemodynamic effects of uterine contractions by M-mode and pulsed-Doppler echocardiography. *Am J Obstet Gynecol*. Oct 1989;161(4):974–7.

24. Stones RW, Paterson CM, Saunders NJ. Risk factors for major obstetric haemorrhage. *Eur J Obstet Gynecol Reprod Biol*. Jan 1993;48(1):15–8.

25. Stergiopoulos K, Shiang E, Bench T. Pregnancy in patients with pre-existing cardiomyopathies. *J Am Coll Cardiol*. Jul 19 2011;58(4):337–50.

26. Balci A et al. Prospective validation and assessment of cardiovascular and offspring risk models for pregnant women with congenital heart disease. *Heart*. Sep 2014;100(17):1373–81.

27. Samiei N et al. Echocardiographic evaluation of hemodynamic changes in left-sided heart valves in pregnant women with valvular heart disease. *Am J Cardiol*. Oct 1 2016;118(7):1046–52.

28. Nishimura RA et al. 2014 AHA/ACC guideline for the management of patients with valvular heart disease: Executive summary: A report of the American College of Cardiology/American Heart Association Task Force on Practice Guidelines. *J Am Coll Cardiol*. Jun 10 2014;63(22):2438–88.

29. Zoghbi WA et al. Recommendations for noninvasive evaluation of native valvular regurgitation: A Report from the American Society of Echocardiography developed in collaboration with the Society for Cardiovascular Magnetic Resonance. *J Am Soc Echocardiogr*. Apr 2017;30(4):303–71.

30. Baumgartner H et al. Echocardiographic assessment of valve stenosis: EAE/ASE recommendations for clinical practice. *J Am Soc Echocardiogr*. Jan 2009;22(1):1–23. quiz 101–102.

31. Lancellotti P et al. Recommendations for the echocardiographic assessment of native valvular regurgitation: An executive summary from the European Association of Cardiovascular Imaging. *Eur Heart J Cardiovasc Imaging*. Jul 2013;14(7):611–44.

32. Hameed A et al. The effect of valvular heart disease on maternal and fetal outcome of pregnancy. *J Am Coll Cardiol*. Mar 1 2001;37(3):893–9.

33. Lesniak-Sobelga A, Tracz W, KostKiewicz M, Podolec P, Pasowicz M. Clinical and echocardiographic assessment of pregnant women with valvular heart diseases—Maternal and fetal outcome. *Int J Cardiol*. Mar 2004;94(1):15–23.

34. Mahli A, Izdes S, Coskun D. Cardiac operations during pregnancy: Review of factors influencing fetal outcome. *Ann Thorac Surg*. May 2000;69(5):1622–6.

35. John AS et al. Cardiopulmonary bypass during pregnancy. *Ann Thorac Surg*. Apr 2011;91(4):1191–6.

36. Stout KK, Otto CM. Pregnancy in women with valvular heart disease. *Heart*. May 2007;93(5):552–8.

37. Baumgartner H et al. 2017 ESC/EACTS Guidelines for the management of valvular heart disease. *Eur Heart J*. Sep 21 2017;38(36):2739–91.

38. Baumgartner H et al. Echocardiographic assessment of valve stenosis: EAE/ASE recommendations for clinical practice. *Eur J Echocardiogr*. Jan 2009;10(1):1–25.

39. van Hagen IM et al. Pregnancy outcomes in women with rheumatic mitral valve disease: Results from the Registry of Pregnancy and Cardiac Disease. *Circulation*. Feb 20 2018;137(8):806–16.

40. Silversides CK, Colman JM, Sermer M, Siu SC. Cardiac risk in pregnant women with rheumatic mitral stenosis. *Am J Cardiol*. Jun 1 2003;91(11):1382–5.

41. Avila WS et al. Pregnancy in patients with heart disease: Experience with 1,000 cases. *Clin Cardiol*. Mar 2003;26(3):135–42.

42. Elassy SM, Elmidany AA, Elbawab HY. Urgent cardiac surgery during pregnancy: A continuous challenge. *Ann Thorac Surg*. May 2014;97(5):1624–9.

43. Baumgartner H et al. ESC Guidelines for the management of grown-up congenital heart disease (new version 2010). *Eur Heart J*. Dec 2010;31(23):2915–57.

44. Orwat S et al. Risk of Pregnancy in moderate and severe aortic stenosis: From the Multinational ROPAC Registry. *J Am Coll Cardiol*. Oct 18 2016;68(16):1727–37.

45. Silversides CK, Colman JM, Sermer M, Farine D, Siu SC. Early and intermediate-term outcomes of pregnancy with congenital aortic stenosis. *Am J Cardiol*. Jun 1 2003;91(11):1386–9.

46. Yap SC et al. Risk of complications during pregnancy in women with congenital aortic stenosis. *Int J Cardiol*. May 23 2008;126(2):240–6.

47. Lui GK et al. Heart rate response during exercise and pregnancy outcome in women with congenital heart disease. *Circulation*. Jan 25 2011;123(3):242–8.

48. Ohuchi H et al. Cardiopulmonary variables during exercise predict pregnancy outcome in women with congenital heart disease. *Circ J*. 2013;77(2):470–6.

49. Bhargava B, Agarwal R, Yadav R, Bahl VK, Manchanda SC. Percutaneous balloon aortic valvuloplasty during pregnancy: Use of the Inoue balloon and the physiologic antegrade approach. *Cathet Cardiovasc Diagn*. Dec 1998;45(4):422–5.

50. Ramsey PS, Hogg BB, Savage KG, Winkler DD, Owen J. Cardiovascular effects of intravaginal misoprostol in the mid-trimester of pregnancy. *Am J Obstet Gynecol*. Nov 2000;183(5):1100–2.

51. Lind J, Wallenburg HC. The Marfan syndrome and pregnancy: A retrospective study in a Dutch population. *Eur J Obstet Gynecol Reprod Biol*. Sep 2001;98(1):28–35.

52. Montoya ME, Karnath BM, Ahmad M. Endocarditis during pregnancy. *South Med J*. Nov 2003;96(11):1156–7.

53. Nishimura RA et al. 2017 AHA/ACC Focused Update of the 2014 AHA/ACC Guideline for the Management of Patients with Valvular Heart Disease: A Report of the American College of Cardiology/American Heart Association Task Force on Clinical Practice Guidelines. *Circulation*. Jun 20 2017;135(25):e1159–95.

54. Khairy P, Ouyang DW, Fernandes SM, Lee-Parritz A, Economy KE, Landzberg MJ. Pregnancy outcomes in women with congenital heart disease. *Circulation*. Jan 31 2006;113(4):517–24.

55. Drenthen W et al. Predictors of pregnancy complications in women with congenital heart disease. *Eur Heart J*. Sep 2010;31(17):2124–32.

56. Donnelly JE, Brown JM, Radford DJ. Pregnancy outcome and Ebstein's anomaly. *Br Heart J*. Nov 1991;66(5):368–71.

57. Hameed AB, Goodwin TM, Elkayam U. Effect of pulmonary stenosis on pregnancy outcomes—A case-control study. *Am Heart J*. Nov 2007;154(5):852–4.

58. Warnes CA et al. ACC/AHA 2008 Guidelines for the Management of Adults with Congenital Heart Disease: Executive Summary: A report of the American College

of Cardiology/American Heart Association Task Force on Practice Guidelines (writing committee to develop guidelines for the management of adults with congenital heart disease). *Circulation*. Dec 2 2008;118(23):2395–451.

59. Drenthen W et al. Non-cardiac complications during pregnancy in women with isolated congenital pulmonary valvar stenosis. *Heart*. Dec 2006;92(12):1838–43.

60. Bruce CJ, Connolly HM. Right-sided valve disease deserves a little more respect. *Circulation*. May 26 2009;119(20):2726–34.

61. Lima FV, Yang J, Xu J, Stergiopoulos K. National trends and in-hospital outcomes in pregnant women with heart disease in the United States. *Am J Cardiol*. May 15 2017;119(10):1694–700.

62. Owens A, Yang J, Nie L, Lima F, Avila C, Stergiopoulos K. Neonatal and maternal outcomes in pregnant women with cardiac disease. *J Am Heart Assoc*. Nov 6 2018;7(21):e009395.

63. van Hagen IM et al. Incidence and predictors of obstetric and fetal complications in women with structural heart disease. *Heart*. Oct 2017;103(20):1610–8.

64. Greutmann M, Pieper PG. Pregnancy in women with congenital heart disease. *Eur Heart J*. Oct 1 2015;36(37):2491–9.

65. Windram JD, Colman JM, Wald RM, Udell JA, Siu SC, Silversides CK. Valvular heart disease in pregnancy. *Best Pract Res Clin Obstet Gynaecol*. May 2014;28(4):507–18.

66. Wolfe DS et al. Addressing maternal mortality: The pregnant cardiac patient. *Am J Obstet Gynecol*. 2019;220(2):167.

67. Silversides CK et al. Pregnancy outcomes in women with heart disease: The CARPREG II Study. *J Am Coll Cardiol*. May 29 2018;71(21):2419–30.

68. Bredy C et al. New York Heart Association (NYHA) classification in adults with congenital heart disease: Relation to objective measures of exercise and outcome. *Eur Heart J Qual Care Clin Outcomes*. Jan 1 2018;4(1):51–8.

69. Holland R, Rechel B, Stepien K, Harvey I, Brooksby I. Patients' self-assessed functional status in heart failure by New York Heart Association class: A prognostic predictor of hospitalizations, quality of life and death. *J Card Fail*. Feb 2010;16(2):150–6.

70. Clark SL. Cardiac disease in pregnancy—Some good news. *BJOG*. Oct 2015;122(11):1456.

71. Heuvelman HJ et al. Pregnancy outcomes in women with aortic valve substitutes. *Am J Cardiol*. Feb 1 2013;111(3):382–7.

72. van Hagen IM et al. Pregnancy in women with a mechanical heart valve: Data of the European Society of Cardiology Registry of Pregnancy and Cardiac Disease (ROPAC). *Circulation*. Jul 14 2015;132(2):132–42.

73. Ladouceur M et al. Educational needs of adolescents with congenital heart disease: Impact of a transition intervention programme. *Arch Cardiovasc Dis*. May 2017;110(5):317–24.

74. Roos-Hesselink JW, Cornette J, Sliwa K, Pieper PG, Veldtman GR, Johnson MR. Contraception and cardiovascular disease. *Eur Heart J*. Jul 14 2015;36(27):1728–34, 1734a–1734b.

75. Roos-Hesselink JW et al. Organisation of care for pregnancy in patients with congenital heart disease. *Heart*. Dec 2017;103(23):1854–9.

12

Cardiomyopathies in Pregnancy

Joan Briller

KEY POINTS

- Cardiomyopathies are a diverse group of disorders characterized by structural abnormalities of the heart muscle, many of which have a genetic component
- Counseling on risk of recurrence and review of symptoms suggestive of heart failure exacerbation are recommended in the preconception period and continued throughout pregnancy

- Medications should be switched to those compatible with pregnancy and breastfeeding
- Delivery planning requires a multidisciplinary team approach
- Well-compensated cardiomyopathy patients may become symptomatic during the postpartum period

What Is a Cardiomyopathy?

The cardiomyopathies are a diverse group of disorders characterized by structural abnormalities of the heart muscle, many of which have a genetic component. Abnormalities may be *anatomic* (dilatation, thickened, or stiff musculature), *histologic* (manifested by fiber disarray, fibrofatty dysplasia, or fibrosis) or *functional* (systolic or diastolic dysfunction). Nonischemic cardiomyopathies have several phenotypes that include dilated, hypertrophic, restrictive, arrhythmogenic right ventricular, and unclassified. Each of these types may have familial and non-familial forms [1–3]. Several classificatory schemes exist, but the most recently endorsed is the MOGE(S) system which incorporates morphofunctional phenotype (M), organ involved (O), genetic inheritance (G), etiologic annotation (E), and functional status [1–4]. Examples of major nonischemic cardiomyopathies are shown in Box 12.1.

Dilated cardiomyopathies (DCM) are characterized by left ventricular (LV) enlargement and impaired systolic function. Dilated cardiomyopathy commonly presents in the third and fourth decade of life, which underscores concerns during reproductive years [5]. Etiologies include genetic defects, infections, and toxins. For many, the underlying cause is unknown and labeled idiopathic [2]. Peripartum cardiomyopathy (PPCM) is a specific form of DCM which is associated with pregnancy and usually classified under the idiopathic group.

Hypertrophic cardiomyopathies (HCM) differ in that they are characterized by ventricular hypertrophy and pressure overload but may not result in systolic dysfunction [2].

BOX 12.1   EXAMPLES OF MAJOR NONISCHEMIC CARDIOMYOPATHIES

- Dilated
  - Idiopathic
    - Includes PPCM
  - Genetic
    - Familial DCM
  - Chemotherapy
    - Anthracyclines
    - Doxorubicin
    - Trastuzumab
  - Toxin/substance abuse
    - Alcoholic
    - Cocaine
  - Myocarditis
    - HIV
    - Viral
    - Chagas
  - Stress induced (Takutsubo)
- Hypertrophic
- Restrictive
  - Amyloid
- Infiltrative
  - Sarcoid
- ARVC/D
- Ventricular non-compaction

Heart failure (HF), in contrast, is a clinical syndrome resulting from impaired LV ejection or filling [6]. HF may be secondary to other underlying pathology such as ischemic disease, hypertensive disease, congenital heart disease, or valvular heart disease in addition to the cardiomyopathies.

How Does Pregnancy Affect Cardiomyopathy?

Adaptation to the physiologic requirements of pregnancy can challenge women with CMP. Women with baseline reduced cardiac reserve may not be able to accommodate demands to increase cardiac output by 30%–50%. Pregnancy is a state of volume overload [7,8]. Increased volume load may exacerbate associated valve lesions such as mitral regurgitation or increased ventricular filling pressure precipitating overt HF. Pregnancy-related alterations in hemodynamic, hormonal, and autonomic systems lead to atrial and ventricular stretch, which may increase arrhythmia burden when combined with the normal increased heart rate during pregnancy [9]. Pregnancy-associated CMP complications and management strategies are shown in Table 12.1.

How Frequently Are Pregnancies Associated with Cardiomyopathy?

The precise frequency of cardiomyopathy during pregnancy is not known and varies with geographic location, population, and specific cardiomyopathy. The European Registry on Pregnancy and Heart Disease (ROPAC) enrolled 1321 women with structural heart disease from 2001–2011. Cardiomyopathy was present in 7% [10]. DCM was seen in 32%, PPCM in 25%, hypertrophic nonobstructive cardiomyopathy in 16%, hypertrophic obstructive cardiomyopathy in 11%, and 5% other forms [10]. HF was the most common cardiovascular event during pregnancy in ROPAC [11]. In the United States, DCM predominated, usually attributed to peripartum cardiomyopathy, followed by hypertrophic etiologies [12,13]. In a CARPREG II study of outcomes in 1938 pregnancies in women with heart disease, at least mild ventricular dysfunction was present 13.6% but not all were secondary to cardiomyopathy, as the most common cardiac diagnosis was congenital heart disease [14]. Pregnancy-associated HF hospitalizations represented 112 cases per 100,000 pregnancy hospitalizations in a National Inpatient Sample analysis from 2001–2011. Cardiomyopathy was the most common comorbidity responsible for 39.7% of HF hospitalizations antepartum, 70.8% of HF during delivery hospitalizations, and 34.5% of postpartum hospitalizations [15]. The reported incidence of PPCM in the United States is approximately 1:1000 to 1:4000 live births [16]. Analysis of the National Inpatient Sample database suggests an increasing PPCM frequency over time with incidence rising from 8.5 to 11.8 per 10,000 live births [17]. There is marked geographic variation with regard to incidence. PPCM is more common in the southern United States and has been reported to occur as frequently as 1:300 live births in Haiti and 1:100 live births in Nigeria [18,19].

TABLE 12.1

Management Strategies for Cardiomyopathy

Primary Issue	Usual Management	Pregnancy Considerations
Systolic dysfunction	Beta-blockers, Ace-i, ARB, ARNi, MRA, diuretics, ivabradine Advanced intervention: LVAD, transplant	Review medications for safety in pregnancy and during lactation If medications are discontinued due to safety, commence alternatives Serial BNPs, echo Hydralazine/nitrates Consider digoxin, consider bromocriptine for PPCM
HCM/ diastolic dysfunction	Beta-blockers, CCB, diuretics, occasionally disopyramide	Serial BNPs, echo, beta-blockers, CCB, diuretics
Mitral regurgitation	Treat ↓ LVSF, mitral clip for some If LVOTO: septal myomectomy or ablation	Adjust meds as above depending on etiology May be well tolerated with HCM
Atrial arrhythmias	Beta-blockers, CCB, cardioversion, anticoagulation for afib/AFl, rate versus rhythm control strategy, ablation	Increased arrhythmias in pregnancy Consider need for anticoagulation and cardioversion, occasional fluoro-less ablation
Ventricular arrhythmias	Beta-blockers, antiarrhythmic therapy, ICD	Increased arrhythmias in pregnancy Surveillance, wearable defibrillator Consider ICD placement if indicated
Genetic CMP	Family screening, assess SCD risk	Family screening, genetic counseling

Abbreviations: Ace-i, angiotensin-converting enzyme inhibitor; ARB, angiotensin receptor blocker; ARNi, angiotensin receptor-neprilysin inhibitor; MRA, mineralocorticoid receptor antagonist; BNP, brain natriuretic peptide; PPCM, peripartum cardiomyopathy; CCB, nondihydropyridine calcium channel blocker; LVSF, left ventricular systolic function; HCM, hypertrophic cardiomyopathy; CMP, cardiomyopathy; LVOTO, left ventricular outflow tract obstruction; Afib/AFL, atrial fibrillation/atrial flutter; ICD, implantable cardiac defibrillator; SCD, sudden cardiac death.

Dilated Cardiomyopathies

The prevalence of DCM in the United States is estimated at 36/100,000 population [6]. Etiology is diverse, ranging from familial cardiomyopathies which are felt to represent approximately 20%–35% of DCM to toxin exposure from substance abuse (e.g., alcohol, cocaine) to prior cancer therapy for childhood leukemia/lymphoma or breast cancer. Idiopathic DCM, which comprises about 50% of DCM, is diagnosed when detectable causes of cardiomyopathy other than genetic have been excluded [6]. Alcoholic cardiomyopathy, another leading cause of DCM, is diagnosed in the setting of heavy alcohol consumption for more than 10 years in the absence of another identified cause. Women represent approximately 14% of alcoholic cardiomyopathy [20]. Cancer patients receiving chemotherapy, especially anthracyclines, or chest radiation therapy are at risk of ventricular dysfunction. In a review of over 1800 survivors of childhood cancer, only 5.8% had overt LV dysfunction but over a third had reduced global longitudinal strain, a more subtle measure of ventricular dysfunction than ejection fraction, diastolic dysfunction, or both [21].

Pregnancy outcomes with DCM are based on a small cohort series [20,22–25]. Grewal examined outcomes in 36 pregnancies in 32 women with DCM. The majority (86%) had idiopathic DCM, the remainder chemotherapy induced. Thirty-nine percent of pregnancies were associated with at least one adverse maternal event. Moderate to severe LV dysfunction and poor functional status were the main determinants of adverse outcome. Neonatal events were also highest in women with increased cardiac risk factors. Sixteen-month event-free survival was worse in women who had a pregnancy than in women who did not [22].

Familial Dilated Cardiomyopathy

Family-based studies suggest a familial relationship in 20%–35% of patients diagnosed with DCM [26]. Most are transmitted as autosomal dominants, although all inheritance patterns are described. Genetic studies have identified mutations in more than 30 genes [26]. Estimated incidence is approximately 1:2500 [1]. Most patients will have an initial diagnosis of idiopathic cardiomyopathy. Diagnosis of familial DCM requires presence of LV dilatation and impaired systolic function in one or both ventricles in two or more closely related family members [27]. Mutation-specific genetic testing is recommended for family members when a DCM causative mutation is found in the index case even in the absence of symptoms [5]. Clinical manifestations of familial DCM are similar to other idiopathic DCM. General risks to be considered include progressive LV dysfunction which can be severe enough to require transplantation, arrhythmias including sudden cardiac death and, if pregnancy is pursued, transmission to offspring. Outcome data on pregnancy in women with familial DCM is extrapolated from a small cohort series of women with idiopathic DCM [20,22–25,28].

Peripartum Cardiomyopathy

PPCM is a form of DCM in association with pregnancy in the absence of structural heart disease or another explanation for DCM. Criteria for diagnosis include LV enlargement and dysfunction (typically an ejection fraction <45%) presenting toward the end of pregnancy or in the months postdelivery in a woman without previously known structural heart disease [16,29]. Diagnosis is confirmed by transthoracic echocardiography.

Risk factors for development of PPCM are well known. In the United States, the incidence is strikingly higher in African Americans [16]. Preeclampsia and hypertension (chronic or gestational), age greater than 30, multiple gestations, and higher gravidity and parity are other risk factors [16,30–33]. Current research suggests that an imbalance in angiogenic factors promotes PPCM in susceptible individuals. Both prolactin and soluble FMs-like tyrosine kinase (sFlt1) have been implicated in its development [34,35]. Several studies suggest familial clustering. Moreover, genetic evaluation of DNA in women with PPCM found truncating variants in 15%, many in the TTN gene which is important in cardiac muscle function similar to a DCM cohort. Presence of a TTN gene mutation correlated with lower ejection fractions at 1-year follow-up [36].

Maternal prognosis is variable but may be better than many other forms of cardiomyopathy [16,37,38]. Mortality is higher, presence of cardiac arrest or shock, and length of stay are significantly longer in patients with PPCM than normal pregnancy. PPCM deliveries were more likely to be by cesarean [33]. Factors suggesting worse prognosis include degree of LV dilatation, worse ejection fraction at presentation, associated RV dysfunction, abnormal cardiac biomarkers, family history of heart failure, and low cholesterol [39–43]. Outcomes are significantly worse in African Americans [39,44–46]. Most women improve in the first 6 months postpartum but delayed recovery has also been reported [38,39]. In the Investigations of Pregnancy-Associated Cardiomyopathy (IPAC) registry, 71% of women had recovered to an ejection fraction >50% by 1 year, mortality was 4%, advanced mechanical support was performed in 4%, and transplantation in 1%. There is a wide variation in published outcomes ranging from 2% in a German registry to 13% in a recent South African study [16,38]. Longer-term mortality is less well known [38].

Neonatal outcomes in PPCM are also worse. Babies were born earlier, smaller, more likely to be small for gestational age, and APGAR scores were lower [47]. In the EURObservational Research Programme (EORP), the neonatal death rate was 3.1% [48].

Should PPCM Patients Receive Bromocriptine?

Bromocriptine stimulates hypothalamic dopaminergic receptors inhibiting prolactin production suggesting a potential role in therapy [49]. A randomized trial in 20 South African women showed improved ventricular recovery as proof in concept [50]. A nonrandomized German registry found bromocriptine use twice as common in women with recovered function, although advanced HF interventions were similar regardless of bromocriptine use [42]. Further interest has been stimulated by a multicenter trial in 63 women with ejection fractions less than 35% who were randomized to 1 week versus 8 weeks of bromocriptine, finding a nonsignificant trend toward greater recovery in the 8-week therapy group, but both groups improved. No women required advanced interventions, right ventricular function improved, and there were no deaths at 6 months [51,52]. A major limitation to the study was lack of a placebo arm. Small numbers of patients, the validity of comparing outcomes in the German study to historical controls in the IPAC registry which had a large number of African Americans known to have worse outcomes, concerns about hypertensive or thrombotic complications with bromocriptine, and loss of the ability to lactate have dampened enthusiasm for use in the United States in the absence of a larger placebo-controlled trial [16,53]. European guidelines have recommended consideration of bromocriptine in addition to guideline directed medical therapy [54]. If bromocriptine is used for treatment, anticoagulation is recommended [51]. *Although approved for other indications, bromocriptine is not FDA approved in the United States for treatment of PPCM at the time of writing.*

Do We Need to Anticoagulate Women with PPCM?

Thromboembolic complications in patients with DCM are estimated at 1%–3% per year and correlate with the degree of LV dysfunction, presence of atrial fibrillation, or presence of thrombus during cardiac imaging [6]. Thromboembolic complications in PPCM are considerably higher: 6.6% and 6.8% in a National Inpatient Sample and in EORP [17,48]. Other studies noted thrombi in more than 20% of patients with PPCM [55]. Precise recommendations for anticoagulation are based on expert opinion and vary but generally recommend anticoagulation for those with significant LV dysfunction (ranging from 30%–40%) at least until the thrombophilia of pregnancy has resolved in the absence of another indication [5,16,48,54,56,57].

Should a Woman with a Diagnosis of PPCM Breastfeed?

Controversy exists about safety of breastfeeding with PPCM. Breastfeeding prolongs postpartum prolactin elevation. Since prolactin has been proposed in the pathogenesis of PPCM, there are fears this will worsen likelihood of recovery. Additional concerns include hemodynamic requirements of breastfeeding and transfer of HF medications to the infant in breast milk. Fifteen percent of women in the IPAC registry breastfed without observed differences in myocardial recovery despite elevated prolactin levels [39]. A retrospective internet survey noted improved recovery in the two-thirds of women who breastfed [58]. However, it is unknown if there was a selection bias for breastfeeding in healthier women or those with better EFs. In another observational study of recurrent pregnancies in women with PPCM, a high percentage of women lactated and there were similar rates of recurrence in those who did or did not breastfeed [59]. Nevertheless, current ESC guidelines discourage breastfeeding for women with the most severe HF (NYHA class III/IV) [54].

What Is the Risk of PPCM Recurrence with a Subsequent Pregnancy?

Many women with PPCM desire another child. Recurrence risk estimations are derived from retrospective analysis of women with subsequent pregnancies. These typically divide women into those with recovered function in comparison with continued LV dysfunction. In the largest study, deterioration was seen in 21% of gravidas with recovered function in comparison with

TABLE 12.2

Clinical Predictors Suggestive of HF Exacerbation in PPCM

Symptom/Sign	0 Points	1 Point	2 Points
Orthopnea	None	Need to elevate head only	Need to elevate body >45°
Dyspnea	None	When climb ≥8 stairs	Walking level
Unexplained cough	None	Nighttime	Day and night
Pitting edema	None	Below knee	Above and below knee
Weight gain (9th Mo)	≤2 lb/week	2–4 lb/week	>4 lb/week
Palpitations	None	When lying down	Any position day and night

Source: From Fett, JD. *Crit Pathw Cardiol.* 2011;10(1):44–45. With permission.
Scoring and Action:
0–2 Low risk, observe
3–4 Mild risk, consider BNP
≥5 High risk, BNP, echo

44% of those with persistent dysfunction [60]. Similar results are noted in other publications and a meta-analysis [59,61–63]. Some women may have subnormal cardiac reserve even in the setting of improved function. Additional risk stratification might be considered using dobutamine or exercise stress prior to proceeding [63,64]. Most believe full recovery is associated with improved outcomes and lower mortality with a subsequent pregnancy, but all patients have a risk of deterioration [38,59,61]. Fett developed a simple periodic self-assessment tool validated on PPCM patients helpful in identifying women who would relapse, shown in Table 12.2. Elevated scores should prompt additional evaluation with biomarkers or transthoracic echocardiography. All women with PPCM had scores greater than 5 and controls less than 4 [65,66].

Hypertrophic Cardiomyopathy

Hypertrophic cardiomyopathy (HCM) is characterized by LV hypertrophy in the absence of another explanatory cardiac or systemic disease [67]. The hypertrophy is often asymmetric with wall thickness >15 mm, but multiple patterns of hypertrophy have been described [67]. Many patients have a normal life expectancy and unremarkable clinical course. However, a subset develop HF related to outflow tract obstruction, diastolic dysfunction, myocardial ischemia, and mitral regurgitation. A small percentage develop systolic HF. Arrhythmia risks include atrial fibrillation, ventricular tachycardia, and sudden cardiac death.

HCM is the most common genetic cardiac disease with estimated prevalence as high as 1:200 using the newest techniques such as cardiac magnetic resonance and genetic testing [68]. HCM is typically caused by mutations in sarcomere genes that encode components of the myocardial contraction. Inheritance is in an autosomal dominant pattern in the vast majority with variable expression and age-related penetrance. Over 1500 mutations in 11 genes have been described as of 2015 [69]. HCM is estimated to be present in about 1:1000 pregnancies [54].

Diagnosis is usually made by a combination of ECG and echocardiography, with increasing use of cardiac magnetic resonance imaging since late gadolinium enhancement provides additional information about myocardial fiber disarray, fibrosis, and sudden death risk [67,70].

Symptomatic patients may present with fatigue, dyspnea, chest pain, palpitations, pre-syncope, or syncope. LV hypertrophy often occurs at the expense of cavity size, reducing stroke volume. Left ventricular outflow obstruction may be dynamic and worsen with exercise or reduced systemic vascular resistance of pregnancy; however, this may be offset by the increased volume of pregnancy. Left atrial enlargement or increased filling pressure can worsen mitral regurgitation and exacerbating arrhythmias such as atrial fibrillation. Despite this, many women with HCM often tolerate pregnancy well [28]. With contemporary management, mortality is very low (0.5% or less) [71,72]. Major adverse cardiac events were present in 23%–29% [71,72], including arrhythmias (atrial and ventricular) or HF usually occurring in the third trimester or postpartum. Issues to be addressed with pregnancy include genetic counseling about risk of transmission, medication adjustment, risk of arrhythmia or sudden death, and development of HF.

Rare Cardiomyopathies

Arrhythmogenic Right Ventricular Cardiomyopathy

Arrhythmogenic right ventricular cardiomyopathy (ARVC/D), sometimes called arrhythmogenic RV dysplasia, is a rare inherited cardiomyopathy transmitted as an autosomal dominant disorder characterized by fibro-fatty tissue replacement in the right ventricle leading to right ventricular dilatation and dysfunction. The left ventricle is also frequently involved. Disruption of normal myocardium increases electrical instability, so arrhythmias are a prominent problem [73]. Prevalence is estimated to be 1:2000 to 1:5000 [73]. ARVC/D is an important cause of sudden cardiac death [1]. Diagnosis is based on echocardiogram or CMR. Information on outcomes during pregnancy is limited. In a single-center French study of 60 pregnancies in 23 women, major adverse cardiovascular events were rare: two (3%) sustained arrhythmias, neither during delivery or postpartum (3%) but no HF exacerbations. Beta-blocker therapy was common (16.7%) and associated with lower birth weights. Preterm delivery and cesarean rates were low, but premature sudden death was seen in five children before age 25 (10%) [74].

Left Ventricular Noncompaction

Left ventricular noncompaction (LVNC) is an uncharacterized type of cardiomyopathy that results in a distinctive spongy appearance of the myocardium due to increased trabeculations and deep myocardial recesses that communicate with the LV cavity increasing the risk for thromboembolism particularly

in pregnancy. Diagnosis is made by echocardiography, cardiac magnetic resonance imaging, or occasionally LV angiography. Clinical manifestations of LVNC include HF (systolic or diastolic), atrial and ventricular arrhythmias, thromboembolic cerebral vascular events, and sudden cardiac death [75]. There are only a few case series of women with LVNC and pregnancy. There are no specific therapies, and general guidelines for management of CMP during pregnancy should be followed with the caveat that patients with LVNC have increased thromboembolic risk which may be enhanced with pregnancy [5,28].

Restrictive Cardiomyopathy

Restrictive cardiomyopathies are characterized by the presence of "restrictive filling pattern in the presence of normal or reduced diastolic volumes, normal or reduced systolic volumes, and normal wall thickness" and may represent various pathologies rather than a distinct entity [2]. Primary restrictive cardiomyopathy may be inherited due to genetic mutations in cardiac proteins, such as troponin, or non-inherited, such as in infiltrative disorders including hemochromatosis, amyloidosis, or sarcoid or radiation exposure [2]. There are only rare case reports of pregnancy outcomes with restrictive cardiomyopathy [76–78]. Some recommend that pregnancy be avoided in symptomatic patients [28].

Pregnancy Care for Women with Cardiomyopathy (Box 12.2)

Pre-pregnancy counseling is mandatory in all women with known cardiomyopathy or at risk of developing cardiomyopathy [54,79]. This allows for estimation of maternal and fetal risk, assessment of potential transmission to offspring for heritable conditions, and modifications of medications compatible with pregnancy. Assessment should include:

1. Detailed medical history including prior cardiac events such as overt HF or arrhythmia, family history, stability of symptoms over time, and medication history
2. Physical exam for volume status and associated valvular insufficiency
3. A 12-lead ECG
4. Echocardiography
5. Other modalities such as magnetic resonance imaging as indicated
6. Baseline exercise tolerance and functional status may be estimated by stress testing
7. Additional testing with regard to arrhythmia risk may be warranted
8. A referral for genetics counseling should be made if a heritable disease is present

Estimation of cardiac risk can then be assessed using mWHO or CARPREG II criteria. Assessment of mWHO risk with regard to cardiomyopathy is shown in Table 12.3 [54]. If decision is

BOX 12.2 CHECKLIST FOR CARDIOMYOPATHY IN PREGNANCY

- Baseline cardiomyopathy history
  - Year commenced
  - How diagnosis was made
  - Etiology of cardiomyopathy
  - Medications currently taking
  - Date of last visit with cardiologist
    - Name, contact information
  - Date of last ECHO
  - Current NYHA functional class
  - Anticoagulation   yes/no/agent/level
- Individualized risk
  - Low
  - High
  - Comorbidities yes/no
  - What are the comorbidities
- Medications
  - Heart failure pregnancy regimen
  - Anticoagulation
- Diagnostic test
  - Echocardiogram   yes/no
    - Repeat every [ ] weeks
  - B-type natriuretic peptide
    - Repeat every [ ] weeks
  - EKG   yes/no
  - CXR   yes/no
  - Other tests   yes/no
    - Arrhythmia monitoring
- Fetus
  - Risk for anomalies   yes/no
  - Detailed fetal anatomy ultrasound   yes/no
  - Fetal echocardiogram   yes/no
  - Serial growth   yes/no
  - Antepartum fetal heart rate testing
- Consultations
  - Cardiology   yes/no
  - Maternal-fetal medicine yes/no
  - Anesthesiology   yes/no
  - Genetics   yes/no
  - Neonatology   yes/no
  - Other   yes/no
- Multidisciplinary meeting for delivery planning in the early third trimester
  - Recent cardiac studies
  - Echo
  - Holter/rhythm monitor
  - Biomarkers (BNP or Nt-proBNP)
  - Location for delivery
  - Planned delivery mode
  - Need for telemetry
  - SBE prophylaxis
  - Central line
  - Two larger bore IVs
  - Arterial line
  - IV with filters   yes/no
- VTE prophylaxis
- Strict fluid management
- Other precautions
- Multidisciplinary team notification
  - List contact information
- Postpartum
  - VTE prophylaxis
  - Medication review
  - Desires tubal ligation
  - Contraceptive plan
  - Patient education on when to seek care
  - Follow-up with heart failure team
  - Rehabilitation
  - Transportation support
  - Social work support
  - Depression screening

made to proceed with a pregnancy, cardiac medications should be adjusted to reduce fetal adverse effects. If pregnancy is not planned, effective contraception should be utilized.

Pregnancy heart team/multidisciplinary team should be identified consisting of a cardiologist, obstetrician/maternal-fetal medicine specialist, and obstetric anesthesiologist versed in management of heart disease in pregnancy. Other members may include neonatologist, geneticist, electrophysiologist, or cardiothoracic surgeon.

Goals of guideline-directed medial therapy are outlined in in Box 12.3. A chart of recommended medical therapy is shown in Table 12.4. *Beta-blockers are generally considered safe with the caveat that fetal growth should be monitored. ACE inhibitors, angiotensin receptor blockers, neprilysin inhibitors, and ivabradine are contraindicated* [80]. Fluid and sodium restriction is recommended for all patients, and loop diuretics for symptomatic relief of pulmonary congestion or significant edema. Digoxin can also be added for symptomatic improvement. Antihypertensive therapy is also recommended for hypertensive patients. Serial echocardiograms, serial measurement of natriuretic peptides, and fetal ultrasounds should be followed during pregnancy [54]. Brain natriuretic peptide (BNP) levels appear to be stable in uncomplicated pregnancy although may also be increased in hypertensive disorders of pregnancy [81,82]. A self-assessment tool for decompensation with PPCM has been validated (see Table 12.2) [66].

Delivery Planning

For women with PPCM, it is unknown if early delivery will diminish progression or prevent development of LV dysfunction, but earlier delivery should be considered in the setting of worsening heart function or HF. Otherwise timing of delivery should be determined by obstetric factors, such as fetal growth or development of preeclampsia, using a team approach [38,54]. Vaginal delivery is preferred with spinal/epidural delivery [54]. In a Canadian review of women with DCM, most deliveries were vaginal, and the most frequent form of

TABLE 12.3

mWHO Classification for Cardiomyopathies in Pregnancy

mWHO Class	Condition	Risk Level	Event Rate	Care Level	Minimum Follow-Up	Delivery Location
II–III	Mildly ↓ LVSF (EF >45%) Hypertrophic CMP	Intermediate mortality/moderate to severe morbidity	Event rate 10%–19%	Referral hospital	Bimonthly	Referral hospital if stable
III	Moderately ↓ LVSF (EF 30%–45%) PPCM with recovered function Ventricular arrhythmias	Significantly ↑ mortality or severe morbidity	Event rate 19%–27%	Expert center	Monthly to bimonthly	Expert center
IV	PPCM with residual LV dysfunction HCM with severe LVOTO Severely ↓ LVSF (EF <30%) Moderately ↓ RVSF	Extremely high risk of mortality or severe morbidity Pregnancy not recommended Options counseling including pregnancy termination should be discussed	Event rate 40%–100%	If decision to proceed care as for mWHO III	Monthly	Expert center

Source: Adapted from Regitz-Zagrosek V et al. *Eur Heart J.* 2018:77(3):245–326.

Abbreviations: LVSF, left ventricular systolic function; EF, ejection fraction; PPCM, peripartum cardiomyopathy; CMP, cardiomyopathy; HCM, hypertrophic cardiomyopathy; LVOTO, left ventricular outflow tract obstruction.

BOX 12.3   GOALS OF GUIDELINE-DIRECTED MEDICAL THERAPY (GDMT) FOR CARDIOMYOPATHY

- Close follow-up
- Fluid management
  - Diuresis/fluid restriction for volume overload
  - Salt restriction
- Vasodilators
- Beta-blockade
- Treatment of hypertension
- Inotropic/advance heart failure intervention if required
- Exercise

---

anesthesia was epidural [22]. In a recent review of recurrent pregnancy in women with PPCM, a majority of the patients (56%) delivered by cesarean but mostly for obstetric indications [59]. Lower-risk HCM patients have no contraindication to a vaginal delivery, and cesarean should be performed for an obstetric indication.

During delivery, noninvasive telemetry monitoring is useful to assess for arrhythmias, point-of-care echocardiogram can give information about volume status, and arterial line pulse wave analysis may provide information on cardiac output and stroke volume variation. Placement of a Swan-Ganz catheter remains the gold standard for measuring cardiac output and filling pressure but has not been shown to have mortality benefit and is not frequently used during delivery, although may be used for patient stabilization and assessment. Whether a patient should be monitored in L&D or the ICU is patient and institution dependent. If medications are being titrated for optimization of hemodynamic status or are rarely used in L&D, this may be more readily achieved in an ICU; alternatively, if urgent delivery is anticipated, this may be more readily performed on L&D with a "borrowed" cardiac/critical-care nurse monitoring parameters on L&D.

Conclusion

The cardiomyopathies encompass a wide spectrum of diseases with genetic and phenotypic overlap. All patients are at risk of decompensation, especially for symptomatic HF and arrhythmias during pregnancy. Overlap of normal symptoms of pregnancy can mimic symptoms of HF so it is important to maintain a high index of suspicion for cardiac decompensation. Management is symptomatic based on guideline-directed medical therapy regardless of etiology in the setting of DCM, with special considerations for PPCM and with modification of medications as required during pregnancy. Goals of therapy are maintenance of normal volume status, treatment of arrhythmias, and prevention of thromboembolic complications. Pre-pregnancy counseling should be performed when possible focusing on maternal functional status and ventricular function and optimization of medical therapy. When a genetic etiology is known, patients should be informed about the risk of transmission to offspring based on the inheritance pattern. During pregnancy and postpartum, a multidisciplinary team approach is imperative. Transthoracic echocardiography and measurement of plasma natriuretic peptides, along with careful history and frequent reassessment, are the mainstays of follow-up during pregnancy and the puerperium.

TABLE 12.4

Common Therapies for Cardiomyopathy

Commonly Used	Indication	Maternal Caution	Fetal Caution
Beta-blockers	Improve neurohormonal axis Reduce mortality	Avoid initiation or up-titration with ADHF	IUGR, SGA, bradycardia
Ace-i/ARB/ARNi	↓ Afterload and preload; ↓ Morbidity, mortality, and hospitalizations	Hypotension, cough, angioedema, ↑ potassium, ↓ renal function	Teratogenic Renal agenesis, limb contractures, skull or lung hypoplasia, death
Diuretics	↓ Lung congestion, ↓ preload; improved symptoms	Electrolyte abnormalities Hypotension, hypovolemia, azotemia	Maternal overdiuresis can result in ↓ placental perfusion, neonatal ↓ Na+
Selected Therapies			
Hydralazine/nitrates	↓ Afterload and preload	First line during pregnancy or other contraindication to Ace-I, ARB, ARNi Lupus-like syndrome, reflex tachycardia	Fetal thrombocytopenia
Aldosterone antagonist	Mortality and morbidity benefit if NYHA class II-IV function on beta-blocker/Ace-i/ARB	Little data in pregnancy; generally not used	Little data in humans Spironolactone has anti-androgenic effects T1 Eplerenone had adverse effects in animal reproduction studies
Ivabradine	Symptomatic HF with EF <35% and HR >70 bpm on maximum beta-blocker	No data during human pregnancy; not recommended to use	Animal reproduction studies have shown adverse effects
Digoxin	Persistent symptoms despite therapy; no mortality benefit	Narrow therapeutic index Generally considered safe with pregnancy	Transmitted to fetus Low birth weight but has been used for fetal arrhythmias
Antiarrhythmic therapy	Serious arrhythmias and SCD prevention Amiodarone Disopyramide in HCM to ↓ LVOTO	Amiodarone: ↓ or ↑ thyroid function, pulmonary toxicity, liver abnormalities, proarrhythmia generally related to cumulative dose Disopyramide: Uterine contractions, placental abruption, prolonged QT	Amiodarone: Congenital goiter, thyroid disorders (hypothyroidism), QT prolongation, neurodevelopmental abnormalities, prematurity Use only after other therapy fails Fetal effects unrelated to duration of use or dose
Anticoagulation	LV thrombus, atrial fibrillation	Increased bleeding risk, DOAC not recommended during pregnancy	Potential for warfarin embryopathy, spontaneous bleeding
ICD	Prevention of SCD	Successful pregnancies reported with ICD in place If cesarean delivery, adjustments to prevent inappropriate function from electrical interference	Radiation exposure if implantation during pregnancy Life-threatening fetal arrhythmias unlikely with discharge
Biventricular pacing	Cardiac resynchronization	Same as above	Unknown
Inotropes	Persistent/palliation with refractory HF; similar indications during pregnancy	Increased arrhythmias, tachycardia	Unknown; maternal well-being benefit deciding factor
LVAD/ transplantation	Advanced HF interventions	Pregnancy not recommended with LVAD, although rare case reports; requires anticoagulation Risk of rejection with transplantation, adequacy of transplanted heart to support pregnancy	Teratogenicity of immunosuppressive agents

Abbreviations: IUGR, intrauterine growth retardation; SGA, small for gestational age; Ace-I, angiotensin-converting enzyme inhibitor; ARB, angiotensin receptor blocker; ARNi, angiotensin receptor-neprilysin inhibitor; Na+, sodium; NYHA, NYHA functional class; T1, first trimester; HF, heart failure; EF, ejection fraction; HR, heart rate; SCD, sudden cardiac death; ICD, implantable cardiac defibrillator; HCM, hypertrophic cardiomyopathy; LVOTO, left ventricular outflow tract obstruction; DOAC, direct oral anticoagulant; LVAD, left ventricular assist device.

REFERENCES

1. Maron BJ et al. Contemporary definitions and classification of the cardiomyopathies: An American Heart Association Scientific Statement from the Council on Clinical Cardiology, Heart Failure and Transplantation Committee; Quality of Care and Outcomes Research and Functional Genomics and Translational Biology Interdisciplinary Working Groups; and Council on Epidemiology and Prevention. *Circulation.* 2006;113(14):1807–16.

2. Elliott P et al. Classification of the cardiomyopathies: A position statement from the European Society of Cardiology Working Group on Myocardial and Pericardial Diseases. *Eur Heart J.* 2008;29(2):270–6.

3. Richardson P et al. Report of the 1995 World Health Organization/International Society and Federation of Cardiology task force on the definition and classification of cardiomyopathies. *Circulation.* 1996;93(5):841–2.

4. Arbustini E et al. The MOGE(S) classification for a phenotype-genotype nomenclature of cardiomyopathy: Endorsed by the World Heart Federation. *J Am Coll Cardiol.* 2013;62(22):2046–72.

5. Bozkurt B et al. Current diagnostic and treatment strategies for specific dilated cardiomyopathies: A scientific statement from the American Heart Association. *Circulation.* 2016;134(23):e579–646.

6. Yancy CW et al. 2013 ACCF/AHA Guideline for the Management of Heart Failure: Executive Summary: A Report of the American College of Cardiology Foundation/American Heart Association Task Force on Practice Guidelines. *Circulation.* 2013;62(16):e147–239.

7. Elkayam U, Gleicher N. Hemodynamics and cardiac function during normal pregnancy and the puerperium. In: Elkayam U (ed.) *Cardiac Problems in Pregnancy Diagnosis and Management of Maternal and Fetal Heart Disease,* 1998, Wiley-Liss, Inc, New York, pp. 3–20.

8. Ouzounian JG, Elkayam U. Physiologic changes during normal pregnancy and delivery. *Cardiol Clin.* 2012;30(3):317–29.

9. Ferrero S, Colombo BM, Ragni N. Maternal arrhythmias during pregnancy. *Arch Gynecol Obstet.* 2004;269(4):244–53.

10. Roos-Hesselink JW et al. Outcome of pregnancy in patients with structural or ischaemic heart disease: Results of a registry of the European Society of Cardiology. *Eur Heart J.* 2013;34(9):657–65.

11. Ruys TP et al. Heart failure in pregnant women with cardiac disease: Data from the ROPAC. *Heart* 2014;100(3):231–8.

12. Hameed AB et al. Pregnancy-related cardiovascular deaths in California: Beyond peripartum cardiomyopathy. *Am J Obstet Gynecol.* 2015;213(3):379.e1–10.

13. Briller J, Koch AR, Geller SE. Maternal cardiovascular mortality in Illinois, 2002–2011. *Obstet Gynecol.* 2017;129(5):819–26.

14. Silversides CK et al. Pregnancy outcomes in women with heart disease: The CARPREG II study. *J Am Coll Cardiol.* 2018;71(21):2419–30.

15. Mogos MF, Piano MR, McFarlin BL, Salemi JL, Liese KL, Briller JE. Heart failure in pregnant women: A concern across the pregnancy continuum. *Circ Heart Fail.* 2018;11(1):e004005.

16. Arany Z, Elkayam U. Peripartum cardiomyopathy. *Circulation.* 2016;133(14):1397–409.

17. Kolte D et al. Temporal trends in incidence and outcomes of peripartum cardiomyopathy in the United States: A nationwide population-based study. *J Am Heart Assoc.* 2014;3(3):e001056.

18. Fett JD, Christie LG, Carraway RD, Murphy JG. Five-year prospective study of the incidence and prognosis of peripartum cardiomyopathy at a single institution. *Mayo Clinic Proc.* 2005;80(12):1602–6.

19. Isezuo SA, Abubakar SA. Epidemiologic profile of peripartum cardiomyopathy in a tertiary care hospital. *Ethn Dis.* 2007;17(2):228–33.

20. Boyle S et al. Dilated cardiomyopathy in pregnancy: Outcomes from an Australian Tertiary Centre for Maternal Medicine and review of the current literature. *Heart Lung Circul.* 2019;28(4):591–7.

21. Armstrong GT et al. Comprehensive echocardiographic detection of treatment-related cardiac dysfunction in adult survivors of childhood cancer: Results from the St. Jude Lifetime Cohort Study. *J Am Coll Cardiol.* 2015;65(23):2511–22.

22. Grewal J et al. Pregnancy outcomes in women with dilated cardiomyopathy. *J Am Coll Cardiol.* 2009;55(1):45–52.

23. Siu SC et al. Prospective multicenter study of pregnancy outcomes in women with heart disease. *Circulation.* 2001;104(5):515–21.

24. Bernstein PS, Magriples U. Cardiomyopathy in pregnancy: A retrospective study. *Am J Perinatol.* 2001;18(3):163–8.

25. Avila WS et al. Pregnancy in patients with heart disease: Experience with 1,000 cases. *Clin Cardiol.* 2003;26(3):135–42.

26. Hershberger RE, Siegfried JD. Update 2011: Clinical and genetic issues in familial dilated cardiomyopathy. *J Am Coll Cardiol.* 2011;57(16):1641–9.

27. Burkett EL, Hershberger RE. Clinical and genetic issues in familial dilated cardiomyopathy. *J Am Coll Cardiol.* 2005;45(7):969–81.

28. Krul SP, van der Smagt JJ, van den Berg MP, Sollie KM, Pieper PG, van Spaendonck-Zwarts KY. Systematic review of pregnancy in women with inherited cardiomyopathies. *Eur J Heart Fail.* 2011;13(6):584–94.

29. Sliwa K et al. Current state of knowledge on aetiology, diagnosis, management, and therapy of peripartum cardiomyopathy: A position statement from the Heart Failure Association of the European Society of Cardiology Working Group on peripartum cardiomyopathy. *Eur J Heart Fail.* 2010;12(8):767–78.

30. Bello N, Rendon IS, Arany Z. The relationship between pre-eclampsia and peripartum cardiomyopathy: A systematic review and meta-analysis. *J Am Coll Cardiol.* 2013;62(18):1715–23.

31. Elkayam U. Clinical characteristics of peripartum cardiomyopathy in the United States: Diagnosis, prognosis, and management. *J Am Coll Cardiol.* 2011;58(7):659–70.

32. Elkayam U et al. Pregnancy-associated cardiomyopathy: Clinical characteristics and a comparison between early and late presentation. *Circulation.* 2005;111(16):2050–5.

33. Kao DP, Hsich E, Lindenfeld J. Characteristics, adverse events, and racial differences among delivering mothers with peripartum cardiomyopathy. *JACC Heart Fail.* 2013;1(5):409–16.

34. Hilfiker-Kleiner D et al. A cathepsin D-cleaved 16 kDa form of prolactin mediates postpartum cardiomyopathy. *Cell* 2007;128(3):589–600.

35. Patten IS et al. Cardiac angiogenic imbalance leads to peripartum cardiomyopathy. *Nature* 2012;485(7398):333–8.

36. Ware JS et al. Shared genetic predisposition in peripartum and dilated cardiomyopathies. *N Engl J Med.* 2016;374(26):2601–2.

37. Felker GM et al. Underlying causes and long-term survival in patients with initially unexplained cardiomyopathy. *N Engl J Med.* 2000;342(15):1077–84.

38. Sliwa K et al. Long-term prognosis, subsequent pregnancy, contraception and overall management of peripartum cardiomyopathy: Practical guidance paper from the Heart Failure Association of the European Society of Cardiology Study Group on Peripartum Cardiomyopathy. *Eur J Heart Fail.* 2018;20(6):951–62.

39. McNamara DM et al. Clinical Outcomes for Peripartum Cardiomyopathy in North America: Results of the IPAC Study (Investigations of Pregnancy-Associated Cardiomyopathy). *J Am Coll Cardiol.* 2015;66(8):905–14.

40. Blauwet LA et al. Predictors of outcome in 176 South African patients with peripartum cardiomyopathy. *Heart.* 2013;99(5):308–13.

41. Blauwet LA et al. Right ventricular function in peripartum cardiomyopathy at presentation is associated with subsequent left ventricular recovery and clinical outcomes. *Circul Heart Fail.* 2016;9(5).

42. Haghikia A et al. Phenotyping and outcome on contemporary management in a German cohort of patients with peripartum cardiomyopathy. *Basic Res Cardiol.* 2013;108(4):366.

43. Hu CL et al. Troponin T measurement can predict persistent left ventricular dysfunction in peripartum cardiomyopathy. *Heart.* 2007;93(4):488–90.

44. Harper MA, Meyer RE, Berg CJ. Peripartum cardiomyopathy: Population-based birth prevalence and 7-year mortality. *Obstet Gynecol.* 2012;120(5):1013–9.

45. Goland S, Modi K, Hatamizadeh P, Elkayam U. Differences in clinical profile of African-American women with peripartum cardiomyopathy in the United States. *J Card Fail.* 2013;19(4):214–8.

46. Irizarry OC et al. Comparison of clinical characteristics and outcomes of peripartum cardiomyopathy between African American and non-African American women. *JAMA Cardiol.* 2017;2(11):1256–60.

47. Gunderson EP, Croen LA, Chiang V, Yoshida CK, Walton D, Go AS. Epidemiology of peripartum cardiomyopathy: Incidence, predictors, and outcomes. *Obstet Gynecol.* 2011;118(3):583–91.

48. Sliwa K et al. Clinical characteristics of patients from the worldwide registry on peripartum cardiomyopathy (PPCM): EURObservational Research Programme in conjunction with the Heart Failure Association of the European Society of Cardiology Study Group on PPCM. *Eur J Heart Fail.* 2017;19(9):1131–41.

49. Spark RF, Pallotta J, Naftolin F, Clemens R. Galactorrhea-amenorrhea syndromes: Etiology and treatment. *Ann Intern Med.* 1976;84(5):532–7.

50. Sliwa K et al. Evaluation of bromocriptine in the treatment of acute severe peripartum cardiomyopathy: A proof-of-concept pilot study. *Circulation.* 2010;121(13):1465–73.

51. Hilfiker-Kleiner D et al. Bromocriptine for the treatment of peripartum cardiomyopathy: A multicentre randomized study. *Eur Heart J.* 2017;38(35):2671–9.

52. Haghikia A et al. Bromocriptine treatment in patients with peripartum cardiomyopathy and right ventricular dysfunction. *Clin Res Cardiol.* 2019;108(3):290–7.

53. Ersboll AS, Arany Z, Gustafsson F. Bromocriptine for the treatment of peripartum cardiomyopathy: Comparison of outcome with a Danish cohort. *Eur Heart J.* 2018;39(37): 3476–7.

54. Regitz-Zagrosek V et al. 2018 ESC Guidelines for the management of cardiovascular diseases during pregnancy. *Eur Heart J.* 2018:77(3):245–326.

55. Talle MA, Buba F, Anjorin CO. Prevalence and aetiology of left ventricular thrombus in patients undergoing transthoracic echocardiography at the University of Maiduguri Teaching Hospital. *Adv Med.* 2014;2014:731936.

56. Bauersachs J et al. Current management of patients with severe acute peripartum cardiomyopathy: Practical guidance from the Heart Failure Association of the European Society of Cardiology Study Group on peripartum cardiomyopathy. *Eur J Heart Fail.* 2016;18(9):1096–105.

57. Elkayam U, Goland S, Pieper PG, Silverside CK. High-risk cardiac disease in pregnancy: Part II. *J Am Coll Cardiol.* 2016:68(5):502–16.

58. Safirstein JG, Ro AS, Grandhi S, Wang L, Fett JD, Staniloae C. Predictors of left ventricular recovery in a cohort of peripartum cardiomyopathy patients recruited via the internet. *Int J Cardiol.* 2012;154(1):27–31.

59. Codsi E, Rose CH, Blauwet LA. Subsequent pregnancy outcomes in patients with peripartum cardiomyopathy. *Obstet Gynecol.* 2018;131(2):322–7.

60. Elkayam U et al. Maternal and fetal outcomes of subsequent pregnancies in women with peripartum cardiomyopathy. *N Engl J Med.* 2001;344(21):1567–71.

61. Elkayam U. Risk of subsequent pregnancy in women with a history of peripartum cardiomyopathy. *J Am Coll Cardiol.* 2014;64(15):1629–36.

62. Guldbrandt Hauge M, Johansen M, Vejlstrup N, Gustafsson F, Damm P, Ersboll AS. Subsequent reproductive outcome among women with peripartum cardiomyopathy: A nationwide study. *BJOG.* 2018;125(8):1018–25.

63. Fett JD, Fristoe KL, Welsh SN. Risk of heart failure relapse in subsequent pregnancy among peripartum cardiomyopathy mothers. *Int J Gynaecol Obstet.* 2010;109(1):34–6.

64. Lampert MB, Weinert L, Hibbard J, Korcarz C, Lindheimer M, Lang RM. Contractile reserve in patients with peripartum cardiomyopathy and recovered left ventricular function. *Am J Obstet Gynecol.* 1997;176(1 Pt 1):189–95.

65. Fett JD. Personal commentary: Monitoring subsequent pregnancy in recovered peripartum cardiomyopathy mothers. *Crit Pathw Cardiol.* 2009;8(4):172–4.

66. Fett JD. Validation of a self-test for early diagnosis of heart failure in peripartum cardiomyopathy. *Crit Pathw Cardiol.* 2011;10(1):44–5.

67. Authors/Task Force m, Elliott PM et al. 2014 ESC Guidelines on diagnosis and management of hypertrophic cardiomyopathy: The Task Force for the Diagnosis and Management of Hypertrophic Cardiomyopathy of the European Society of Cardiology (ESC). *Eur Heart J.* 2014;35(39):2733–79.

68. Semsarian C, Ingles J, Maron MS, Maron BJ. New perspectives on the prevalence of hypertrophic cardiomyopathy. *J Am Coll Cardiol.* 2015;65(12):1249–54.

69. Ingles J, Burns C, Barratt A, Semsarian C. Application of genetic testing in hypertrophic cardiomyopathy for preclinical disease detection. *Circ Cardiovasc Genet.* 2015;8(6):852–9.

70. Aquaro GD et al. Usefulness of delayed enhancement by magnetic resonance imaging in hypertrophic cardiomyopathy as a marker of disease and its severity. *Am J Cardiol.* 2010;105(3):392–7.

71. Schinkel AF. Pregnancy in women with hypertrophic cardiomyopathy. *Cardiol Rev.* 2014;22(5):217–22.

72. Goland S et al. Pregnancy in women with hypertrophic cardiomyopathy: Data from the European Society of Cardiology initiated Registry of Pregnancy and Cardiac disease (ROPAC). *Eur Heart J.* 2017;38(35):2683–90.

73. Corrado D, Thiene G. Arrhythmogenic right ventricular cardiomyopathy/dysplasia: Clinical impact of molecular genetic studies. *Circulation.* 2006;113(13):1634–7.

74. Gandjbakhch E et al. Pregnancy and newborn outcomes in arrhythmogenic right ventricular cardiomyopathy/dysplasia. *Int J Cardiol.* 2018;258:172–8.

75. Bhatia NL, Tajik AJ, Wilansky S, Steidley DE, Mookadam F. Isolated noncompaction of the left ventricular myocardium in adults: A systematic overview. *J Card Fail.* 2011;17(9):771–8.

76. Sugishita K et al. Postpartum complete atrioventricular block due to cardiac sarcoidosis: Steroid therapy without permanent pacemaker. *Int Heart J.* 2008;49(3):377–84.

77. Ertekin E, Roos-Hesselink JW, Moosa S, Sliwa K. Two cases of cardiac sarcoidosis in pregnant women with supraventricular arrhythmia. *Cardiovasc J Afr.* 2015;26(2):96–100.

78. Nayak UA, Shekhar SP, Sundari N. A rare case of pregnancy with restrictive cardiomyopathy. *J Cardiovasc Echogr.* 2016;26(2):65–7.

79. Stergiopoulos K, Shiang E, Bench T. Pregnancy in patients with pre-existing cardiomyopathies. *J Am Coll Cardiol.* 2011;58(4):337–50.

80. Halpern DG, Weinberg CR, Pinnelas R, Mehta-Lee S, Economy KE, Valente AM. Use of medication for cardiovascular disease during pregnancy: JACC state-of-the-art review. *J Am Coll Cardiol.* 2019;73(4):457–76.

81. Hameed AB, Chan K, Ghamsary M, Elkayam U. Longitudinal changes in the B-type natriuretic peptide levels in normal pregnancy and postpartum. *Clin Cardiol.* 2009;32(8):E60–2.

82. Moghbeli N et al. N-terminal pro-brain natriuretic peptide as a biomarker for hypertensive disorders of pregnancy. *Am J Perinatol.* 2010;27(4):313–9.

13

Vascular Disease and Dissection in Pregnancy

Melinda B. Davis

KEY POINTS

- Pregnancy increases the risk or aortic dissection by 25-fold above the baseline for the general population
- The most common risk factor for aortic aneurysm and dissection is hypertension that is most frequently encountered in the third trimester of pregnancy
- Spontaneous coronary artery dissection is the most common cause of myocardial infarction in pregnancy

---

Introduction

Women with vascular diseases are at increased risk for complications during pregnancy and the early postpartum period. Unfortunately, the initial presentation for women with underlying vascular disease may be with a catastrophic complication, such as aortic or coronary dissection, and may present during pregnancy. Women at risk for vascular complications include those with connective tissue disorders, such as Marfan syndrome, Ehlers-Danlos syndrome (EDS), and Loeys-Dietz syndrome; other disorders associated with aortopathy, such as bicuspid aortic valve (BAV) and Turner syndrome; and other systemic vascular disorders such as fibromuscular dysplasia. These conditions pose high risk of maternal, obstetric, and fetal complications, and appropriate management requires multiple subspecialties. In some situations, pregnancy is contraindicated. This chapter will address vascular disorders that may affect women during childbearing; major complications, including coronary and aortic dissections; and considerations for preconception counseling, antepartum, labor and delivery, and postpartum care. Genetic counseling and prenatal diagnosis of offspring should be considered.

Epidemiology

Vascular complications that occur in young women of childbearing age are most commonly related to underlying conditions. Many of these diseases may be undiagnosed in young women during pregnancy but only come to attention after an acute presentation of vascular dissection [1,2]. The true prevalence of vascular disorders and dissections in pregnancy is likely to be underestimated due to low suspicion and missed opportunities for diagnosis.

The incidence of aortic dissection in the normal population is approximately 6 per 100,000 individuals per year. Women with vascular diseases have higher risk. In the absence of pregnancy, the incidence of aortic dissection is 170 per 100,000 in Marfan syndrome [3], 36 per 100,000 in Turner syndrome [4], and 31 per 100,000 in BAV [5]. Pregnancy increases the risk 25-fold [6]. Clearly, aortic dissection can have devastating consequences. In a study of maternal mortality in the Netherlands, half of the total maternal deaths (3 per 100,000 deliveries) were attributed to aortic dissection [7]. Aortic dissections can occur in the first trimester (5%), second trimester (10%), third trimester (50%), and postpartum (20%) [8].

Spontaneous coronary artery dissection (SCAD) may account for 1%–4% of all acute coronary syndromes, but 35% of cases in women under age 50 [9]. SCAD is the most common cause of pregnancy-associated myocardial infarction, accounting for 43% of cases [10]. Pregnancy-associated SCAD portends worse outcomes with higher troponin, lower LV function, more congestive heart failure, and cardiogenic shock [11,12]. Most cases occur during late pregnancy or early postpartum, with the highest incidence being the first week postpartum; however, pregnancy-associated SCAD has been reported as little as 2 weeks after conception and >12 months postpartum, especially in women who are breastfeeding [2,13].

Vascular Disorders

Several vascular disorders cause increased risk of cardiovascular complications during pregnancy, and many have underlying genetic abnormalities. Women who present with vascular complications should undergo workup for the presence of underlying vascular diseases, and be offered genetic counseling when appropriate. Additional risk factors for aortic dissection include prior history of cardiac surgery and cardiac catheterization. Stressors that can increase the vascular wall stress and precipitate vascular dissections include hypertension, pheochromocytoma, cocaine and other stimulant drugs, weight-lifting and intense Valsalva, trauma, deceleration injury, intense emotional stress, and labor and delivery. *The most common risk factor for aortic aneurysm and dissection is hypertension.* Specific vascular disorders include Marfan syndrome, EDS, BAV, Turner syndrome, and fibromuscular dysplasia (Table 13.1).

Marfan Syndrome

Marfan syndrome is an autosomal dominant disorder caused by various mutations in the gene (*FBN-1* on chromosome 15) that encode for extracellular matrix protein fibrillin I [14,15]. Marfan syndrome has an estimated incidence of 1 in 5000 and involves skeletal, ocular, and cardiovascular systems. Most patients have cardiovascular involvement, and the presence of aortic dilatation confers high risk for morbidity and mortality. Valvular disease, including aortic regurgitation and prolapse of the mitral and tricuspid valves, can lead to arrhythmias and heart failure, and premature rupture of membranes can occur during pregnancy [16,17]. Clinical heterogeneity, even among individuals with the same genetic mutation, can add to the complexity of diagnosis. The original diagnostic criteria, known as the *Ghent Nosology*, was published in 1996, which was later revised to include many patients who do not have the fibrillin 1 mutation. The diagnosis can be challenging, and a multidisciplinary team should be involved, including clinical genetics. The diagnosis is sometimes only considered after a life-threatening complication occurs during pregnancy [17,18].

Vascular Ehlers-Danlos Syndrome

Vascular Ehlers-Danlos syndrome (EDS) (type IV) is inherited in an autosomal dominant pattern related to mutations in the *COL3A1* gene. Patients with EDS are at high risk of early death due to arterial, intestinal, and uterine rupture. Arterial complications occur in an unpredictable manner, even without arterial dilatation, and surgical repair is challenging due to the friable nature of the vascular tissue. Vascular EDS poses a high risk of obstetric complications, and deaths can occur from arterial dissection or uterine rupture. In a study of 81 pregnancies, 12 women died (14.8%) [19]. A subsequent study of 565 pregnancies reported arterial dissection in 9.2%, uterine rupture in 2.6%, and maternal deaths in 6.5% [20]. Other obstetric complications in women with all types of EDS include separation of the symphysis pubis, severe postpartum hemorrhage, and preterm delivery. Pregnancy is considered contraindicated in women with vascular EDS due to the high risk of mortality, but shared decision making is essential, and women who choose to pursue pregnancy should be followed by a multidisciplinary team at a specialized center [20,21].

Bicuspid Aortic Valve

Bicuspid aortic valve (BAV) is one of the most common congenital heart defects and is present in about 1% of the population. BAV is associated with histopathologic abnormalities of the ascending aorta leading to dilation and aneurysm [22]. Among young patients <40 years with aortic dissection, BAV was present in 9% [23]. Patients with BAV should be screened for the coexistence of aortic coarctation by clinical examination and imaging, since coarctation can compound the risk of aortic aneurysms [24]. First-degree relatives of patients with BAV should also be offered screening echocardiogram to assess for valve disease and aortopathy (class IIa) [24].

Turner Syndrome

Turner syndrome is caused by the loss of part or all of the X chromosome and occurs in 1 in 2500 girls. Pregnancy in women with Turner syndrome can occur spontaneously in women with mosaic pattern (0.5%–10%), but otherwise occurs with assisted fertility treatment. Women should undergo cardiovascular evaluation prior to beginning fertility therapy [25] because Turner syndrome is associated with congenital heart disease, aortic dilatation, hypertension, diabetes, and atherosclerotic disease, as well as preeclampsia [26]. Blood pressure control and diabetes management are important. During pregnancy, the risk of death from aortic dissection may be 2%, and the risk may increase with concomitant BAV and/or aortic coarctation [27].

Fibromuscular Dysplasia

Fibromuscular dysplasia (FMD) is a vascular disease associated with arterial tortuosity, stenosis, and aneurysms in any arterial bed, but most commonly in the renal arteries, carotid arteries, and intracranial arteries [28]. Coronary dissections and aortic aneurysms can occur. Patients who present with SCAD are frequently diagnosed with FMD in another arterial circulation. Due to the high incidence of arterial aneurysms and dissections, every patient with FMD is recommended to undergo one-time head-to-pelvis cross-sectional imaging with CTA or MRA. FMD should also be suspected in young women with hypertension, severe persistent headache, TIA or stroke, aneurysms, renal infarction, or in the presence of an abdominal or carotid bruit [29].

Vascular Complications during Pregnancy

The hemodynamic stress of pregnancy (increase in blood volume, heart rate, stroke volume, and cardiac output) [30,31], partially offset by decreased peripheral vascular resistance and diastolic blood pressure, may contribute to increased risk of vascular complications during pregnancy. In addition, histologic changes in the aorta that predispose to vascular fragility that are related to the hormonal changes of pregnancy include decreased acid mucopolysaccharides, loss of normal corrugation of elastic fibers, and fragmentation of the aortic reticulin fibers [32,33]. The hemodynamic and hormonal changes increase susceptibility to vascular dissections, particularly in women with preexisting abnormal structure of the vasculature related to connective tissue diseases or fibromuscular dysplasia. Labor and delivery may cause increased aortic and coronary shear stress. Complications can occur at any time during pregnancy, but after the second trimester or postpartum are the highest risk [34]. Among women with SCAD, the highest incidence occurs in the first month postpartum, particularly in the first week, suggesting a contribution from uterine contraction and the massive increase in blood volume post-delivery [12].

Women with vascular diseases can suffer from several types of complications during pregnancy, including myocardial infarction, cardiogenic shock, hemorrhage, heart failure, arrhythmias, and venous thromboembolism. Two of the most feared complications are aortic dissection and coronary artery dissection.

TABLE 13.1

Vascular Diseases, Phenotypes, Genetic Mutations, and Considerations for Pregnancy

Vascular Disease	Clinical Phenotype	Vascular Features	Genetic Mutations	Consider Prophylactic Surgery before Pregnancy	Management	Follow-Up Surveillance Postpartum
Marfan syndrome	• Aortic dilatation • Ectopia lentis • Various characteristic musculoskeletal abnormalities, as well as skin, lung, and CNS	• Aortic dilatation (in 60%–80% of patients) and often starts initially at root	FBN1	≥45 mm aortic diameter (or less if other risk factors)	• Beta-blockers • Consider addition of ARB (but contraindicated in pregnancy) • ? Limited data suggests avoiding CCB	• Echo and CT/MRI initially; 6 months • If stable and echo correlates with CT/MRI, CT/MRI every 3–5 years (or more often if screening descending/abdominal aorta) • If stable and <45 mm, then annual imaging • If ≥45 mm, more often (every 6 months)
Loeys-Dietz	• Craniofacial (hypertelorism, bifid uvula, cleft palate)	• Arterial tortuosity • Dissection often at aortic root, but widespread arterial involvement	TGFBR1 TGFBR2 SMAD3 TGFB2 TGFB3	≥45 mm aortic diameter (or less if other risk factors)	• Consider prophylactic surgery • Consider ARBs and/or beta-blockers	• Annual MRI (or CT) from cerebral to pelvic circulation
Vascular Ehlers-Danlos (type IV)	• Thin translucent skin • Easy bruising • Facial features (tight skin, pinched nose, thin lips) • Rupture of visceral organs	• Dilatation of aorta may not precede dissection • Entire aorta and branches at risk	COL3A1 – Type III procollagen	Pregnancy considered contraindicated. Surgery reserved for life-threatening complications or high-risk aneurysms	• Celiprolol or other beta-blockers may reduce risk of aortic dissection	• Annual carotid and abdominal US • Consider thoracic aortic surveillance
Familial TAAD	• Non-syndromic • Variable associations (i.e., patent ductus arteriosus, livedo reticularis, etc.)	• Some may have dissection without preceding dilatation	ACTA2 MYH11 TGFBR2 MYLK PRKG1	≥50 mm aortic diameter; however, lack of data and attention to family history is needed	• May consider beta-blocker, but limited data	• Consider routine serial screening • Screen at risk relatives
Turner syndrome	• Short stature • Premature ovarian failure • Metabolic syndrome (obesity, glucose intolerance, hyperlipidemia) • Hypertension	• Associated with BAV in 30% and coarctation of the aorta in 12% • Dilatation often at root/ascending aorta	45XO karyotype	ASI ≥27 mm/m²	• Index the aorta diameter for BSA • Consider ARBs/ACEi and/or beta-blockers	• TTE/MRI surveillance based on aortic dimensions
Bicuspid aortic valve	• Present in 2% of the population	• Dilatation of the ascending aorta, independent of valve function	NOTCH1	≥50 mm aortic diameter (some consider if >45 mm; or if ≥5 mm increase per year)	• Consider beta-blockers during pregnancy if aorta dilated	• MRI or CT to evaluate entire aorta • Screen first-degree relatives • Follow-up imaging customized to the individual
Fibromuscular dysplasia (FMD)	• Idiopathic disease of the arterial walls leading to aneurysm, tortuosity, and dissection	• Aneurysms can occur in renal, carotid, intracranial, mesenteric, coronary arteries and aorta	May be sporadic PHACTR1	Not applicable	• Manage hypertension	• Follow-up imaging customized to the individual • Patients with SCAD need postpartum imaging from brain to pelvis to assess for FMD

Note: Additional risk factors for aortic aneurysms: family history of aortic dissection, growth rate ≥3 mm/year, hypertension. Factors that may influence the decision to proceed with prophylactic aortic repair surgery include severe mitral or aortic regurgitation and other indications for cardiac surgery such as coronary artery bypass grafting.

Abbreviations: CNS, central nervous system; CCB, calcium channel blocker; TGFBR1, TGF-beta receptor 1; TGFBR2, TGF-beta receptor 2; SMAD3, SMAD family member 3; TGFB2, TGF-beta 2 ligand; TGFB3, TGF-beta 3 ligand; ACTA2, smooth muscle alpha-2-actin; MYH11, smooth muscle myosin heavy chain; TGFBR2, TGF-beta receptor 2; MYLK, myosin light-chain kinase; PRKG1, type I cGMP-dependent protein kinase regulating smooth muscle cell relaxation; BSA, body surface area; ARB, angiotensin receptor blocker; ACEi, angiotensin converting enzyme inhibitor.

Aortic Dissection

Aortic dissection occurs when an interruption in the medial layer of the aorta allows intramural hemorrhage and propagation of blood, resulting in a sudden, severe, tearing type of pain with radiation to the back. The dissection can propagate to the aortic valve causing aortic regurgitation, or blood may enter the pericardial space causing cardiac tamponade. If branch vessels are involved, ischemia of the coronary, carotid, spinal, or visceral arteries can occur.

Precise classification of thoracic aortic dissections is important. The Stanford classification scheme includes type A dissections (involving the ascending aorta) and type B dissections (involving the descending aorta, and not the ascending aorta) (Figure 13.1). The DeBakey classification scheme describes dissections in the ascending aorta, arch, and descending aorta (type I); those that are confined to the ascending aorta (type II); and those that involve the descending aorta (type III). Early and accurate diagnosis of aortic dissection is essential (Figure 13.2).

Symptoms of Aortic Dissection

1. *Pain*: Abrupt, acute onset of pain in the chest or back occurs in 90% of patients characterized as sharp, knife-like, worst-ever pain, unlike any pain previously experienced, that leads patients to seek medical attention within minutes to hours. Symptom constellation correlates to the involved segments of the aorta. Symptoms may also include those of heart failure, stroke, acute coronary syndrome, pericardial tamponade, or abdominal pain. Painless dissection is uncommon but can occur.
2. *Syncope*: Loss of consciousness occurs in 5%–10% and often indicates involvement of the brachiocephalic vessels or cardiac tamponade [35].

Physical Exam Findings of Aortic Dissection

1. *Pulse and blood pressure deficit*: Bilateral pulses should be rapidly examined at bedside. Impaired blood flow to peripheral vessels can manifest as asymmetric or decreased pulsations in carotid, brachial, radial, or femoral pulses. Systolic blood pressure in bilateral arms may differ by >20 mmHg.
2. *Blood pressure*: While hypertension is a risk factor for developing aortic dissection, hypotension occurs in 12% of patients with type A ascending aorta dissections [36] and may be due to acute aortic regurgitation, cardiac tamponade, or malperfusion of the brachiocephalic vessels resulting in low brachial cuff pressures.
3. *Heart murmur*: Aortic regurgitation causes a diastolic decrescendo murmur and occurs when the aortic dissection extends to involve the aortic valve and complicates half to two-thirds of ascending dissections [36]. Other associated findings include wide pulse-pressure, hypotension, and/or heart failure.
4. *Focal neurologic deficits*: When branch arteries are involved in the dissection, neurologic deficits can include stroke or altered consciousness (from carotid artery involvement), hoarseness (from compression of the laryngeal nerve), or acute paraplegia (from spinal cord ischemia).

Diagnostic Testing for Aortic Dissection

Initial Testing

1. *Electrocardiogram (ECG)*: If the aortic dissection has extended to include the coronary arteries, findings consistent with acute myocardial infarction may be present, but this is not always evident on the ECG [37].

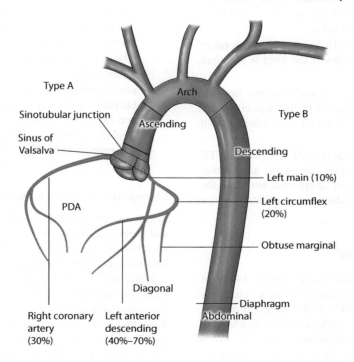

FIGURE 13.1 Classification of aortic anatomy and coronary anatomy with incidence of dissection.

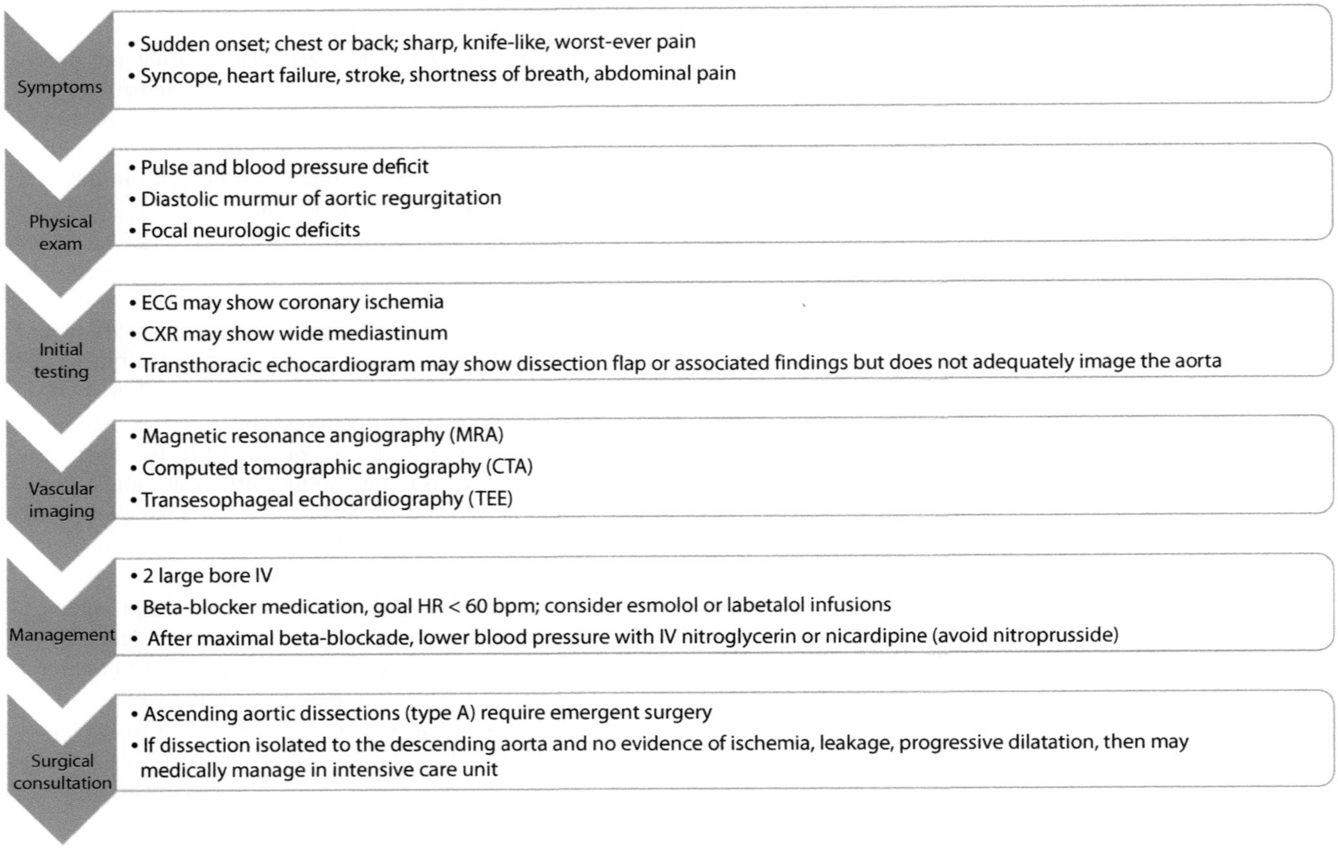

Symptoms	• Sudden onset; chest or back; sharp, knife-like, worst-ever pain • Syncope, heart failure, stroke, shortness of breath, abdominal pain
Physical exam	• Pulse and blood pressure deficit • Diastolic murmur of aortic regurgitation • Focal neurologic deficits
Initial testing	• ECG may show coronary ischemia • CXR may show wide mediastinum • Transthoracic echocardiogram may show dissection flap or associated findings but does not adequately image the aorta
Vascular imaging	• Magnetic resonance angiography (MRA) • Computed tomographic angiography (CTA) • Transesophageal echocardiography (TEE)
Management	• 2 large bore IV • Beta-blocker medication, goal HR < 60 bpm; consider esmolol or labetalol infusions • After maximal beta-blockade, lower blood pressure with IV nitroglycerin or nicardipine (avoid nitroprusside)
Surgical consultation	• Ascending aortic dissections (type A) require emergent surgery • If dissection isolated to the descending aorta and no evidence of ischemia, leakage, progressive dilatation, then may medically manage in intensive care unit

FIGURE 13.2 Algorithm for diagnosis and management of aortic dissection.

2. *Chest radiograph (CXR)*: Widening of the aortic silhouette may be seen on CXR but sensitivity is limited, and additional imaging is needed.

3. *D-dimer*: A low or negative D-dimer may be helpful in ruling out an aortic dissection if the level is less than 500 ng/mL [38].

4. *Troponin*: An elevated troponin level indicates myocardial ischemia from propagation of the dissection into the coronary arteries or subendocardial ischemia from hypotension.

5. *Transthoracic echocardiogram (TTE)*: A surface TTE may demonstrate a dissection flap at the aortic root, aortic valve regurgitation, or tamponade but lacks the necessary specificity and does not adequately image the entire aorta.

Diagnostic Vascular Imaging

1. *Magnetic resonance angiography (MRA)*: MRA of the aorta with gadolinium contrast has a sensitivity and specificity of 95%–100% [39]. MRA can only be used in hemodynamically stable patients with adequate monitoring. Although gadolinium contrast is often avoided during pregnancy, there are times when the benefit outweighs the risk [40,41].

2. *Computed tomographic angiography (CTA)*: The advantage of CTA is the widespread availability and speed. During pregnancy, ionizing radiation is often avoided but may be needed for the diagnosis of aortic dissection, which carries high mortality for both the mother and fetus.

3. *Transesophageal echocardiography (TEE)*: TEE can be useful during pregnancy or in hemodynamically unstable patients who cannot safely be transported to a scanner. However, limitations include operator availability, level of expertise, and the need for esophageal intubation requiring sedation, which may worsen hypotension.

Management of Acute Aortic Dissection

Aortic dissection of the ascending aorta is a surgical emergency and early consultation is necessary. Descending aortic dissections may also require emergency surgery, particularly if there is involvement of branch vessels or other evidence of malperfusion.

Initial medical management includes large bore intravenous access and continuous monitoring for heart rate and blood pressure, preferably with an arterial line. Standard treatment of aortic dissection involves controlling the heart rate to <60 beats per minute and systolic blood pressure to between 100–120 mmHg. Involvement of a maternal-fetal medicine specialist is needed to monitor the effects on the fetus. Beta-blockers decrease both hypertension and the pulsatile wall stress that can increase shear forces. Esmolol or labetalol infusions are first-line choices. If the systolic blood pressure is still >100 mmHg after maximal beta-blockade with heart rate <60 beats per minute, infusion of vaso-dilators such as nitroglycerin or nicardipine can further lower the blood pressure. Nitroprusside can cause fetal cyanide toxicity and should be avoided. Additional management includes IV opioids for pain control and a foley catheter to monitor urine output and renal perfusion. Only patients who do not require emergent/urgent surgery or stent-grafting can be managed medically in an intensive care unit. Transfer to a center with readily available surgical services may be necessary.

If acute type A dissection occurs during pregnancy, the surgical strategy depends on the gestational age of the fetus. Before 28 weeks' gestation, cardiac surgery with the fetus in utero is typically recommended. If the fetus is viable, a primary cesarean section followed directly by surgical repair of the aorta can be considered.

For type B dissection, the initial management strategy typically involves strict antihypertensive treatment. Surgery is indicated for type B dissections if there is evidence of leakage, rupture, progressive aortic dilatation, uncontrolled hypertension, compromise of an arterial trunk, extension of the dissection while on adequate medical therapy, or continued or recurrent pain.

Spontaneous Coronary Artery Dissection

Spontaneous coronary artery dissection (SCAD) occurs when an intimal tear or bleeding of the vasa vasorum causes an intramedial hemorrhage and a false lumen that fills with intramural hematoma and expands under pressure. SCAD can occur with or without atherosclerosis. The most frequently affected vessel is the left anterior descending artery in approximately 40%–70% of cases [13,42] (Figure 13.1). Dissection often occurs in a single coronary artery, but multiple vessels and noncontiguous segments can be involved [10,43]. Patients may present with STEMI, NSTEMI, or life-threatening arrhythmias.

Symptoms of SCAD

Diagnosis of an acute coronary syndrome and SCAD should be considered in any pregnant woman with chest pain or other angina equivalents, particularly in the absence of classic atherosclerotic risk factors. Signs and symptoms of SCAD are similar to those of acute myocardial infarction, with chest pain in 96% of cases. Other symptoms include pain in the neck, back, one or both arms, nausea and vomiting, diaphoresis, and shortness of breath.

Diagnostic Testing for SCAD

1. *Electrocardiogram* (ECG) should be performed immediately in women with chest pain or other symptoms concerning for acute coronary syndrome. SCAD may manifest as STEMI or NSTEMI. Even without evidence of ischemia on the ECG, a high index of suspicion should be maintained. Often repeat ECG is required to detect dynamic ECG changes and life-threatening arrhythmias.

2. *Troponin* elevation is indicative of coronary ischemia. Troponin should be serially measured in any woman presenting with chest pain or an angina equivalent.

3. *Coronary angiography* is the first-line diagnostic test for ACS, including pregnant women, with attempts to minimize the dose of radiation if possible. Several angiographic types of SCAD can be identified by an experienced operator [9]. Additional imaging techniques include optical coherence tomography and intravascular ultrasound; however, additional instrumentation carries high risk of propagation of the dissection.

4. *Coronary computed tomography angiography* (CCTA) can be considered as a noninvasive approach to diagnosis in women who are at low risk, but may lack sensitivity [9]. CCTA also involves radiation and contrast and may require high doses of beta-blockade.

Management of SCAD

After diagnosis by limited angiography, conservative therapy is often recommended (Figure 13.3). Stable patients with low-risk NSTEMI, normal TIMI grade 3 flow, and no critical stenosis can be treated conservatively. There are limited data to support follow-up stress testing or coronary angiography. Patients presenting with STEMI, NSTEMI with ongoing ischemia, unstable features, or hemodynamic instability should be revascularized with primary percutaneous coronary intervention (PCI) or bypass surgery. Instrumentation of the coronary arteries risks further propagation of the dissection due to fragility of the vessel wall. Other technical challenges include difficulty advancing wires through the true lumen, occlusion of side branches, dissection at the edges of stents, dissection in small caliber distal vessels, and extensive dissections that require long stents resulting in higher risk of stent thrombosis [9,29]. If there is any concern for cardiogenic shock, transfer to a facility with emergency mechanical circulatory support and close monitoring of mother and fetus is necessary. A delivery strategy should be in place in case of deterioration.

Medical management after SCAD includes long-term aspirin, beta-blocker, and 1 year of clopidogrel. Statin medications are used if the patient has dyslipidemia. Beta-blocker treatment has been associated with a lower risk of recurrent SCAD [44].

Management of Women with Vascular Disease

Preconception Management

Preconception counseling is essential for women with vascular disease given the known risks associated with pregnancy. Women need to be counseled differently based on their underlying disease condition. Women with aortopathy should undergo MRI (or CT) of the entire aorta prior to conception. Aortic dimensions for consideration of surgical repair prior to pregnancy are shown in Table 13.1. Additional risk factors include family history of aortic dissection or sudden death, the rate of growth (increase in diameter is ≥5 mm/year), and/or worsening aortic regurgitation [21,45]. Even after aortic replacement, risk for dissection in the distal aorta or other vascular beds remains [46]; however,

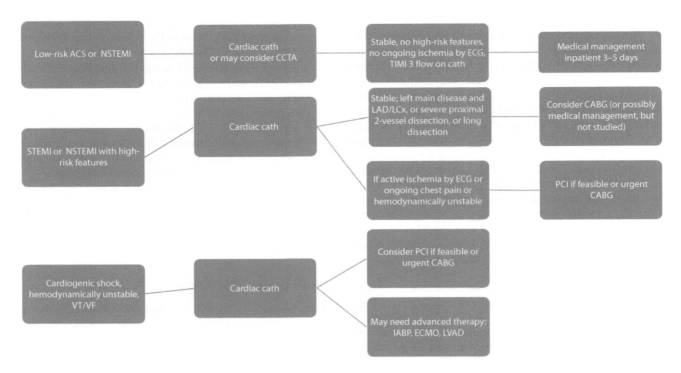

FIGURE 13.3 Algorithm for management of spontaneous coronary artery dissection (SCAD). *Abbreviations*: ACS, acute coronary syndrome; VT/VF, ventricular tachycardia/ventricular fibrillation; CCTA, computed coronary tomography angiography; ECG, electrocardiogram; LAD, left anterior descending; LCx, left circumflex; PCI, percutaneous coronary intervention; CABG, coronary artery bypass grafting; IABP, intra-aortic balloon pump; ECMO, extracorporeal membrane oxygenation; LVAD, left ventricular assist device.

the level of risk is unclear and depends largely on the underlying connective tissue disorder. Preconception counseling should also include discussion of the possible need for cardiothoracic surgery during pregnancy, and education about the symptoms of aortic dissection and the need for emergent medical attention. Pregnancy is not recommended for women with a prior aortic dissection or vascular EDS [21].

For women with SCAD, there are scant data about the safety of subsequent pregnancies, and this is generally considered to be contraindicated, regardless of whether or not the SCAD occurred in association with pregnancy. Women with ejection fraction <40% are at high risk during pregnancy and should be counseled to avoid pregnancy due to risk of heart failure and deterioration in LV function [21].

Medications need to be reviewed during preconception counseling. Angiotensin-converting enzyme inhibitors (ACE) and angiotensin-receptor blocker (ARB) medications are often discontinued as soon as contraception is stopped. Fetal malformations have been linked to first trimester exposure [47], although no increase in risk was reported in a more recent study [48]. Beta-blockers may slow the rate of aortic dilatation and decrease aortic complications, but data are limited [49]. Beta-blockers are typically continued during pregnancy if already prescribed, or may be initiated in women with Marfan syndrome, vascular EDS, heritable thoracic aortic disease, or Loeys-Dietz. Beta-blockers may also be considered for women with BAV or Turner syndrome with aortic dilatation, and for women with history of SCAD. Metoprolol is typically preferred during pregnancy. Counseling should include discussion of the

association between beta-blockers and intrauterine growth restriction [50].

Genetic counseling is important since certain conditions will increase the risk of subsequent complications and there may be a 50% chance of passing an inherited condition to offspring (see Counseling section below). After discussion between the patient and providers, if the maternal or fetal risks are felt to be prohibitive, discussion of effective birth control is essential.

Antepartum Management

Imaging

Surveillance of aortopathies during pregnancy depends on the diameter of the aorta and level of risk. The ESC pregnancy guidelines suggest monitoring by echocardiography every 4–12 weeks throughout pregnancy and 6 months postpartum, more frequently if the aortic diameter is larger or if the underlying diagnosis confers increased risk [21]. The 2010 ACC/AHA thoracic aortic disease guidelines recommend monthly or bimonthly echocardiographic imaging of the ascending aorta until delivery [45]. If the dilatation of the ascending aorta is not well-seen on echocardiography, or if the dilatation is in the aortic arch or the descending or abdominal aorta, serial monitoring should be done using MRI without gadolinium [45]. Measurements of the aortic size will vary depending on the technique used and there may be mild inter-observer variability. Fetal echocardiogram can be performed to diagnose inherited conditions.

Medications

Women with aortopathies, high-risk vascular disorders, or prior SCAD are recommended to take beta-blocker medication during pregnancy, with close follow-up to detect fetal growth restriction. In women with Marfan syndrome, the beta-blocker dose may be adjusted to achieve a reduction in heart rate by at least 20 beats/minute [51]. Strict blood pressure control is important for women with aortic disease; gestational hypertension and preeclampsia may increase the risk of aortic dissection [8].

Surgery during Pregnancy

Acute complications, such as ascending aortic dissection or severe SCAD, may require emergent surgery during pregnancy. Elective surgery could be considered during pregnancy if the aorta is >45 mm and increasing rapidly (class IIA recommendation) [21]. If the fetus is viable, cesarean section can be performed followed directly by cardiothoracic surgery. If the fetus is not yet viable, surgical treatment for the mother is recommended. Several modifications and precautions can be implemented during cardiothoracic surgery to improve fetal outcomes, including the use of continuous fetal monitoring, high-pressure perfusion with pulsatile flow, and avoidance of hypothermia [52]. Cardiac surgery performed during pregnancy generally carries a 3% risk of maternal mortality, up to 30% risk of fetal mortality, and 3%–6% risk of neonatal morbidity [53,54]. An experienced multidisciplinary team should include cardiothoracic surgery, cardiology, obstetrics, maternal-fetal medicine, and cardiac anesthesiology.

Management for Labor and Delivery

Several connective tissue disorders are associated with increased risk of miscarriage and preterm delivery. Women may be advised to be near the delivery center in last month of pregnancy. Management of women at high risk for vascular complications should involve a multidisciplinary team.

Labor and Delivery

The goal during labor and delivery in women with aortopathies is to avoid excessive aortic wall stress. During vaginal delivery, the systolic and diastolic blood pressure increase during each uterine contraction; however, much of these hemodynamic changes are driven by pain and anxiety and mitigated by high-quality anesthesia. Neuraxial anesthesia can be difficult in the setting of dural ectasia or scoliosis, commonly seen in patients with Marfan syndrome, Loeys-Dietz, or EDS. Cesarean delivery carries risks of hemodynamic fluctuations, increased blood loss and hemorrhage, infection, and thromboembolic complications. Although no studies have compared vaginal versus cesarean delivery in women with vascular disorders, cesarean delivery should be considered in women with a history of aortic dissection, vascular EDS, or when the ascending aorta is >45 mm [21]. Vaginal delivery is recommended if the ascending aorta diameter is <40 mm (class I recommendation). If the ascending aorta

diameter is 40–45 mm, vaginal delivery with expedited second stage and regional anesthesia should be considered (class IIA), but cesarean may also be considered (class IIB) [21]. Postpartum hemorrhage after cesarean delivery in women with Marfan syndrome should be anticipated [51]. Women with SCAD may have vaginal delivery with goals of minimal maternal effort, passive second stage of labor, and delayed Valsalva [9]. The ESC guidelines recommend (class I) women with aortic dilatation or history of aortic dissection deliver in an experienced center with a pregnancy heart team and with cardiothoracic surgery availability [21].

Intrapartum Monitoring

Continuous electrocardiogram monitoring can be considered for high-risk patients and concern for myocardial ischemia or arrhythmias. Arterial monitoring can be used to instantly detect blood pressure fluctuations. In high-risk patients, the arterial line should be placed prior to induction of either neuraxial or general anesthesia to mitigate blood pressure fluctuations. A central venous catheter line may be useful for administration of vasoactive drugs, volume resuscitation, and estimating high or low central venous pressure; however, a minority of patients require this level of invasive monitoring, such as those with active dissection, hemodynamic instability, pulmonary edema, or active hemorrhage. Pulmonary artery catheter monitoring is not indicated. If a patient is at high risk for aortic dissection, or if the necessary level of invasive monitoring is not available in the labor and delivery unit, alternative delivery locations such as the cardiac intensive care unit should be explored.

Medications for Labor and Delivery

Certain medications used during labor and delivery for various obstetric indications may be contraindicated or used with caution in women with vascular disorders (Table 13.2). Terbutaline, methylergonovine (Methergine), carboprost tromethamine (Hemabate), and epinephrine can cause hypertension and vasoconstriction and should not be used. Oxytocin (Pitocin) can cause decreased systemic blood pressure and peripheral vascular resistance and should only be used as a dilute solution in a continuous infusion, since a large bolus can cause a sudden decrease in afterload and reflex tachycardia. Magnesium sulfate, if administered in high doses, can cause respiratory depression, hypoxia, and cardiac dysfunction, but can be used with caution.

Postpartum Care

Aortic Disease

Imaging

The first 4–6 weeks postpartum confers a high-risk time for aortic dissection. Depending on the individual's risk and size of the aorta, follow-up could range from weekly visits with imaging to just one postpartum visit. Prior to a subsequent pregnancy, the entire aorta should be imaged, preferably with MRI with gadolinium.

TABLE 13.2

Medications Used during Labor and Delivery and Considerations for Women with Vascular Disease

Medication	Indication	Side Effects	Recommendations
Magnesium sulfate	• Seizure prophylaxis • Neonatal neuroprotection	• High levels can cause respiratory depression, hypoxia, and cardiac dysfunction • Increased risk when used with calcium-channel blocker	Use with caution
Oxytocin (Pitocin)	• Labor augmentation • Prevention of postpartum hemorrhage	• Decrease in mean arterial pressure • Decrease in peripheral vascular resistance • Large bolus can cause sudden decrease afterload and reflex tachycardia	No bolus Can be used cautiously as a dilute solution in a continuous IV infusion
Terbutaline	• Stop premature labor, prolonged or frequent uterine contractions	• Hypertension and tachycardia (1%–10%)	Extreme caution, contraindicated
Methylergonovine (Methergine)	• Stop postpartum hemorrhage	• Vasoconstriction leading to hypertension and myocardial ischemia	Contraindicated
Carboprost tromethamine (Hemabate)	• Prostaglandin used for refractory postpartum uterine bleeding or pregnancy termination	• Hypertension	Avoid in women with vascular disease or aortic aneurysms
Epinephrine	• For combined spinal-epidural anesthesia or epidural	Intense vasoconstriction and hypertension and tachycardia	Avoid in women with aortic disease and coronary dissection

Contraception

Reliable contraception is essential for women at high risk for a subsequent pregnancy. Evidence linking hormonal contraception with aortic dilatation and dissection is unclear. Side effects of hypertension should be treated.

Prognosis and Recurrence

Long-term survival should be considered when counseling about subsequent pregnancy. The natural history of aortic disease tends to involve progressive dilatation over time but reported outcomes are variable and the overall risks depend on the underlying condition, size of the aorta, and associated risk factors. Pre-pregnancy aortic root repair does not eliminate the risk of dissection during pregnancy, and other sites in the aorta can become involved. Unrelated to pregnancy, overall survival among patients with acute aortic dissection has been reported at 37%–88% at 10 years [55–57]. Pregnancy in women with a prior aortic dissection is not advised [21]. Preconception consultation should occur with a cardiologist, geneticist, and obstetrician, and possibly a cardiothoracic surgeon depending on the severity of the aortic aneurysm.

Genetic Counseling

Presentation with aortic disease at a young age suggests a higher risk of genetically mediated thoracic aortic disease. Providers should take a family history for all first-degree relatives related to history of aortic aneurysm, brain aneurysm, aortic dilatation, aortic dissection, and abdominal aortic aneurysm. Consultation with a geneticist is often recommended [45]. The risk of transmission of inherited conditions to the child must be addressed, particularly given the 50% transmission risk with Marfan syndrome, Loeys-Dietz, and vascular EDS, all of which are autosomal dominant conditions. The genetic transmission of BAV

and coarctation are less well defined [58]. If the parental genetic mutation is known, prenatal diagnosis with chorionic villous sampling or amniocentesis can be used to detect the mutation in the fetus. These procedures carry a 1% risk of miscarriage [59] and are only indicated if the results will lead to termination. Alternatively, in vitro fertilization in conjunction with preimplantation genetic diagnosis can be used to select embryos unaffected by a known mutation.

SCAD

Imaging

Postpartum, women with SCAD should undergo full-body cross-sectional imaging (preferably with computed tomographic angiography) to diagnose concomitant fibromuscular dysplasia and diagnose additional dissections or aneurysms [9].

Contraception

The presumed pathophysiologic association of female sex hormones with SCAD has led to concerns about hormonal contraception and hormone replacement therapy in women following SCAD. Avoiding hormonal contraception may be reasonable if other reliable options exist [9,29].

Prognosis and Recurrence

Patients with SCAD have a high rate of recurrence. One prospective study reported recurrent SCAD in 10.4% of patients [44], while another cohort reported a recurrence rate of 17.2%, and the estimated 10-year rate of combined major adverse cardiac events (death, heart failure, myocardial infarction, and SCAD recurrence) was 47% [42]. In a small case series of eight women with subsequent pregnancy after prior SCAD, one woman suffered recurrent SCAD of the left main artery at 9 weeks postpartum resulting in a large MI and emergent CABG [60]. Although the data are limited, many experts advise against pregnancy due to the high risk of recurrence and complications [21]. Women who choose to proceed with pregnancy should be followed closely by a multidisciplinary team that includes maternal-fetal medicine and cardiology specialists [9].

Conclusion

During and after pregnancy, women with vascular diseases are at increased risk for catastrophic complications including aortic and coronary artery dissections. A high index of suspicion should be maintained to prevent missed diagnosis and ensure early and accurate treatment. Aortopathy or SCAD should prompt investigation for underlying connective tissue diseases, and genetic counseling may be appropriate.

Women with vascular diseases are at increased risk for complications during pregnancy and the early postpartum period. Unfortunately, the initial presentation for women with underlying vascular disease may be with a catastrophic complication, such as aortic or coronary dissection, and may occur during pregnancy. Women at risk for vascular complications include those with connective tissue disorders, such as Marfan syndrome, EDS, and Loeys-Dietz syndrome; other disorders associated with aortopathy, such as BAV and Turner syndrome; and systemic vascular disorders, such as fibromuscular dysplasia. These conditions pose high risk of maternal, obstetric, and fetal complications, and appropriate management requires multiple subspecialties. This chapter addresses vascular conditions that affect women during childbearing, with particular attention to major complications including aortic dissection and spontaneous coronary artery dissection. Recommendations for preconception counseling and management during antepartum, labor and delivery, and postpartum have been reviewed. Genetic counseling and prenatal diagnosis of offspring should also be considered.

REFERENCES

1. la Chapelle C, Schutte J, Schuitemaker N, Steegers E, van Roosmalen J. Maternal mortality attributable to vascular dissection and rupture in the Netherlands: A nationwide confidential enquiry. *BJOG An Int J Obstet Gynaecol*. 2012 Jan 1;119(1):86–93.
2. Saw J, Ricci D, Starovoytov A, Fox R, Buller CE. Spontaneous coronary artery dissection: Prevalence of predisposing conditions including fibromuscular dysplasia in a tertiary center cohort. *JACC Cardiovasc Interv*. 2013 Jan 1;6(1):44–52.
3. Jondeau G et al. Aortic event rate in the Marfan population. *Circulation*. 2012 Jan 17;125(2):226–32.
4. Højbjerg Gravholt C et al. Clinical and epidemiological description of aortic dissection in Turner's syndrome. *Cardiol Young*. 2006 Oct 20;16(05):430.
5. Michelena HI et al. Incidence of aortic complications in patients with bicuspid aortic valves. *JAMA*. 2011 Sep 14;306(10):1104.
6. Nasiell J, Lindqvist PG. Aortic dissection in pregnancy: The incidence of a life-threatening disease. *Eur J Obstet Gynecol Reprod Biol*. 2010 Mar 1;149(1):120–1.
7. Huisman CM, Zwart JJ, Roos-Hesselink JW, Duvekot JJ, van Roosmalen J. Incidence and predictors of maternal cardiovascular mortality and severe morbidity in the Netherlands: A prospective cohort study. *PLOS ONE*. 2013 Feb 14;8(2):e56494.
8. Wanga S, Silversides C, Dore A, de Waard V, Mulder B. Pregnancy and thoracic aortic disease: Managing the risks. *Can J Cardiol*. 2016 Jan 1;32(1):78–85.
9. Statement AHAS et al. Spontaneous Coronary Artery Dissection: Current State of the Science a Scientific Statement from the American Heart Association. *Circulation*. 2018;137(19):e523–57.
10. Elkayam U et al. Pregnancy-associated acute myocardial infarction. *Circulation*. 2014 Apr 22;129(16):1695–702.
11. Ito H, Taylor L, Bowman M, Fry ETA, Hermiller JB, Van Tassel JW. Presentation and therapy of spontaneous coronary artery dissection and comparisons of postpartum versus non-postpartum cases. *Am J Cardiol*. 2011 Jun 1;107(11):1590–6.
12. Tweet MS, Hayes SN, Codsi E, Gulati R, Rose CH, Best PJM. Spontaneous coronary artery dissection associated with pregnancy. *J Am Coll Cardiol*. 2017 Jul 25;70(4):426–35.
13. Saw J et al. Spontaneous coronary artery dissection. *Circ Cardiovasc Interv*. 2014 Oct;7(5):645–55.
14. Judge DP, Dietz HC. Marfan's syndrome. *Lancet*. 2005 Dec 3;366(9501):1965–76.
15. Goyal A, Keramati AR, Czarny MJ, Resar JR, Mani A. The genetics of aortopathies in clinical cardiology. *Clin Med Insights Cardiol*. 2017;11:1179546817709787.
16. Goland S, Elkayam U. Cardiovascular problems in pregnant women with Marfan syndrome. *Circulation*. 2009 Feb 3;119(4):619–23.
17. Goland S, Elkayam U. Pregnancy and Marfan syndrome. *Ann Cardiothorac Surg*. 2017 Nov;6(6):642–53.
18. Loeys BL et al. The revised Ghent nosology for the Marfan syndrome. *J Med Genet*. 2010 Jul 1;47(7):476–85.
19. Pepin M, Schwarze U, Superti-Furga A, Byers PH. Clinical and genetic features of Ehlers-Danlos syndrome type IV, the vascular type. *N Engl J Med*. 2000 Mar 9;342(10):673–80.
20. Murray ML, Pepin M, Peterson S, Byers PH. Pregnancy-related deaths and complications in women with vascular Ehlers-Danlos syndrome. *Genet Med*. 2014 Dec 12;16(12):874–80.
21. Regitz-Zagrosek V et al. ESC Guidelines for the management of cardiovascular diseases during pregnancy. *Heart J*. 2018 Sep 7;39(34):3165–241.
22. Braverman AC. Aortic involvement in patients with a bicuspid aortic valve. *Heart*. 2011 Mar 15;97(6):50–613.
23. Januzzi JL et al. Characterizing the young patient with aortic dissection: Results from the international registry of aortic dissection (IRAD). *J Am Coll Cardiol*. 2004 Feb 18;43(4):665–9.
24. Stout KK et al. 2018 AHA/ACC guideline for the management of adults with congenital heart disease. *J Am Coll Cardiol*. 2018 Aug 16;25255.
25. Chevalier N et al. Materno-fetal cardiovascular complications in turner syndrome after oocyte donation: Insufficient prepregnancy screening and pregnancy follow-up are associated with poor outcome. *J Clin Endocrinol Metab*. 2011 Feb 1;96(2):E260–7.

26. Cabanes L et al. Turner syndrome and pregnancy: Clinical practice. Recommendations for the management of patients with Turner syndrome before and during pregnancy. *Eur J Obstet Gynecol Reprod Biol.* 2010 Sep 1;152(1):18–24.

27. Practice Committee of the American Society for Reproductive Medicine. Increased maternal cardiovascular mortality associated with pregnancy in women with Turner syndrome. *Fertil Steril.* 2012 Feb 1;97(2):282–4.

28. Gornik HL et al. First International Consensus on the diagnosis and management of fibromuscular dysplasia. *Vasc Med.* 2019 Jan 16;24(5). doi: 1358863X1882181.

29. Adlam D et al. European Society of Cardiology, acute cardiovascular care association, SCAD study group: A position paper on spontaneous coronary artery dissection. *Eur Heart J.* 2018;39(36):3353–68.

30. Hytten F. Blood volume changes in normal pregnancy. *Clin Haematol.* 1985 Oct;14(3):601–12.

31. Thornburg KL, Jacobson S-L, Giraud GD, Morton MJ. Hemodynamic changes in pregnancy. *Semin Perinatol.* 2000 Feb 1;24(1):11–4.

32. Manalo-Estrella P, Barker AE. Histopathologic findings in human aortic media associated with pregnancy. *Arch Pathol.* 1967 Apr;83(4):336–41.

33. Nolte JE, Rutherford RB, Nawaz S, Rosenberger A, Speers WC, Krupski WC. Arterial dissections associated with pregnancy. *J Vasc Surg.* 1995 Mar 1;21(3):515–20.

34. Immer FF et al. Aortic dissection in pregnancy: Analysis of risk factors and outcome. *Ann Thorac Surg.* 2003 Jul 1;76(1):309–14.

35. Nallamothu BK et al. Syncope in acute aortic dissection: Diagnostic, prognostic, and clinical implications. *Am J Med.* 2002 Oct 15;113(6):468–71.

36. Hagan PG et al. The International Registry of Acute Aortic Dissection (IRAD). *JAMA.* 2000 Feb 16;283(7):897.

37. Bossone E et al. Coronary artery involvement in patients with acute type A aortic dissection: Clinical characteristics and in-hospital outcomes. *J Am Coll Cardiol.* 2003 Mar 19;41(6):235.

38. Suzuki T et al. Diagnosis of acute aortic dissection by D-dimer: The International Registry of Acute Aortic Dissection substudy on biomarkers (IRAD-Bio) experience. *Circulation.* 2009 May 26;119(20):2702–7.

39. Gebker R, Gomaa O, Schnackenburg B, Rebakowski J, Fleck E, Nagel E. Comparison of different MRI techniques for the assessment of thoracic aortic pathology: 3D contrast enhanced MR angiography, turbo spin echo and balanced steady state free precession. *Int J Cardiovasc Imaging.* 2007 Nov 1;23(6):747–56.

40. Bulas D, Egloff A. Benefits and risks of MRI in pregnancy. *Semin Perinatol.* 2013 Oct 1;37(5):301–4.

41. Webb JAW, Thomsen HS, Morcos SK, (ESUR) M of CMSC of ES of UR. The use of iodinated and gadolinium contrast media during pregnancy and lactation. *Eur Radiol.* 2005 Jun 18;15(6):1234–40.

42. Tweet MS et al. Clinical features, management, and prognosis of spontaneous coronary artery dissection. *Circulation.* 2012 Jul 31;126(5):579–88.

43. Lempereur M, Gin K, Saw J. Multivessel spontaneous coronary artery dissection mimicking atherosclerosis. *JACC Cardiovasc Interv.* 2014 Jul 1;7(7):e87–8.

44. Saw J et al. Spontaneous coronary artery dissection. *J Am Coll Cardiol.* 2017 Aug 29;70(9):1148–58.

45. Hiratzka LF et al. 2010 ACCF/AHA/AATS/ACR/ASA/SCA/SCAI/SIR/STS/SVM guidelines for the diagnosis and management of patients with thoracic aortic disease: Executive summary. *JAC.* 2010;55(14):1509–44.

46. Sayama S et al. Peripartum type B aortic dissection in patients with Marfan syndrome who underwent aortic root replacement: A case series study. *BJOG.* 2018 Mar 1;125(4):487–93.

47. Cooper WO et al. Major congenital malformations after first-trimester exposure to ACE inhibitors. *N Engl J Med.* 2006 Jun 8;354(23):2443–51.

48. Bateman BT et al. Angiotensin-converting enzyme inhibitors and the risk of congenital malformations. *Obstet Gynecol.* 2017;129(1):174–84.

49. Koo H-K, Lawrence KA, Musini VM. Beta-blockers for preventing aortic dissection in Marfan syndrome. *Cochrane Database Syst Rev.* 2017 Nov 7;11:CD011103.

50. Ersbøll A, Hedegaard M, Søndergaard L, Ersbøll M, Johansen M. Treatment with oral beta-blockers during pregnancy complicated by maternal heart disease increases the risk of fetal growth restriction. *BJOG.* 2014 Apr 1;121(5):618–26.

51. Elkayam U, Goland S, Pieper PG, Silversides CK. High-risk cardiac disease in pregnancy. *J Am Coll Cardiol.* 2016;68(5):502–16.

52. Reitman E, Flood P. Anaesthetic considerations for non-obstetric surgery during pregnancy. *Br J Anaesth.* 2011 Dec 1;107(suppl_1):i72–8.

53. John AS et al. Cardiopulmonary bypass during pregnancy. *Ann Thorac Surg.* 2011 Apr 1;91(4):1191–6.

54. Arnoni RT et al. Risk factors associated with cardiac surgery during pregnancy. *Ann Thorac Surg.* 2003 Nov 1;76(5):1605–8.

55. Pansini S et al. Early and late risk factors in surgical treatment of acute type A aortic dissection. *Ann Thorac Surg.* 1998 Sep;66(3):779–84.

56. Sabik JF, Lytle BW, Blackstone EH, McCarthy PM, Loop FD, Cosgrove DM. Long-term effectiveness of operations for ascending aortic dissections. *J Thorac Cardiovasc Surg.* 2000 May;119(5):946–62.

57. Chiappini B et al. Early and late outcomes of acute type A aortic dissection: Analysis of risk factors in 487 consecutive patients. *Eur Heart J.* 2005 Jan 1;26(2):180–6.

58. Andreassi MG, Della Corte A. Genetics of bicuspid aortic valve aortopathy. *Curr Opin Cardiol.* 2016 Nov;31(6):585–92.

59. Mujezinovic F, Alfirevic Z. Procedure-related complications of amniocentesis and chorionic villous sampling. *Obstet Gynecol.* 2007 Sep;110(3):687–94.

60. Tweet MS, Hayes SN, Gulati R, Rose CH, Best PJM. Pregnancy after spontaneous coronary artery dissection: A case series. *Ann Intern Med.* 2015 Apr 21;162(8):598.

14

Acute Coronary Syndromes in Pregnancy

Pavan Reddy, Gassan Moady, and Uri Elkayam

KEY POINTS

- The incidence of myocardial infarction in pregnancy is three- to fourfold higher than age-matched nonpregnant women occurring during pregnancy or within 6–12 weeks in the postpartum period
- The most common cause of myocardial infarction in pregnancy is spontaneous coronary artery dissection
- Left anterior descending artery is the most commonly involved vessel in spontaneous coronary artery dissection in pregnancy

- As in nonpregnant women, coronary angiography with the goal of opening the infarct related artery is the standard of care in pregnant women with STEMI and in most high-risk patients with NSTEMI
- Thrombolytic therapy should be avoided in SCAD because of the reported harm and clinical deterioration due to extension of intramural hematoma and dissection

---

Introduction

The term *acute coronary syndrome* (ACS) refers to any group of clinical symptoms compatible with acute myocardial ischemia and includes unstable angina (UA), non-ST segment elevation myocardial infarction (NSTEMI), and ST-segment elevation myocardial infarction (STEMI). Pregnancy-associated myocardial infarction (PAMI) is defined as myocardial infarction (MI) occurring during pregnancy or within 6–12 weeks postpartum [1].

Incidence

Recent systemic review and meta-analysis of population-based studies including over 66 million pregnancies reported a pooled PAMI incidence of 1:30,000 worldwide and the U.S. incidence of 1:20,500 [2]. When compared to nonpregnant women in similar age, the incidence in pregnancy is three- to fourfold higher [2–6].

Etiology of Acute Coronary Syndromes in Pregnancy

In a large series published in 2014 by Elkayam et al., the main mechanisms of PAMI were spontaneous coronary artery dissection (SCAD), accounting for 43% of cases, atherosclerotic plaques in 27%, coronary artery thrombosis without atherosclerosis in 17%, normal coronary arteries in 9%, Takotsubo cardiomyopathy in 2%, and suspected coronary spasm in 1% of the cases [7]. Increased incidence of SCAD in this group of women is likely due to the increased estrogen and progesterone levels in

pregnant women, which tends to accelerate degenerative changes in the vessel wall with the potential for coronary artery dissection [8,9]. The left anterior descending (LAD) artery is the most involved vessel (more than 70%), followed by the left main coronary artery, circumflex, and then the right coronary artery. Involvement of multiple coronary vessels in the dissection process is not an uncommon finding in pregnancy [9].

Risk Factors

Older age is a known risk factor, with over 70% of women with PAMI being older than 30 years and 40% over the age of 35 years. For women older than 40 years of age, the risk of ACS during pregnancy increases by 20% with each advancing year [10]. The incidence of conventional atherosclerotic risk factors is relatively low in the young female population, ranging between 10%–25% [7]. Incidence of PAMI has been also reported to be higher in pregnant women with thrombophilia, history of postpartum infections, anemia requiring transfusions, multiparity, non-Hispanic whites, and African Americans [3,4]. Notably, pregnancy and postpartum periods are known hypercoagulable states in part due to alterations in the coagulation cascade [11]. Table 14.1 summarizes the reported risk factors in women with PAMI.

Complications and Mortality

A recent review of 150 contemporary cases reported 7% maternal and 5% fetal mortality [7]. Top causes of maternal mortality were cardiogenic shock and ventricular arrhythmias. The rate of significant complications was strikingly high and included a markedly reduced LVEF ($\leq$40%) in 54% of the patients. This

TABLE 14.1

Risk Factors for Pregnancy-Associated Myocardial Infarction

Age >30 years
African American race
Hypertension
Diabetes
Obesity
Dyslipidemia
Physical inactivity
Smoking
Cocaine use
Preeclampsia
Thrombophilia
Multiparity
Postpartum hemorrhage
Postpartum infection

TABLE 14.2

Diagnostic Modalities

	Features
Symptoms	Chest pain, shortness of breath
Electrocardiogram	ST segment elevation/depression
	T wave inversion
	Loss of R wave
	New Q wave
Biomarker	Elevated troponin level
Echocardiogram	Wall motion abnormalities

degree of LV dysfunction was associated with a high incidence of heart failure, cardiogenic shock, ventricular arrhythmias, and mortality. Clinical deterioration required mechanical support, including the use of intra-aortic balloon pump, LV assist device, and extracorporeal membrane oxygenation in 28% of the patients with PAMI due to SCAD [9].

Diagnosis of Myocardial Infarction in Pregnancy

Diagnosis of PAMI is made when STEMI or NTSEMI occur during pregnancy or within 6–12 weeks postpartum. The term ACS encompasses a spectrum of pathology pertaining to the degree of coronary occlusion.

- STEMI is defined as ST elevation or left bundle branch block on ECG with evidence of myocardial injury, i.e., troponin elevation. STEMI almost invariably represents complete acute occlusion of a coronary artery with resultant transmural infarct (involving the entire ventricular wall segment).

- NSTEMI is present when there is troponin elevation but without ST elevation on ECG. ST depression or T wave inversion may or not be present and are not required for diagnosis. Pathologically, NSTEMI often represents subtotal occlusion of a coronary artery resulting in less severe injury (subendocardial).

- Unstable angina is characterized by cardiac chest pain without troponin elevation [12]. UA is denoted as such given the propensity to evolve into more severe forms of MI.

- Angina, considered apart from the ACS spectrum of disease, is defined as chest pain that occurs with stress and is relieved with rest or nitroglycerin [13]. Angina specifically pertains to stable ischemic heart disease for which the treatment mainly involves conservative measures such as lifestyle modifications and anti-anginal medications (i.e., beta-blockers or calcium channel blockers).

Most reported PAMI cases occur either late in pregnancy or in the postpartum period, primarily presenting as STEMI involving the anterior ventricular wall [7–9].

As in nonpregnant women, PAMI is diagnosed when the above definitions of STEMI and NSTEMI are met in the right clinical setting. The leading presenting symptoms are chest pain and dyspnea (Table 14.2) [7–9]. Differential diagnosis includes pulmonary embolism, aortic dissection, and preeclampsia.

Cardiac troponin is still the preferred biomarker for evaluation of acute MI. In general, troponin levels are not altered in normal pregnancy. Mild elevations of cardiac troponin levels may be seen in hypertensive women and individuals with preeclampsia [14,15]. Of note, minor electrocardiographic changes involving the ST segment and T wave have been reported in otherwise healthy pregnant women during labor and delivery [16].

Echocardiogram (ECG) is a very useful tool that is safe in the diagnostic workup of pregnant patients with chest pain or suspected MI. Nearly all patients with MI demonstrate wall motion abnormalities.

Exercise stress test, with or without ECG, can be used in pregnancy to diagnose inducible ischemia after ruling out MI and when the patient's hemodynamic condition is stable. The use of submaximal test (70% of maximal predicted heart rate) is recommended due to previous reports of fetal bradycardia and reduced fetal heart rate variability during maternal moderate to heavy exercise [17].

Computed coronary tomography angiography can be useful for ruling out acute coronary syndrome in questionable cases, but it carries the risk of radiation exposure and has lower sensitivity for lesions in small distal vessels. In addition, for optimal visualization of the coronary tree, high doses of beta-blockers may be needed for lowering heart rate [18].

Management of Myocardial Infarction in Pregnancy

Women with PAMI should be managed in intensive care units. Similar to nonpregnant individuals, coronary angiography with the goal of opening the infarct-related artery is the standard of care in pregnant women with STEMI and in most high-risk patients with NSTEMI.

Medical Therapy

Medical therapy used in MI includes beta-blockers, calcium channel blockers (CCB), nitrates, anticoagulants, statins, and antiplatelet therapy. Beta-blockers should be used when benefits outweigh risks; the use of selective beta-1 agents is preferred due to fewer effects on uterine activity [19,20]. Currently only nifedipine, a dihydropyridine CCB, has been shown to be safe during gestation [21]. Oral and intravenous nitrates have been used during pregnancy for treating hypertension, but careful titration is needed to avoid maternal hypotension [22]. Angiotensin converting enzyme inhibitors and angiotensin receptor blockers are contraindicated during pregnancy due to multiple teratogenic effects [23]. Information about the use of statins during pregnancy is limited, however, there are conflicting reports of teratogenicity [24]. The use of statins has been classified as contraindicated in pregnancy [23]. Both heparin and low molecular weight heparin (LMWH) do not cross the placenta and are considered safe in pregnancy [25]. Use of low-dose aspirin is also considered safe for use in pregnant women. Limited information is available regarding the fetal safety of standard antiplatelet drugs, including clopidogrel (category B), prasugrel (category B) and ticagrelor (category C) [26]. Clopidogrel use was reported in 56 patients in two contemporary studies and should be considered the preferred P2Y12 receptor antagonist in pregnancy [7,9]. Although its use decreased substantially in the era of percutaneous coronary intervention, thrombolytic therapy should be considered in pregnant women in appropriate conditions similar to nonpregnant women. However, caution should be exercised given the lack of controlled clinical trials including pregnant women and the nature of the weak evidence level of the cumulative data available [27]. The role of heparin for SCAD is controversial because of the potential risk of extending the dissection with anticoagulation, which on the other hand may be beneficial for resolving overlying thrombus and improving true lumen patency. Thrombolytic therapy should be avoided in SCAD because of the reported harm and clinical deterioration due to extension of intramural hematoma and dissection [28]. Beta-blockers play an important role in the pharmacological armamentarium for SCAD because of their reducing effect on the coronary arterial wall stress.

Coronary Angiography

Coronary angiography in pregnancy is associated with increased risk of catheter-induced coronary artery dissection, especially in the left main artery; this iatrogenic risk together with the documented high rates of spontaneous healing of the dissected arteries leads to the suggestion of conservative management in stable low-risk patients [9,29]. Nonselective contrast injection in the aortic root, avoidance of deep catheter intubation (especially with the radial approach), and minimal use of low-pressure injections are recommended to decrease the risk of dissection. A suggested algorithm for the treatment of PASCAD is given in Figure 14.1. Fetal radiation exposure remains a significant concern during cardiac catheterization of pregnant women, as the average amount of radiation exposure to the fetus is estimated at 3 mSv. External abdominal shielding, lower magnification, low fluoroscopy frame rates, and using the radial approach are acceptable methods to reduce risk of radiation exposure [26].

Management of Complications

1. *Cardiogenic shock:* PAMI-associated heart failure or cardiogenic shock should be managed according to guideline recommendations [30]. Diuretics and vasodilators such as nitroglycerin are the cornerstone of therapy. Inotropes and mechanical circulatory support should be employed as needed and emergent revascularization with either PCI or CABG should be considered.

2. *Arrhythmias:* In managing arrhythmias with associated hemodynamic compromise, electrical cardioversion is a reasonable option in all stages of pregnancy. In cases where a trial of medications is possible, caution must be exercised to avoid teratogenic medications [23]. Lidocaine is classified as a category B medication and should be considered first among medical therapy options. Amiodarone is category D and therefore should be avoided except in life-threatening situations refractory to safer medications. In cases of symptomatic bradycardia, medications such as atropine, epinephrine, and dopamine are considered safe. Transvenous pacing is thought to be safe with minimal risk of radiation exposure to the fetus.

3. Recurrent angina or acute MI occurs in 20% patients and is managed along the same principles outlined in Figure 14.1.

Delivery Planning

A multidisciplinary approach is essential in the care of the pregnant patient with PAMI. Multidisciplinary team members generally consist of an obstetrician, cardiologist, anesthesiologist, and neonatologist. Delivery details discussed at the meeting should include time of delivery, mode of delivery, location, and type of monitoring, and should be shared with all patient care providers. Patient care should be individualized and based on the risk factors, extent of myocardial damage, gestational age, and risk of anticipated complications.

Mode of Delivery

The mode of delivery in a patient with pregnancy-associated MI should be determined by obstetric considerations and the clinical status of the mother. Vaginal delivery can be accomplished relatively safely in the stable patient with a non-SCAD pregnancy–associated acute myocardial infarction (AMI) when measures aimed to reduce cardiac workload and oxygen demands are taken [8]. Assisted vaginal delivery is recommended to avoid excessive maternal efforts and prolonged labor.

1. *Optimize cardiac output:* Positioning the patient in the left lateral position can help to improve cardiac output during labor and delivery. In addition, the patient's pain, fear, and apprehension, which may lead to tachycardia and hypertension and thus to increase in myocardial oxygen demand, should be prevented and treated. Vital signs as well as oxygen saturation, electrocardiogram, and fetal heart rate should be monitored continuously.

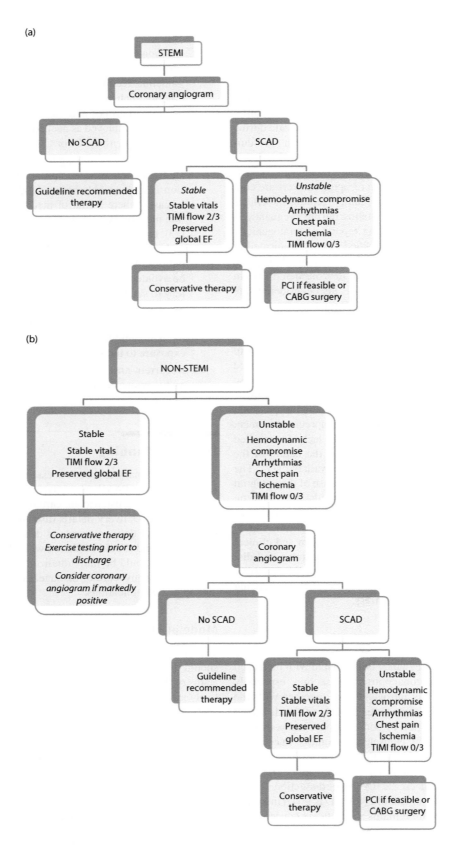

FIGURE 14.1 Suggested algorithms for the management of patients with PAMI: (a) STEMI; (b) non-STEMI. *Abbreviations:* STEMI, ST-segment elevation MI; SCAD, spontaneous coronary dissection; VS, vital signs; TIMI flow 0, complete coronary artery occlusion; TIMI flow 1, penetration of the obstruction by contrast but no distal perfusion; TIMI flow 2, perfusion of the entire artery but delayed flow; TIMI flow 3, full perfusion, normal flow; PCI, percutaneous coronary intervention; CABG, coronary artery bypass graft.

For prevention or treatment of myocardial ischemia during labor, intravenous nitroglycerin, beta-blockers, and calcium antagonists can be used. It should be noted that nitroglycerin and calcium antagonists have some tocolytic effects and may prolong labor. Cesarean section delivery is advisable in women with MI due to SCAD in order to avoid increase in coronary wall stress and recurrent dissection.

2. *Pain relief:* Neuraxial analgesia and anesthesia are preferred for both vaginal and cesarean delivery. Anesthesia-related hypotension can be minimized with use of low-dose local anesthetic techniques, administration of intravenous fluid, and careful titration of vasoconstrictors. Neuraxial anesthesia can be performed safely in women receiving low-dose aspirin, but clopidogrel should be discontinued 5–7 days prior to the procedure, intravenous unfractionated heparin 4–6 hours after (and verifying a normal aPTT), and LMWH ≥24 hours before performing neuraxial anesthesia [31].

Recurrence Risk in Future Pregnancy

Limited information is available regarding the risk of pregnancy in women with a history of AMI. Pregnancy is generally well tolerated in asymptomatic patients with normal ejection fraction, but may be associated with complications such as arrhythmias, heart failure, and chest pain, especially in patients with prior history of angina, heart failure, and LV dysfunction. Mortality is rare, and most of these complications are manageable [32–35]. Patients with a history of MI should ideally be evaluated prior to the subsequent pregnancy. Such an evaluation should include a detailed history and physical examination, an ECG, and exercise testing. Cardiac drugs which are contraindicated during pregnancy including angiotensin-converting enzyme inhibitors or angiotensin receptor blockers, aldosterone receptor antagonists, statins, ivabradine, and new oral anticoagulants should be discontinued prior to pregnancy or as soon as pregnancy is diagnosed.

Women with evidence for ongoing myocardial ischemia, heart failure, or severe LV dysfunction prior to pregnancy should be advised against pregnancy, and those who are already pregnant should consider early pregnancy termination. Information on the risk of subsequent pregnancy in women with a history of pregnancy-associated SCAD is also anecdotal [36]. However, because of the high incidence of recurrent SCAD reported in women with SCAD in prior pregnancy and pregnancy-related vulnerability of the coronary arteries, subsequent pregnancy does not seem advisable [7,9].

REFERENCES

1. Honigberg MC, Scott NS. Pregnancy-Associated myocardial infarction. *Cur Treat Options Cardiovasc Med.* 2018;20:58.
2. Gibson P, Narous M, Firoz T, Chou D, Barreix M, Say L, James M. Incidence of myocardial infarction in pregnancy: A systematic review and meta-analysis of population-based studies. *Eur Heart J Qual Care Clin Outcomes.* 2017;3:198–207.
3. Ladner HE, Danielsen B, Gilbert WM. Acute myocardial infarction in pregnancy and the puerperium: A population-based study. *Obstet Gynecol.* 2005;105:480–4.
4. James AH, Jamison MG, Biswas MS, Brancazio LR, Swamy GK, Myers ER. Acute myocardial infarction in pregnancy: A United States population-based study. *Circulation.* 2006;113:1564–71.
5. Mulla ZD, Wilson B, Abedin Z, Hernandez LL, Plavsic SK. Acute myocardial infarction in pregnancy: A statewide analysis. *J Registry Manag.* 2015;42:12–7.
6. Petitti DB, Sidney S, Quesenberry CP Jr, Bernstein A. Incidence of stroke and myocardial infarction in women of reproductive age. *Stroke.* 1997;28:280–3.
7. Elkayam U, Jalnapurkar S, Barakkat MN, Khatri N, Kealey AJ, Mehra A, Roth A. Pregnancy-associated acute myocardial infarction: A review of contemporary experience in 150 cases between 2006 and 2011. *Circulation.* 2014;129:1695–702.
8. Roth A, Elkayam U. Acute myocardial infarction associated with pregnancy. *J Am Coll Cardiol.* 2008;52:171–80.
9. Havakuk O, Goland S, Mehra A, Elkayam U. Pregnancy and the risk of spontaneous coronary artery dissection: An analysis of 120 contemporary cases. *Circ Cardiovasc Interv.* 2017;10.
10. Bush N et al. Myocardial infarction in pregnancy and postpartum in the UK. *Eur J Prev Cardiol.* 2013;20:12–20.
11. James AH. Pregnancy and thrombotic risk. *Crit Care Med.* 2010;38:S57–63.
12. Amsterdam EA et al. 2014 AHA/ACC Guideline for the Management of Patients with Non-ST-Elevation Acute Coronary Syndromes: A report of the American College of Cardiology/American Heart Association Task Force on Practice Guidelines. *J Am Coll Cardiol.* 2014;64:e139–228.
13. Fihn SD et al. 2012 ACCF/AHA/ACP/AATS/PCNA/SCAI/STS Guideline for the diagnosis and management of patients with stable ischemic heart disease: A report of the American College of Cardiology Foundation/American Heart Association Task Force on Practice Guidelines, and the American College of Physicians, American Association for Thoracic Surgery, Preventive Cardiovascular Nurses Association, Society for Cardiovascular Angiography and Interventions, and Society of Thoracic Surgeons. *J Am Coll Cardiol.* 2012;60:e44–e164.
14. Pergialiotis V, Prodromidou A, Frountzas M, Perrea DN, Papantoniou N. Maternal cardiac troponin levels in pre-eclampsia: A systematic review. *J Matern Fetal Neonatal Med.* 2016;29:3386–90.
15. Aydin C, Baloglu A, Cetinkaya B, Yavuzcan A. Cardiac troponin levels in pregnant women with severe pre-eclampsia. *J Obstet Gynaecol.* 2009;29:621–3.
16. Mathew JP, Fleisher LA, Rinehouse JA, Sevarino FB, Sinatra RS, Nelson AH, Prokop EK, Rosenbaum SH. ST segment depression during labor and delivery. *Anesthesiology.* 1992;77:635–41.
17. Avery ND, Stocking KD, Tranmer JE, Davies GA, Wolfe LA. Fetal responses to maternal strength conditioning exercises in late gestation. *Can J Appl Physiol.* 1999;24:362–76.
18. Sabarudin A, Sun Z. Beta-blocker administration protocol for prospectively ECG-triggered coronary CT angiography. *World J Cardiol.* 2013;5:453–8.
19. Hurst AK, Hoffman R, Frishman WH. The use of beta-adrenergic blocking agents in pregnancy and lactation. In: Elkayam U (ed). *Cardiac Problems in Pregnancy: Diagnosis and Management of Maternal and Fetal Heart Disease,* 3rd ed. Wiley-Liss; 1998.

20. Magee LA, Elran E, Bull SB, Logan A, Koren G. Risks and benefits of beta-receptor blockers for pregnancy hypertension: Overview of the randomized trials. *Eur J Obstet Gynecol Reprod Biol.* 2000;88:15–26.

21. Childress CH, Katz VL. Nifedipine and its indications in obstetrics and gynecology. *Obstet Gynecol.* 1994;83:616–24.

22. Qasqas SA, McPherson C, Frishman WH, Elkayam U. Cardiovascular pharmacotherapeutic considerations during pregnancy and lactation. *Cardiol Rev.* 2004;12:240–61.

23. Halpern DG, Weinberg CR, Pinnelas R, Mehta-Lee S, Economy KE, Valente AM. Use of medication for cardiovascular disease during pregnancy: JACC State-of-the-Art review. *J Am Coll Cardiol.* 2019;73:457–76.

24. Lecarpentier E, Morel O, Fournier T, Elefant E, Chavatte-Palmer P, Tsatsaris V. Statins and pregnancy: Between supposed risks and theoretical benefits. *Drugs.* 2012;72:773–88.

25. Yarrington CD, Valente AM, Economy KE. Cardiovascular management in pregnancy: Antithrombotic agents and antiplatelet agents. *Circulation.* 2015;132:1354–64.

26. Ismail S, Wong C, Rajan P, Vidovich MI. ST-elevation acute myocardial infarction in pregnancy: 2016 update. *Clin Cardiol.* 2017;40:399–406.

27. Gartman EJ. The use of thrombolytic therapy in pregnancy. *Obstet Med.* 2013;6:105–11.

28. Saw J, Mancini GBJ, Humphries KH. Contemporary review on spontaneous coronary artery dissection. *J Am Coll Cardiol.* 2016;68:297–312.

29. Tweet MS, Hayes SN, Codsi E, Gulati R, Rose CH, Best PJM. Spontaneous coronary artery dissection associated with pregnancy. *J Am Coll Cardiol.* 2017;70:426–35.

30. Ibanez B et al. 2017 ESC Guidelines for the management of acute myocardial infarction in patients presenting with ST-segment elevation: The Task Force for the management of acute myocardial infarction in patients presenting with ST-segment elevation of the European Society of Cardiology (ESC). *Eur Heart J.* 2018;39(2):119–77.

31. Horlocker TT, Vandermeulen E, Kopp SL, Gogarten W, Leffert LR, Benzon HT. Regional Anesthesia in the Patient Receiving Antithrombotic or Thrombolytic Therapy: American Society of Regional Anesthesia and Pain Medicine Evidence-Based Guidelines (Fourth Edition). *Reg Anesth Pain Med.* 2018;43:263–309.

32. Vinatier D, Virelizier S, Depret-Mosser S, Dufour P, Prolongeau JF, Monnier JC, Decoulx E, Theeten G. Pregnancy after myocardial infarction. *Eur J Obstet Gynecol Reprod Biol.* 1994;56:89–93.

33. Frenkel Y, Barkai G, Reisin L, Rath S, Mashiach S, Battler A. Pregnancy after myocardial infarction: Are we playing safe? *Obstet Gynecol.* 1991;77:822–5.

34. Tedoldi CL, Manfroi WC. Myocardial infarction and subsequent pregnancy. *Arq Bras Cardiol.* 2000;74:347–50.

35. Janion-Sadowska A, Sadowski M, Zandecki L, Kurzawski J, Polewczyk A, Janion M. Pregnancy after myocardial infarction and coronary artery bypass grafting—Is it safe? *Postepy Kardiol Interwencyjnej.* 2014;10:29–31.

36. Tweet MS, Hayes SN, Gulati R, Rose CH, Best PJ. Pregnancy after spontaneous coronary artery dissection: A case series. *Ann Intern Med.* 2015;162:598–600.

15

Pulmonary Hypertension in Pregnancy

Nisha Garg and Stephanie Martin

KEY POINTS

- Pulmonary hypertension is defined as an elevated mean pulmonary arterial pressure $\geq$25 mmHg at rest confirmed by right heart catheterization
- Pulmonary hypertension in pregnancy should be managed closely by a pulmonary hypertension specialist as part of a multidisciplinary team approach at an appropriate level of maternal care

- Pregnancy is contraindicated in all patients with pulmonary hypertension
- Epoprostenol is the most commonly used drug for pulmonary hypertension in pregnancy
- Both BNP and pro-BNP levels have been shown to correlate with survival in patients with pulmonary hypertension

---

Introduction

Pulmonary hypertension is one of the highest risk medical conditions encountered in pregnancy. This rare, progressive condition has a prevalence of 9.7 cases per 100,000 that preferentially affects young women of child-bearing age [1] with a female to male ratio of almost 2:1 [2,3]. The physiologic burden of pregnancy in pulmonary hypertension is an area of great concern and is associated with high rates of maternal and fetal morbidity and mortality. Given the complexity of pulmonary hypertension in pregnancy, it is important to manage it with a multidisciplinary approach.

Definition

Pulmonary hypertension is defined as an elevated mean pulmonary arterial pressure (mPAP) $\geq$25 mmHg at rest confirmed by right heart catheterization, and is considered severe when mPAP is $\geq$50 mmHg [4].

Pulmonary hypertension encompasses a group of diseases with various pathophysiologies, including pulmonary arterial hypertension (PAH), pulmonary hypertension related to left heart disease, pulmonary hypertension related to lung disease, chronic thromboembolic pulmonary hypertension, and pulmonary hypertension with unclear and/or multifactorial mechanisms. PAH is characterized by precapillary pulmonary hypertension, that is, pulmonary artery wedge pressure of <15 mmHg and pulmonary vascular resistance of >3 Wood units in the absence of underlying lung parenchymal or thromboembolic/vascular disease [4]. The World Health Organization (WHO) has classified pulmonary hypertension into five groups based upon etiology (Table 15.1).

Genetic Factors

Familial or inherited PAH constitutes less than 10% of cases. Mutations in two genes in the transforming growth factor beta-receptor pathway, BMPR2 and activin-like kinase 1, have been linked to this condition, with the majority (50%–90%) attributed to BMPR2 mutations. Familial PAH is characterized by incomplete penetrance, however when expressed it is associated with earlier onset and more severe disease.

Drugs

Drug-induced PAH is associated with certain appetite suppressants that increase serotonin release, such as fenfluramine and dexfenfluramine. Pulmonary hypertension is also associated with use of illicit drugs such as cocaine and methamphetamine.

Connective Tissue Diseases

Certain connective tissue diseases are associated with a primary pulmonary arteriopathy. This most commonly occurs in patients with CREST syndrome, or the limited cutaneous form of systemic sclerosis. At autopsy, up to 80% of patients have histologic evidence of pulmonary arterial hyperplasia, however less than 10% actually develop clinical disease.

Autoimmune Disorders

Pulmonary hypertension has also been associated with other autoimmune disorders such as systemic lupus erythematosus, mixed connective tissue disease, and rheumatoid arthritis.

TABLE 15.1

World Health Organization Classifications of Pulmonary Hypertension

		Etiologies
Group 1	Pulmonary arterial hypertension	Idiopathic Hereditary Drug/toxin-induced Associated with: • Connective tissue diseases • HIV infection • Portal hypertension • Congenital heart disease • Schistosomiasis
Group 2	Pulmonary hypertension due to left heart disease	Left ventricular systolic dysfunction Left ventricular diastolic dysfunction Valvular disease Cardiomyopathies Left heart inflow/outflow tract obstruction Pulmonary vein stenosis
Group 3	Pulmonary hypertension due to lung disease and/or hypoxia	Chronic obstructive pulmonary disease Interstitial lung disease Restrictive/obstructive lung disease Sleep-disordered breathing
Group 4	Chronic thromboembolic pulmonary hypertension	Chronic thromboembolic pulmonary hypertension Other pulmonary artery obstructions
Group 5	Pulmonary hypertension with unclear multifactorial mechanisms	Hematologic disorders • Hemolytic anemia • Myeloproliferative disorders • Splenectomy Systemic disorders • Sarcoidosis • Pulmonary histiocytosis • Lymphangioleiomyomatosis • Neurofibromatosis Metabolic disorders • Thyroid disorders • Glycogen storage disease Fibrosing mediastinitis Chronic renal failure with or without dialysis

Source: Adapted from Galiè N et al. Comments on the 2015 ESC/ERS Guidelines for the Diagnosis and Treatment of Pulmonary Hypertension. *Rev Esp Cardiol.* 2016;69(2):102–8.

Infections

In patients with HIV, studies have suggested an incidence of pulmonary hypertension of 0.5%, which is significantly higher than the general population. In these cases, the development of pulmonary hypertension appears to be independent of CD4 count or opportunistic infections, and is directly proportional to the duration of HIV infection. The mechanism of action of PAH in HIV patients is unclear, and routine screening is not recommended.

Portal Hypertension

Pulmonary artery hypertension also appears to be associated with portal hypertension with an estimated prevalence of 2%–6%, and the risk of developing disease increases with the duration of portal hypertension.

Pulmonary Arterial Hypertension

Finally, PAH is a well-recognized complication of uncorrected congenital heart disease involving increased pulmonary blood flow and systemic to pulmonary shunts. Common examples include unrepaired ventricular or atrial septal defects, and patent ductus arteriosus. These conditions may progress into Eisenmenger syndrome, that is, the reversal of left-to-right shunt flow due to elevation of pulmonary artery pressures above that of systemic pressures. Pulmonary hypertension is a known complication of sickle cell disease, with an estimated prevalence of 10%–30%. The etiology of pulmonary hypertension in these patients is felt to be pulmonary vasculopathy, but also may be secondary to thromboembolic events, restrictive lung disease, and/or left heart disease [5].

Diagnosis

The diagnosis of pulmonary hypertension is established based on clinical presentation, physical examination, and the results of diagnostic testing summarized in Table 15.2.

Symptoms

Clinical manifestations of pulmonary hypertension can be non-specific and include exertional dyspnea and fatigue. The condition is progressive, and therefore symptoms typically worsen over time. *As the disease progresses, increasing pulmonary pressures lead to right heart failure and symptoms become more pronounced. These include chest pain, syncope, peripheral edema, and right upper quadrant pain due to hepatic congestion.* Because of the nonspecific nature of early symptoms, delays are common, and the diagnosis of pulmonary hypertension may not even be established prior to pregnancy. In fact, 24% of pulmonary hypertension due to congenital heart disease is diagnosed during pregnancy, often presenting in the second or third trimester with shortness of breath [8,9].

Physical Examination

Findings of pulmonary hypertension include increased P2, prominent a-wave in the jugular venous pulse, right-sided S4, and right-sided murmurs.

Diagnostic Testing

Further evaluation includes EKG and B-type natriuretic peptide (BNP) level. If these are normal, then pulmonary hypertension is unlikely [10]. Both BNP and pro-BNP levels have been shown to correlate with survival, and possibly with right ventricular enlargement and dysfunction [5].

If pulmonary hypertension is suspected, an echocardiogram is indicated. Echocardiography can estimate pulmonary artery pressures. Additional findings on echocardiogram related to severe pulmonary hypertension include right ventricular enlargement and tricuspid regurgitation. However, it is important to recognize that echocardiography is a screening tool and does not definitively diagnose pulmonary hypertension. It may especially have a higher false positive rate in detecting pulmonary hypertension in pregnant patients [11,12]. This may be related to

TABLE 15.2

Diagnosis of Pulmonary Hypertension

History	Physical Examination	Diagnostic Tests

Fatigue
Weakness
Shortness of breath
Dry cough
Hemoptysis
Exercise-induced nausea/vomiting
Hoarseness
Wheezing
Chest pain
Syncope
Abdominal distention
Ankle edema
	• Loud pulmonary component of second heart sound (P2)
	• Third heart sound (S3)
	• Left parasternal lift
	• Systolic murmur of tricuspid regurgitation
	• Diastolic murmur of pulmonary regurgitation
	• Elevated jugular venous pressure
	• Hepatomegaly
	• Ascites
	• Peripheral edema
		☐ EKG
		  Tall P waves—P pulmonale, right axis deviation, right ventricular hypertrophy, prolonged QTc, atrial arrhythmias—flutter/fibrillation in 25% patients with longstanding disease [6]
		☐ CXR
		  Central pulmonary arterial dilation with peripheral "pruning" of vessels
		☐ Pulmonary function test
		  Reduced lung volume
		  Decreased lung diffusion capacity
		  Peripheral airway obstruction
		☐ Sleep study
		  Nocturnal hypoxemia and central sleep apnea 70%–80% [7]
		☐ Arterial blood gas
		  Hypoxemia with normal/decreased arterial carbon dioxide pressure
		☐ Echocardiography
		  Elevated pulmonary artery systolic pressure
		  Dilated right ventricle
		  Flattening of the interventricular septum
		☐ Ventilation/perfusion lung scan
		☐ High resolution computed tomography and pulmonary angiography
		☐ Cardiac magnetic resonance imaging
		☐ Laboratory
		  • Hepatitis serology
		  • HIV
		  • ANA, dsDNA, anti-Ro, U3 RNP, U1 RNP
		  • Antiphospholipid antibodies
		  • NT pro-BNP
		☐ Abdominal ultrasound
		☐ Right heart catheterization with vasoreactivity testing
		☐ Minute walk test
		☐ Cardiopulmonary exercise testing

the increased blood volume and decrease in systemic vascular resistance that are associated with pregnancy. This may lead to an increase in size of the inferior vena cava, thus exaggerating the estimated right atrial pressure and pulmonary artery systolic pressure. *Right heart catheterization is required for definitive diagnosis of pulmonary hypertension and to accurately determine the severity.* However, cardiac catheterization is an invasive procedure that carries a 1%–5% risk of complications including pneumothorax, bleeding, and infection [11]. Therefore, the indications for right heart catheterization are based on initial echocardiographic findings. If echocardiogram shows findings suggestive of pulmonary hypertension (elevated peak tricuspid regurgitation velocity, flattening of the interventricular septum, increased pulmonary artery diameter, etc.), then further investigation of pulmonary hypertension with right heart catheterization is indicated [3,10].

Pregnancy Risks and Antepartum Care

Pulmonary hypertension in pregnancy carries a high maternal mortality rate estimated at 17%–33%, which represents an improvement in recent years, particularly in patients with severe pulmonary hypertension and Eisenmenger syndrome [13]. Mortality is mostly the result of the inability of the right ventricle to accommodate the increased pulmonary artery pressure, leading to right heart failure [2]. The risk of right heart failure is particularly high during the intrapartum and postpartum periods due to the changes in intravascular volume and pressure during these stages [14]. A retrospective review of 49 pregnant women with pulmonary hypertension reported a mortality of 16% [2]. Nearly all of these fatalities occurred in the postpartum period, with the primary cause of death being heart failure, followed by sudden death and thromboembolism. In addition, fetal risks include mortality (11%–28%), premature birth, and growth restriction [14] (Table 15.3). Because of the excess maternal morbidity and mortality risks, pregnancy is contraindicated in patients with PAH. Women who choose to continue pregnancy despite these risks should be followed closely throughout the pregnancy by a multidisciplinary team with expertise in this

area [9]. Better outcomes are anticipated in patients who maintain a long-term favorable response to calcium channel blockers (CCBs) [15]. Poor outcomes have been reported in patients with decreased lung diffusion capacity at <45% of normal [3].

Management Strategies

A management approach proposed by the ESC/ERS for patients with pulmonary hypertension is outlined below [3].

- *Step I*
  - Avoid pregnancy
  - Influenza and pneumococcal vaccines
  - Supervised exercise training
  - Psychosocial support
  - Treatment adherence
  - Genetic counseling
  - Travel accommodations
  - Supportive therapy—anticoagulants, diuretics, oxygen, digoxin
  - Referral to expert center for vasoreactivity testing
- *Step II*
  - Therapy with high-dose CCBs in vasoreactive patients and other approved drugs for treatment of pulmonary hypertension in non-vasoreactive patients
- *Step III*
  - Assess response to initial therapy
  - Combination drugs and lung transplantation are considered for refractory cases

Medications

Medical management of pulmonary hypertension in pregnancy should be done carefully by a pulmonary hypertension specialist as part of a multidisciplinary team approach [9]. Management is guided by the etiology of the pulmonary hypertension, severity of disease, and the functional status. Most pregnant women with pulmonary hypertension are treated with a prostanoid, usually epoprostenol. Other medication classes include phosphodiesterase 5-inhibitors and CCBs (Table 15.4). Data on the benefits of each option are primarily limited to the nonpregnant patient. It is important to note that endothelin receptor antagonists (bosentan, macitentan, ambrisentan) and guanylate cyclase stimulants (riociguat) are contraindicated in pregnancy due to concern for teratogenicity [16]. As a result, access to these medications is restricted for female patients and must be through a registry with outlined contraception and sterilization recommendations [16].

Prostanoids

Prostanoids have no known teratogenic effects and are often utilized in pregnant patients with pulmonary hypertension. They are potent pulmonary vasodilators, and may also enhance right ventricular function [17]. They are available in parenteral or inhaled formulations. Currently available parenteral prostaglandins

TABLE 15.3

Maternal and Fetal Complications in Pulmonary Hypertension

Maternal Complications	Fetal Complications
Right heart failure	Preterm birth
Bronchial artery rupture—hemoptysis	Growth restriction
Pulmonary artery dilation leading to	Fetal demise
• Dissection/rupture	
• Left recurrent laryngeal nerve compression (hoarseness)	
• Compression of left main coronary artery (ischemia)	
• Compression of large airways (wheezing)	
Maternal mortality	

TABLE 15.4

Medical Therapy for Pulmonary Hypertension*

Medication	Mechanism of Action	Comments	Examples
Prostanoids	• Potent vasodilator • Inhibits platelet aggregation • Antiproliferative effects	Indicated in patients who are deteriorating and/or with worsening functional class (WHO functional class III/IV)	Parenteral/inhaled: Epoprostenol Treprostinil Iloprostol Oral: Selexipag
Phosphodiesterase 5-inhibitors	• Pulmonary vasodilator • Antiproliferative effects	Usually used in combination with a prostanoid	Sildenafil Tadalafil *(no reports of use in pregnancy)*
Calcium channel blockers	• Peripheral/pulmonary vasodilator	Those with acute response to inhaled vasodilators via vasoreactivity testing are candidates	Nifedipine Diltiazem Amplodipine *Note: Avoid Verapamil*
Endothelin receptor agonists	Pulmonary vasodilator	*Contraindicated in pregnancy*	Bosentan Macitentan Ambrisentan
Guanylate cyclase stimulants	Pulmonary vasodilator	*Contraindicated in pregnancy*	Riociguat

* See further reference [3].

include epoprostenol, treprostinil, and iloprost [17]. Selexipag is a selective prostacyclin receptor agonist that is available in an oral formulation. It has recently been approved in the United States for treatment of PAH and has been shown to decrease pulmonary vascular resistance and improve morbidity [3]. Pre-pregnancy use of these medications may be an indicator of more severe disease [17].

Typical indications for starting prostaglandin treatment include worsening functional class (WHO functional class III or IV) and deteriorating right ventricular function. Earlier introduction of targeted therapy has also been described, with daily nebulized iloprost being administered in the first trimester in patients in WHO functional class II [9]. In patients who are deteriorating, have worsening functional class, or have inadequate clinical response, treatment should be escalated with rapid conversion to parenteral forms (such as IV epoprostenol) or with addition of a phosphodiesterase 5-inhibitor [9,17]. Continuous IV epoprostenol use is expensive and cumbersome, as it requires an indwelling central venous catheter and continuous infusion pump and requires daily preparation [3]. However, it has been shown to improve cardiac indices, functional class, and is the only therapy for PAH that has been shown to prolong survival [3,5]. A meta-analysis of three randomized control trials of epoprostenol showed a risk reduction for mortality of 70%, and long-term efficacy has also been shown [3,18,19].

Phosphodiesterase 5-Inhibitors

Phosphodiesterase 5-inhibitors have been utilized successfully in pregnancies complicated by pulmonary hypertension, either alone or in combination with prostanoids [8,9,17]. Sildenafil and tadalafil may be used in pregnancy, although data are limited. Side effects are usually mild to moderate and are related to vasodilation (headaches, flushing, epistaxis) [3].

Calcium Channel Blockers

CCBs are useful in certain patients with pulmonary hypertension for vasodilation of the pulmonary vasculature. Upon

initial diagnosis of pulmonary hypertension, many patients will undergo vasoreactivity testing. Patients who are responders are candidates for treatment with CCBs, and these patients have a substantially improved prognosis compared to patients without an acute vasodilator response [17,20,21]. In certain patients, CCBs may be dangerous because of their nonselective vasodilatory effects, leading to decreased systemic vascular resistance. The most commonly used CCBs in patients with pulmonary hypertension are long-acting nifedipine, diltiazem, or amlodipine. Verapamil should be avoided due to its potential negative inotropic effects [5].

Diuretics

Diuretics are used to manage signs of right ventricular fluid overload, such as elevated jugular venous pressure, lower extremity edema, and abdominal distension or ascites [5]. Diuretics may be administered orally or intravenously; however, renal function and serum electrolytes should be monitored.

Supplemental Oxygen

Supplemental oxygen is recommended to maintain oxygen saturation above 90%, since hypoxemia is a potent vasoconstrictor [5]. Data are lacking on the ideal SpO_2 target during pregnancy for patients with pulmonary hypertension, but it should be maintained at least 90%.

Anticoagulation

Patients with pulmonary hypertension may already be on anticoagulation, which should continue during the pregnancy. Candidates for anticoagulation are those with pulmonary hypertension associated with congenital cardiac shunts in the absence of significant hemoptysis, or those with associated connective tissue disorders. In pulmonary hypertension associated with portal hypertension, anticoagulation is not recommended for patients with increased risk of bleeding [13].

In patients with advanced or decompensated PAH, right heart failure can occur. This is a potentially lethal process, which may require escalation to more aggressive therapies including atrial septostomy, extracorporeal membrane oxygenation (ECMO), and lung and/or heart transplantation [3].

Considerations in Pregnancy

Preconception Counseling

All women with known pulmonary hypertension should be offered preconception counseling from a specialist, often a maternal-fetal medicine physician. Because cardiopulmonary disease in pregnancy is associated with such morbidity and mortality, experts have classified cardiac conditions into four risk-stratified categories, modeled after the WHO classification of risk for contraceptive options (Table 15.5) [22,23].

Pulmonary hypertension is classified as WHO class IV [22]. Therefore, these women should be counseled accordingly about the very high risk of maternal mortality and morbidity, and offered appropriate contraception. After patients are counseled about their risk associated with pregnancy, should they still decide to conceive, medical optimization should be pursued. Many commonly prescribed medications for cardiac conditions have teratogenic potential and/or suspected adverse fetal effects. These should be discontinued or changed prior to conception, as the greatest risk for medication-related birth defects is from exposure during the first trimester [23]. Examples include warfarin, angiotensin-converting enzyme inhibitors, angiotensin II receptor blockers, atenolol, and amiodarone. Patients should also be prescribed a prenatal vitamin that includes sufficient folic acid supplementation. Finally, all patients with hereditary or idiopathic pulmonary hypertension should be offered genetic counseling, as these types can be associated with known genetic mutations [17]. Preconception counseling should include discussions regarding expectations for the antepartum, intrapartum, and postpartum period (discussed below).

First Trimester

Once pregnancy is diagnosed, the patient should be counseled regarding the risks of continuing the pregnancy including maternal and fetal morbidity and mortality. Pregnancy termination and appropriate contraception should be offered for all women with pulmonary hypertension regardless of functional class, given the high maternal mortality rates [13]. Given the risks of anesthesia, termination procedures should be performed in a tertiary center that is experienced in the management of patients with

pulmonary hypertension and has potential for advanced life support capabilities. Most series suggest pregnancy termination may be accomplished with minimal risk of maternal mortality, however some recent series report mortality rates approaching 50% [2,15,24].

If the decision is made to continue the pregnancy, management should be carefully coordinated with a multidisciplinary team that includes a pulmonary hypertension specialist, cardiologist, high-risk obstetrician, anesthesiologist, and neonatologist [9]. The following should be obtained:

- Genetics consultation
- Baseline echocardiogram
- BNP/NT pro-BNP level
- Medications review

If the patient is already taking targeted medications for pulmonary hypertension that are considered safe in pregnancy, she should be advised to continue them. However, those with teratogenic potential should be substituted with more appropriate alternatives for use in pregnancy.

Second Trimester

Major cardiovascular changes occur during the second trimester, including volume expansion and an increase in cardiac output. Because patients with pulmonary hypertension may have difficulty accommodating to these changes, right ventricular volume overload and failure often tends to occur during this time. Follow-up echocardiogram and repeat BNP levels should be obtained every 2–4 weeks [17]. If the patient develops symptoms of right heart failure (dyspnea, dizziness, chest pain, syncope), there is a need for prompt evaluation and treatment. Patients are frequently hospitalized in the late second trimester due to worsening of symptoms, as discussed above. In the Registry of Pregnancy and Cardiac Disease (ROPAC) cohort of 151 patients with pulmonary hypertension in pregnancy, 50% of them required at least one hospitalization, the majority for cardiac indications, with the median gestational age at admission being 27 weeks [24].

Third Trimester

By the third trimester, maternal cardiac output and plasma volume have increased by 30%–50% above baseline. The main concern during this time is preparation for delivery. Repeat echocardiograms and BNP levels should be obtained as indicated [17]. Importantly, consider administering betamethasone

TABLE 15.5

Risk Stratification of Cardiac Conditions in Pregnancy

	WHO Class I	WHO Class II	WHO Class III	WHO Class IV
Pregnancy risk	Average risk	Small increased risk of mortality and morbidity	Significant increased risk of mortality and morbidity	Pregnancy contraindicated; very high risk of maternal mortality and morbidity

for fetal benefit given the high risk of preterm delivery for maternal indications.

Delivery Planning

- *Multidisciplinary team*: As with prenatal care, intrapartum care should be multidisciplinary and include the obstetrician, maternal-fetal medicine specialist, anesthesiologist, intensivist, and pulmonary hypertension specialist.
- *Monitoring*: Continuous cardiovascular monitoring during labor and delivery or during cesarean delivery is of utmost importance. It should include telemetry, pulse oximetry, and blood pressure assessment. In some patients, invasive assessment with central venous pressure catheter and/or arterial line may be required.
- *Timing/mode of delivery*: The decision of timing of delivery and mode of delivery remain controversial, and ultimately should be individualized to each case. Both vaginal and cesarean deliveries pose potential risks for the patient to deteriorate. Elective preterm cesarean delivery (between 32–36 weeks) has been advocated in patients with severe pulmonary hypertension, as this may offer the benefit of known availability of resources and personnel, as well as control of location and potential for delivery prior to maternal decompensation [17,25].

Vaginal delivery typically requires the Valsalva maneuver, increasing intrathoracic pressure and decreasing venous return. This may lead to decreased cardiac output. In addition, labor-induced vasovagal responses have similar effects on venous return and can lead to cardiopulmonary collapse. For these reasons, many experts recommend cesarean delivery, though there is little evidence to support this recommendation. The European Society of Cardiology favors a planned cesarean or vaginal delivery over emergent cesarean delivery [13]. The Pulmonary Vascular Research Institute recommends cesarean delivery, as this bypasses the hemodynamic complications associated with labor, including decreased venous return with pain and Valsalva [17]. However, non-obstetric surgery in patients with pulmonary hypertension is associated with increased risks, including mortality, so it is reasonable to extrapolate that cesarean section may carry similar risks.

In the ROPAC registry of the European Society of Cardiology, of the 151 pregnancies complicated by pulmonary hypertension, 63% of patients underwent cesarean section—90% of these were planned, mainly for cardiac indications. Of the five maternal deaths in the series, none occurred following vaginal birth, two occurred after emergency cesarean delivery, two occurred after scheduled cesarean delivery, and one occurred after pregnancy termination. In addition, peripartum heart failure occurred in 3.8% of vaginal deliveries compared to 13% of cesarean deliveries [24]. In a recent retrospective review of 49 pregnant patients with pulmonary hypertension, 61% of them were allowed a trial of labor with a 76% success rate. Of those, 52% had an assisted second stage, thereby minimizing maternal Valsalva efforts. Mortality rates were higher in the cesarean delivery group (18%) compared to the vaginal delivery group (5%). Interestingly, the greatest mortality risk appears to be for patients with severe pulmonary hypertension in WHO group 1 who undergo intrapartum cesarean delivery. This suggests that those patients may have a higher likelihood for decompensation in labor and may be better candidates for scheduled cesarean delivery.

Current evidence suggests the greatest maternal risk follows an intrapartum cesarean delivery. Ultimately, the decision for mode of delivery should be individualized based on the patient's obstetric history, likelihood of successful vaginal delivery, type and severity of pulmonary hypertension, functional status, and hemodynamic indices.

Anesthesia

The choice of anesthesia during delivery is extremely important in patients with pulmonary hypertension. Adequate pain control during labor and delivery minimizes the significant changes in heart rate and cardiac output. The goals of anesthesia for patients undergoing cesarean delivery should be to avoid increased pulmonary vascular resistance, decreased systemic vascular resistance, and increased venous return, all while maintaining normal cardiac function and oxygenation [26].

Indiscriminate use of fluid bolus administration should be avoided, with focus on gradual onset of analgesia and/or anesthesia. Neuraxial anesthesia is generally preferred over general anesthesia due to concerns for increased maternal mortality risks with general anesthesia compared to neuraxial anesthesia [8,15,19]. General anesthetics may depress cardiac contractility, and positive pressure ventilation increases pulmonary vascular resistance [8]. In the ROPAC registry, patients receiving general anesthesia were four times more likely to die compared with patients receiving neuraxial anesthesia [24]. However, these results should be interpreted cautiously, as a selection bias may be shown toward a sicker population requiring general anesthesia. Some have reported on the successful use of general anesthesia in these patients with good maternal outcome [27]. However, if severe right heart failure is present, general anesthesia is often unavoidable [1].

Importantly, single-shot spinal anesthesia is considered contraindicated in patients with pulmonary hypertension because of the risk of rapid rise in block height and subsequent systemic hypotension [17,28,29]. Therefore, epidural anesthesia with incremental doses is often advocated as the best regional technique [1,17,26,28]. However, with the development of modern techniques and technologies, many anesthesiologists prefer using a combined spinal-epidural technique because of its superior sensory block compared with epidural alone, with no conceivable additional risk of hypotension when a very low dose is used spinally [17,28,30].

Medications

Certain medications that are used in the peripartum period should be used with caution in patients with pulmonary hypertension. Carboprost (PGF2α) is often used as a uterotonic medication for management of uterine atony; however, it may lead to bronchoconstriction or worsening pulmonary hypertension. Beta blockers are commonly employed antihypertensive medications that should be used cautiously in patients with heart failure.

See Table 15.6 for a summary of principles of management of pregnant patients with pulmonary hypertension.

TABLE 15.6

Principles of Management of Pulmonary Hypertension in Pregnancy [9,13,17,25–27]

Measure	Comments
Establish multidisciplinary team early in the course of pregnancy	Pulmonary hypertension specialist, cardiologist, MFM, anesthesiologist, neonatologist, geneticist
Discontinue ERA immediately	Risk of teratogenicity
Discontinue vitamin K antagonists and replace with low molecular weight heparin	Risk of teratogenicity with vitamin K antagonists; avoid oral anticoagulants in pregnancy
Initiate prostanoids +/− PDE 5-inhibitors as mainstay of treatment	Also CCB if determined to be responders to acute vasodilators
Arrange regular follow-up visits at monthly intervals	Including clinic, echocardiogram, and BNP evaluation. Increase frequency to weekly visits in third trimester
Elective preterm delivery at 32–36 weeks	Via vaginal delivery with assisted second stage, or scheduled cesarean delivery
Neuraxial anesthesia during delivery	CSE or epidural anesthesia, with GETA as a last resort. Single-shot spinal is contraindicated
ICU monitoring postpartum	Postpartum period poses greatest risk for maternal decompensation
Contraception planning	LARC or BTL at time of delivery. Estrogen-containing methods contraindicated

Abbreviations: PH, pulmonary hypertension; MFM, maternal fetal medicine; ERA, endothelin receptor antagonists; CCB, calcium channel blockers; BNP, brain natriuretic peptide; CSE, combined spinal epidural; GETA, general endotracheal anesthesia; ICU, intensive care unit; LARC, long-acting reversible contraception; BTL, bilateral tubal ligation.

Fetal and Neonatal Outcomes

Rates of pregnancy loss and neonatal complications are higher in patients with pulmonary hypertension. Women with more severe forms of the disease have the highest risk of an adverse fetal or neonatal outcome. The most common complications include pregnancy loss, decreased birth weight or fetal growth restriction, preterm birth, and congenital cardiac disease [8,24,28,31,32].

Postpartum

The postpartum period poses the greatest risk for maternal decompensation in women with pulmonary hypertension. The first postpartum week is a particularly vulnerable period, and the majority of maternal deaths occur during this time [2,8,24,32]. Therefore, these patients should be monitored closely in the intensive care unit for several days. Providers should remain vigilant for any signs of right heart failure and treat appropriately with diuretics. Pharmacologic prophylaxis for venous thromboembolism prevention is required in the postpartum period.

Contraception

All patients with a diagnosis of pulmonary hypertension should be counseled against pregnancy. A discussion of the contraceptive options should take place and preferably implemented prior to the patient's discharge to home. Common options are briefly reviewed (see Chapter 5).

- Long-acting reversible contraceptive (LARC) methods, such as intrauterine devices or subdermal hormonal implants, and permanent sterilization may be the most appropriate options with the lowest maternal risks.
- Permanent sterilization at time of cesarean delivery (if indicated).

- Estrogen-containing contraception is not recommended because of the increased risk of venous thromboembolic events (Medical Eligibility Criteria Category 4) [33]. In addition, exogenous estrogens may contribute to the pathogenesis of pulmonary hypertension [17].
- Progestin-only pills are not contraindicated, however have a relatively high "typical use" failure rate and are therefore are not an ideal choice.
- Injectable progestins (depo-provera) are Medical Eligibility Criteria Category 1 and therefore acceptable, although some evidence suggests risk of thrombotic events may be increased [17,33].

A recent meta-analysis reviewed eight studies and showed that depo-provera was associated with a twofold increase risk of venous thromboembolism. This same analysis showed no increased risk with progestin-only pills [34].

Clinical Implications:

- Bosetan may reduce the efficacy of oral contraceptives
- Intrauterine device placement may lead to vasovagal reaction poorly tolerated by a patient with pulmonary hypertension [22]

Follow-Up

Once patients are discharged from the hospital, they should be followed closely as an outpatient by a pulmonary hypertension specialist.

Conclusion

Pulmonary hypertension in pregnancy is a potentially life threatening condition that should be managed in a specialty center with a multidisciplinary team experienced in the care of such patients. Pregnancy is considered a contraindication in patients with pulmonary hypertension; however, if pregnancy is pursued, patients should be monitored closely for signs of deterioration and treated appropriately by experienced professionals.

REFERENCES

1. Duarte AG et al. Management of pulmonary arterial hypertension during pregnancy: A retrospective, multicenter experience. *Chest.* 2013;143(5):1330–6.
2. Meng M et al. Pulmonary hypertension in pregnancy. *Obstet Anesth Dig.* 2009;19(3):160.
3. Galiè N et al. Comments on the 2015 ESC/ERS Guidelines for the Diagnosis and Treatment of Pulmonary Hypertension. *Rev Esp Cardiol.* 2016;69(2):102–8.
4. Hoeper MM et al. Definitions and diagnosis of pulmonary hypertension. *J Am Coll Cardiol.* 2013;62. doi: 10.1016/j.jacc.2013.10.032.
5. McLaughlin VV et al. ACCF/AHA 2009 Expert Consensus Document on Pulmonary Hypertension. *J Am Coll Cardiol.* 2009;53(17):1573–619.
6. Escribano-Subias P et al. Survival in pulmonary hypertension in Spain: Insights from the Spanish registry. *Eur Respir J.* 2012;40(3):596–603.
7. Jilwan FN, Escourrou P, Garcia G, Jaïs X, Humbert M, Roisman G. High occurrence of hypoxemic sleep respiratory disorders in precapillary pulmonary hypertension and mechanisms. *Chest.* 2013;143(1):47–55.
8. Bédard E, Dimopoulos K, Gatzoulis MA. Has there been any progress made on pregnancy outcomes among women with pulmonary arterial hypertension? *Eur Heart J.* 2009;30(3):256–65.
9. Kiely DG et al. Improved survival in pregnancy and pulmonary hypertension using a multiprofessional approach. *BJOG An Int J Obstet Gynaecol.* 2010;117(5):565–74.
10. Hoeper MM, Ghofrani H-A, Grünig E, Klose H, Olschewski H, Rosenkranz S. Pulmonary hypertension. *Deutch Arztebl Int.* 2017;114(5):73–84.
11. Penning S, Robinson KD, Major CA, Garite TJ. A comparison of echocardiography and pulmonary artery catheterization for evaluation of pulmonary artery pressures in pregnant patients with suspected pulmonary hypertension. *Am J Obstet Gynecol.* 2001;184:1568–70.
12. Wylie BJ, Epps KC, Gaddipati S, Waksmonski CA. Correlation of transthoracic echocardiography and right heart catheterization in pregnancy. *J Perinat Med.* 2007;35(6):497–502.
13. Regitz-Zagrosek V et al. ESC Guidelines on the management of cardiovascular diseases during pregnancy: The Task Force on the Management of Cardiovascular Diseases during Pregnancy of the European Society of Cardiology (ESC). *Eur Heart J.* 2011;32(24):3147–97.
14. Olsson KM, Channick R. Pregnancy in pulmonary arterial hypertension. *Eur Respir Rev.* 2016;25(142):431–7.
15. Jaïs X et al. Pregnancy outcomes in pulmonary arterial hypertension in the modern management era. *Eur Respir J.* 2012;40(4):881–5.
16. NIOSH List of Antineoplastic and Other Hazardous Drugs in Healthcare Settings, 2016. (Supersedes 2014-138). 2016. doi:10.26616/NIOSHPUB2016161
17. Hemnes AR et al. Statement on pregnancy in pulmonary hypertension from the Pulmonary Vascular Research Institute. *Pulm Circ.* 2015;5(3):435–65.
18. Barst RJ et al. A comparison of continuous intravenous epoprostenol (Prostacyclin) with conventional therapy for primary pulmonary hypertension. *N Engl J Med.* 2002;334(5):296–301.
19. Rubin LJ et al. Treatment of primary pulmonary hypertension with continuous intravenous prostacyclin (epoprostenol). Results of a randomized trial. *Ann Intern Med.* 1990;112(7):485–91.
20. Sitbon O et al. Long-term response to calcium-channel blockers in non-idiopathic pulmonary arterial hypertension. *Eur Heart J.* 2010;31(15):1898–907.
21. Rich S, Kaufmann E, Levy PS. The effect of high doses of calcium-channel blockers on survival in primary pulmonary hypertension. *N Engl J Med.* 1992;327(2):76–81.
22. Thorne S et al. Pregnancy and contraception in heart disease and pulmonary arterial hypertension. *J Fam Plan Reprod Heal Care.* 2006;32(2):75–81.
23. Clapp MA, Bernstein SN. Preconception counseling for women with cardiac disease. *Curr Treat Options Cardiovasc Med.* 2017;19(9).
24. Sliwa K et al. Pulmonary hypertension and pregnancy outcomes: Data from the Registry Of Pregnancy and Cardiac Disease (ROPAC) of the European Society of Cardiology. *Eur J Heart Fail.* 2016;18(9):1119–28.
25. Konstantinides S V. Trends in pregnancy outcomes in patients with pulmonary hypertension: Still a long way to go. *Eur J Heart Fail.* 2016;18(9):1129–31.
26. Lin D, Lu JK. Anesthetic management in pregnant patients with severe idiopathic pulmonary arterial hypertension. *Int J Obstet Anesth.* 2014;23(3):288–9.
27. O'Hare R, Mc Loughlin C, Milligan K, McNamee D, Sidhu H. Anaesthesia for Caesarean section in the presence of severe primary pulmonary hypertension. *Br J Anaesth.* 1998;81(5):790–2.
28. Bonnin M et al. Severe pulmonary hypertension during pregnancy mode of delivery and anesthetic management of 15 consecutive cases. *Anesthesiology.* 2005;102.
29. Weeks SK, Smith JB. Obstetric anaesthesia in patients with primary pulmonary hypertension. *Can J Anaesth.* 1991;38(7):814–6.
30. Duggan AB, Katz SG. Combined spinal and epidural anaesthesia for caesarean section in a parturient with severe primary pulmonary hypertension. *Anaesth Intensive Care.* 2003;31(5):565–9.
31. Kampman MAM et al. Maternal cardiac function, uteroplacental Doppler flow parameters and pregnancy outcome: A systematic review. *Ultrasound Obstet Gynecol.* 2015;46(1):21–8.
32. Weiss BM, Zemp L, Seifert B, Hess OM. Outcome of pulmonary vascular disease in pregnancy: A systematic overview from 1978 through 1996. *J Am Coll Cardiol.* 1998;31(7):1650–7.
33. Curtis K, Tepper NK, Jatlaoui TC, Berry-Bibee E, Horton LG. U.S. medical eligibility criteria for contraceptive use, 2016. *MMWR Recomm Rep.* 2016;65(3):1–103.
34. Mantha S, Karp R, Raghavan V, Terrin N, Bauer KA, Zwicker JI. Assessing the risk of venous thromboembolic events in women taking progestin-only contraception: A meta-analysis. *BMJ.* 2012;345(7872). doi: 10.1136/bmj.e4944.

16

Arrhythmias in Pregnancy

Dana Senderoff Berger and Lee Brian Padove

KEY POINTS

- Only 10% of symptomatic episodes of palpitations in pregnancy are due to an arrhythmia
- Premature ventricular or atrial contractions are seen in 59% of symptomatic and 50% of asymptomatic pregnant women
- The incidence of arrhythmia is highest among pregnant women with underlying heart disease
- Symptoms of arrhythmia in pregnancy often mimic normal pregnancy symptoms
- Extent of evaluation should be based on frequency and severity of symptoms, risk factors, and physical examination findings

---

Introduction

Palpitations account for 16% of the outpatient medical visits [1] and cardiac arrhythmias seen in 60% of otherwise healthy young adults [2]. Arrhythmias are relatively uncommon in pregnancy as evidenced by the prevalence rate of 166 per 100,000 hospital admissions [5]. Interestingly, palpitations in pregnancy often do not correspond to arrhythmias [4], with only 10% of symptomatic episodes of palpitations due to an arrhythmia [3]. Arrhythmias and palpitations occur more frequently during pregnancy probably due to the hemodynamic, hormonal, and autonomic changes [6]. Pregnancy may precipitate new-onset arrhythmia or can exacerbate preexisting stable arrhythmia. The vast majority of arrhythmias are benign in a structurally normal heart [5]; however, they may be related to an underlying structural cardiac defect, which if diagnosed in a timely manner may decrease the associated mortality and/or morbidity.

Common Causes of Palpitations in Pregnancy

Tachycardia is common in pregnancy given the physiologic changes that occur during a normal pregnancy (see Chapter 3). Bradycardia, on the other hand, is uncommon, occurring only in 1% of pregnant patients presenting with cardiac complaints. Benign ectopic beats are seen in 59% of symptomatic and 50% of asymptomatic pregnant women [3,4], and the most common sustained arrhythmia in pregnancy is supraventricular tachycardia. Arrhythmias may range from more benign ectopic beats to more serious ones such ventricular tachycardia (Table 16.1) [3].

TABLE 16.1

Overview of Arrhythmias in Pregnancy [8–11]

Arrhythmia	Frequency	Treatment	Prognosis
Premature atrial contractions	Most common in pregnancy Usually asymptomatic	Beta-blockers for symptom control only	Excellent
Supraventricular tachycardia	Most common sustained arrhythmia	Vagal maneuvers Adenosine Cardioversion Beta-blockers Calcium channel blockers Ibutilide	Good
Atrial fibrillation and flutter	Uncommon Usually underlying structural cardiac defect	Beta-blockers Calcium channel blockers Digoxin Cardioversion Ibutilide Flecainide Anticoagulation	Good
Ventricular Tachycardia	Rare Usually underlying structural cardiac defect	Beta-blockers Cardioversion Flecainide Amiodarone ICD	Fair
Bradycardia and heart blocks	Rare	Pacemaker for symptoms	Good

An Approach to the Pregnant Patient with a Suspected or Known Arrhythmia

Palpitations may represent a physiologic response in pregnancy; however, the goal is to rule out an underlying cardiac disease in a symptomatic patient, as its presence may be associated with adverse maternal and neonatal outcomes. Differential diagnosis is extensive and is summarized in Key Points. Evaluation of a patient with palpitations begins with:

1. Detailed history and physical examination
2. Electrocardiogram (EKG)
3. *Laboratory testing*: Complete blood count (CBC), thyroid function tests, potassium and magnesium levels
4. Rhythm monitoring in select patients
5. Echocardiogram in select patients

Specific diagnosis can be achieved in one-third of patients with palpitations based solely on a combination of history and

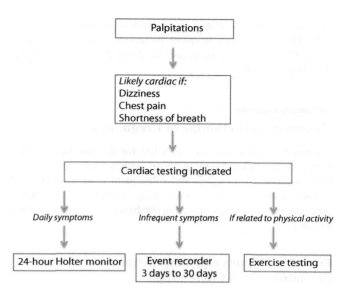

FIGURE 16.1 Approach to the patient with palpitations.

physical examination, limited laboratory testing, and an EKG [17]. Should the patient have a concerning history, physical exam, laboratory, or EKG finding, the obstetrician must refer the patient to cardiology for further evaluation (Box 16.1 and Figure 16.1).

High-Risk Features in Pregnancy That Warrant Evaluation

Most palpitations in pregnancy are self-limiting and benign; however, there is a higher likelihood of an underlying structural cardiac defect if palpitations are accompanied by dizziness, chest pain, shortness of breath or syncope, history of structural/congenital heart disease, or prior cardiac surgery [3,12,13]. If the patient has a prior history of arrhythmia, there is an increased likelihood of recurrent arrhythmias [14] and therefore the patient should be referred to a cardiologist. A family history of sudden death may also identify a patient at risk for a potentially lethal arrhythmia. Physical exam can also help identify palpitations favoring cardiac referral as listed in Box 16.2. However, it is important to be aware of the limitations of physical exam in pregnancy (Chapter 6). In general, high-risk patients include

---

BOX 16.1 DIFFERENTIAL DIAGNOSIS FOR PALPITATIONS IN THE GENERAL POPULATION [17,18]

1. Cardiac (43%)
   a. Arrhythmias
   b. Other cardiac causes
      i. Valvular heart disease including mitral valve prolapse
      ii. Pericarditis
      iii. Heart failure
      iv. Cardiomyopathy
      v. Atrial myxoma
2. Psychiatric (31%)
   a. Anxiety or panic disorder
   b. Depression
   c. Somatization
3. Medications
   a. Sympathomimetics
   b. Vasodilators
   c. Anticholinergics
   d. Beta-blocker withdrawal
   e. Substance use
   f. Cocaine
   g. Amphetamines
   h. Nicotine
4. Other
   a. Vasovagal syncope
   b. Hypoglycemia
   c. Thyrotoxicosis
   d. Pheochromocytoma
   e. Electrolyte imbalance
   f. Pulmonary embolism
   g. Infection
   h. Hemorrhage
   i. High output states including pregnancy

BOX 16.2 PHYSICAL EXAM SIGNS CONCERNING FOR PATHOLOGIC PALPITATIONS WARRANTING REFERRAL TO CARDIOLOGY

- Non-physiologic murmur (any diastolic murmur or holosystolic murmur)
- Marked jugular venous pressure elevation
- Marked edema
- Rales
- Right ventricular heave
- Palpable thrills

sustained arrhythmias and those with structural heart disease [15]. Those with very frequent premature ventricular contractions (PVCs) may also be at risk for developing a reversible cardiomyopathy [16].

Common Arrhythmias in Pregnancy

As noted, arrhythmias may manifest for the first time in pregnancy or be exacerbated in those with underlying structural heart disease. Recognition and subsequent workup in pregnant women at risk is crucial in preventing morbidity and even mortality. Commonly encountered arrhythmias in pregnancy are as follows.

Premature Ventricular Contractions and Premature Atrial Contractions

PVCs and premature atrial contractions (PACs) are common in pregnancy [3,4] and typically run a benign course. The exception may be very frequent PVCs. Rhythm monitoring is indicated to establish the burden of arrhythmia to help guide therapy. PACs are quite common in both symptomatic (59%) and asymptomatic pregnant patients (50%) [3]. However, treatment is only recommended if symptoms are intolerable. Symptoms typically improve or resolve in the postpartum period.

High-burden PVCs (>5%) have an association with maternal cardiac events (but no death) and low birth weight babies [19], while even higher burden (certainly identified in patients with as low as 10% but felt to be more likely >20% [20]) may be associated with PVC mediated cardiomyopathy which is felt to be a reversible.

Atrial Fibrillation

There is an increasing incidence of atrial fibrillation in pregnancy, with recent literature citing it as being the leading cause of hospital admissions among sustained arrhythmias in pregnancy [21]. Risk factors include older age, obstructive sleep apnea, underlying congenital heart disease, and hypertension [21]. Pregnancy-associated atrial fibrillation is also known as *lone atrial fibrillation*, that is, without a prior history of atrial fibrillation outside of pregnancy and no structural heart disease. These episodes of atrial fibrillation are usually self-limited with low risk of embolic events. There appears to be a high variability in the interventions and care in this group [22]. The general basis of treatment of atrial fibrillation is heart rate/rhythm control, and prevention of stroke.

Atrial fibrillation among pregnant patients with structural heart disease may be a marker of increased risk for maternal mortality as well as intrauterine growth restriction [23], which may be predictable based upon the severity of preexisting disease.

Supraventricular Tachycardia

Supraventricular tachycardia (SVT) is reported as the most common sustained arrhythmia in pregnancy [21,22], i.e., 22/100,000 pregnancy related hospitalizations in the United States.

Wolff-Parkinson-White Syndrome

Wolff-Parkinson-White syndrome is characterized by the presence of an extra electrical pathway that provides a source for reentry ("short circuit"). The overall incidence of Wolff-Parkinson-White is not well delineated in the general population, or in pregnancy. In one study, it made up 2.5% of arrhythmias in pregnancy in patients with maternal cardiac disease [21]. The classic resting ECG has a *delta wave*.

Reentrant Arrhythmias

The reentrant arrhythmia is usually *orthodromic*, i.e., narrow QRS complex SVT. Impulse travels from atrium to ventricle and then retrograde through the accessory pathway. Usual agents used to treat SVT can safely be used in pregnancy [8].

On the other hand, if the electrical impulse travels antegrade down the accessory pathway it is called *antidromic*; this can be potentially life threatening with wide QRS complex and special care has to be taken in the selection of medications used [8].

Supraventricular tachycardia during pregnancy had higher adjusted odds for severe maternal morbidity, cesarean delivery, low birth weight, preterm delivery, and fetal abnormalities. This population-based cohort study found that prophylactic ablation pre-pregnancy, while decreasing incidence of SVT during pregnancy, did not seem to change this risk [24].

Ventricular Tachycardia

Ventricular tachycardia (VT) is rare in pregnancy (16 per 100,000 pregnancy-related admissions) [25] and is usually associated with structural heart disease with a reported 1.4% incidence in those with structural heart disease [26]. Patient history with emphasis on prior arrhythmias and syncope along with family history of arrhythmia and/or sudden death should be reviewed. EKG should be done at rest to assess QT interval and if possible, during arrhythmia to identify source/site of origin. The most common source of idiopathic ventricular tachycardia in this age group is right ventricular outflow tract, which is identified by ECG by left bundle branch block pattern and inferior axis deviation.

Ventricular tachycardia if associated with structural heart disease is associated with both increased maternal mortality and poor fetal outcomes [25]. That being said, new-onset ventricular tachycardia in pregnancy is likely of right ventricular outflow tract origin, possibly associated with borderline low magnesium or potassium levels and seems to improve postpartum [27].

Arrhythmias with Genetic Basis

Brugada Syndrome

Brugada syndrome is a rare autosomal dominant genetically transmitted disorder of sodium/calcium channels with varying phenotypic presentations and pathognomonic EKG findings (right bundle like with coved ST segment elevation) that may be intermittent. Its greatest risk is the risk of sudden death and current definitive treatment in the at-risk group is automatic implantable cardioverter defibrillator (AICD) placement [28]. Syncope during pregnancy does not identify a patient as higher risk [29].

In Brugada syndrome, *many medications that an obstetrician, cardiologist, or anesthesiologist might normally use may have dire consequences* and should be avoided, such as bupivicaine, procaine, flecainide, ergonovine, and procainamide. Drugs to preferably avoid include amiodarone, verapamil, ketamine, tramadol, and propranolol. A full list and discussion of these medications can be found on line at www.brugadadrug.com [28].

Congenital Long QT Syndrome

Congenital long QT syndrome is associated with a repolarization abnormality with a significant risk of sudden death. Diagnosis is made by a combination of patient history, family history, and EKG findings. Long QT syndrome can be associated with a significant risk of sudden death in the postpartum period [31]. Patients generally have successful pregnancy and delivery; however, there may be increased risk of sudden death reported up to 9 months postpartum which may be attenuated with use of beta-blockers from delivery through the postpartum period [16,30,31]. Serum potassium and magnesium should be checked and optimized to keep on the high end within the normal range. A calm environment is important. *Avoidance of QT-prolonging drugs both during the pregnancy and during the peripartum and delivery is important. See below for anesthesia considerations. There have been some recommendations to consider assisted delivery to prevent prolonged second stage or Valsalva, which may potentially increase QTC. An up-to-date list of potentially harmful drugs is available at www.crediblemeds.org. Pharmacy consult should be obtained on admission.*

Catecholaminergic Biventricular Tachycardia

Catecholaminergic biventricular tachycardia is a rare genetic disease that has limited data in pregnancy. Many of these patients have AICDs in place and are on beta blockade, the dose of which may need maximization during pregnancy. We have had an experience similar to a report in the literature with a pregnant patient developing worsening tachycardia with subsequent induced cardiomyopathy that improved with the addition of flecainide [32].

Arrhythmogenic Right Ventricular Cardiomyopathy

Arrhythmogenic right ventricular cardiomyopathy is another inherited disease with limited data, but with successful pregnancy outcomes and low incidence of maternal arrhythmias (3%–13% of pregnancies). Interventions reported in one series included adjustment of beta-blockers, short term use of diuretics, and flecainide [33,34].

Bradyarrhythmias

Atrioventricular Conduction Heart Block

Successful pregnancy outcomes have been reported in asymptomatic patients with heart block with or without pacemakers. Therefore, in asymptomatic women without structural heart disease, prophylactic temporary pacing is not necessary [35]. Thaman et al. noted heart block may worsen during pregnancy but also reported two patients in whom heart block resolved postpartum [36].

Transient Postpartum Bradycardia

Transient bradycardia has been reported in postpartum period that does not require intervention [37]. Anecdotally, our experience and case reports in the literature demonstrate that most of these patients had preeclampsia or relatively elevated blood pressures.

Management Options in Pregnancy

For the Cardiologist: Obstetrician's Perspective

The majority of cardiologists are not used to discussions with pregnant patients. Not only is the physiology different [37], but usually the priorities, worries, and concerns of the individuals involved including the future mother, the spouse/loved one, and referring doctors vary considerably from what is generally encountered by a cardiologist. Their concerns include:

1. Fetal morbidity and mortality.
2. Maternal morbidity, days in the hospital, route of delivery, anesthesia, breast feeding, etc. The top priority in the mother's mind is safety of her future baby and reassurance about various testing, even something as simple as EKGs or echocardiography.
3. There is a lack randomized trials or large studies in the pregnant population. Data are often limited to case series, retrospective studies, and some prospective descriptive research.
4. Counseling should be tailored to the specific needs of the pregnant woman.

In general, if symptom treatment is the goal, the first line of treatment is reassurance. If symptoms are disruptive enough to affect lifestyle and nonpharmacologic interventions fail, every effort should be made to use the lowest dose of medications for the shortest duration that will control symptoms. There is limited evidence of antiarrhythmic drugs in pregnancy, therefore providers must weight risks and benefits and take into consideration the stage of pregnancy, severity of the arrhythmia, and possible teratogenicity. Cardiac drugs in pregnancy are discussed in detail in Chapter 20.

Treatment of Specific Arrhythmias

Management of arrhythmias in pregnancy is based on the results extrapolated from observational studies, and generally similar to that in the nonpregnant state.

Frequent PVCs

High burden of PVCs, that is, 20% or greater, is considered an indication for therapy. Beta-blockers are first-line therapy after shared decision making with the patient [25]. If beta-blockade is not effective, flecainide or sotalol may be considered as the next line therapy. It should be noted that beta-blockers are associated with intrauterine growth restriction [39,40]. In addition, there is risk of neonatal hypoglycemia and bradycardia, i.e., 4.3% with beta-blocker exposure group versus 1.2% no exposure and 1.6% versus 0.5%, respectively. Beta-blocker properties are listed in Table 16.2.

TABLE 16.2

Properties of Different Beta-Blockers in Pregnancy
[25,38,41,42]

Type	Selectivity	Dose Adjustment Required?	Comment
Metoprolol	β_1-selective	Yes May require increased frequency of dosing due to increased maternal metabolism in the 2nd and 3rd trimesters	Long history of use in pregnancy and the peripartum period
Propranolol	Nonselective	No	Reports of association with neonatal hypoglycemia and bradycardia; beneficial if hyperthyroidism
Atenolol	β_1-selective		Stronger association with fetal growth restriction than other beta-blockers therefore typically avoided

TABLE 16.3

CHADSVASc Scoring System for Risk Stratification
for Anticoagulation

CHA_2DS_2-VASc	Score
Congestive heart failure	1
Hypertension	1
Age >75 years (n/a to OB)	2
Diabetes	1
Stroke/TIA/thromboembolic	2
Vascular disease (*myocardial infarction, peripheral arterial disease, aortic plaque*)	1
Age 65–74 years (n/a to OB)	1
Sex category (female)	1

Source: From data in Lee MS et al. *J Am Heart Assoc.* 2016;5(4): e003182.

Atrial Fibrillation

The treatment in pregnancy is similar to nonpregnant patients (Figure 16.2). There is no benefit of rhythm control over rate control except when still symptomatic after rate control. In addition, in the majority of those presenting with a structurally normal heart, the first episode of atrial fibrillation typically converts quickly prior to any intervention, or within 24 hours with rate control [10,30]. And although pregnancy is thought to be

a hypercoagulable state, a large retrospective study at Kaiser Permanente Southern California showed no cases of stroke despite low use of aspirin or anticoagulants in a relatively low risk group (average CHADVASC score 1.2) [22]. (See Table 16.3.)

1. *Rate control:* First-line therapy is beta blockade. If hemodynamically stable, *metoprolol* IV 5 mg every 5 minutes up to 15 mg is used for heart rate control. If patient seems relatively dry, with history of poor oral intake, emesis, or marginal blood pressure, intravenous saline boluses are given. Second-line treatment includes intravenous diltiazem or digoxin [10,30]. Intravenous verapamil is typically not recommended due to potential to induce hypotension, which may lead to fetal hypoperfusion [30]. While digoxin has a large amount of safety data, it has a limited role as primary rate control and requires increased dosing in pregnancy and monitoring of levels. Nondihydropyridine calcium channel blockers have limited information, but some use verapamil as a third-line agent.

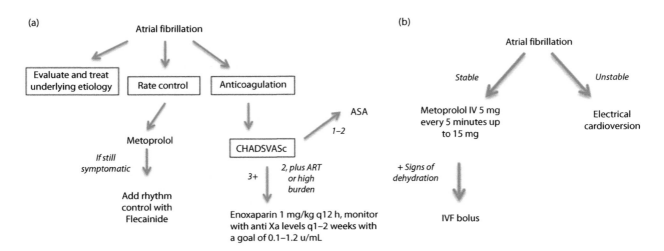

FIGURE 16.2   Management of atrial fibrillation.

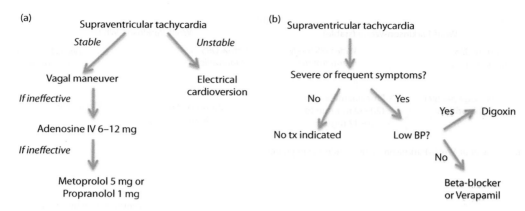

FIGURE 16.3 Management of supraventricular tachycardia in pregnancy.

2. *Rhythm control:* Rhythm control is indicated if patient remains symptomatic despite rate control. *Flecainide* has been used a great deal in the treatment of fetal SVT [20], with overall fetal safety demonstrated; therefore, we recommend it as the primary rhythm control agent in maternal atrial fibrillation with a structurally normal heart. We recommend starting low at 50 mg twice daily and increasing if needed. We usually will load while on maternal telemetry and will check a 12-lead ECG after the third dose. As expected, based on its use in fetal SVT, it does cross the placental barrier. Propafenone and sotalol can also be used in this situation, although propafenone has less data in pregnancy in the literature compared with flecainide, and sotalol is less preferable due to its effects on maternal blood pressure and heart rate. Amiodarone should be avoided due to potential fetal toxicity [30].

3. If hemodynamically unstable, *electrical cardioversion* is the treatment of choice. Synchronized cardioversion is considered safe for the fetus in the same doses used in the nonpregnant state [43]. We typically use anticoagulation, either unfractionated heparin or low molecular weight heparin, if the duration of atrial fibrillation is unclear.

One approach is to use prophylactic aspirin 81 mg in atrial fibrillation that are CHADVASC 1 and most CHADVASC 2 while using full anticoagulation with some patients with CHADVASC score of 2 (ART pregnancies, high burden of atrial fibrillation/PAF) and those with a CHADVASC score 3 or greater. The novel anticoagulants (NOACS) have limited data and thus are not recommended in pregnancy. Warfarin should not be used early in pregnancy due to embryopathy, or near delivery due to potential bleeding complications; however, it can be used second and third trimester. My practice has been to use enoxaparin, starting at 1 mg/kg subcutaneous every 12 hours with monitoring of anti-Xa every 1–2 weeks with monitoring of peak 4–6 hours post dose (goal level .01 to 1.2 u/mL) and trough (>0.6 u/mL) withholding prior to delivery [44].

Supraventricular Tachycardia

If hemodynamically unstable, *electrical cardioversion* is the treatment of choice. For stable patients, first line intervention is

vagal maneuvers, followed quickly if necessary by *adenosine IV 6–12 mg* [30]. If adenosine is ineffective, the patient's history suggests she has been going in and out of the arrhythmia that day, or there is clinical suspicion of hyperthyroidism, intravenous beta-blocker (metoprolol 5 mg or propranolol 1 mg) may be used. If these fail, intravenous procainamide or verapamil may be used [24]. However, as previously stated, verapamil should be avoided if possible due to potential for hypotension and fetal hypoperfusion. Aside from avoidance of verapamil, this management strategy is similar to the nonpregnant patient. The European Society of Cardiology recommends *beta-blocker or verapamil* for preventive therapy in this group [30]. If maternal blood pressure is marginal or relatively low, digoxin is safe and can be used as first line. Dosing with digoxin usually is twice a day during pregnancy and at higher doses than usual while following therapeutic effects and levels. (See Figure 16.3.)

Wolff-Parkinson-White

If stable, therapy is based on whether orthodromic or antidromic. The patient who presents with a *narrow QRS complex SVT* (orthodromic, travels the normal pathway from atrium to ventricle and then retrograde the accessory pathway) can be treated in the same manner as SVT above. If the patient presents with *wide complex tachycardia* (probable antidromic SVT) or extremely rapid atrial fibrillation and is hemodynamically stable, *procainamide* (20–50 mg/min to 10–17 mg/kg) can be used for either heart rate control or conversion. The drip should be continued until therapeutic goals are met (rate control or cardioversion), maximum dose, hypotension, or QRS widens by 50%. In antidromic, *flecainide* can be used to prevent recurrence. Ablation should be undertaken postpartum or if recalcitrant arrhythmias are occurring [22]. (See Figure 16.4.)

Ventricular Tachycardia

If hemodynamic compromised, an *electrical cardioversion* should be performed. If stable, intravenous *lidocaine* may be used. Beta blockade with *metoprolol* is most commonly used for chronic prophylaxis. Amiodarone should be preserved for when no other options are available. Idiopathic RVOT can be treated with metoprolol or verapamil. If these fail, flecainide may be used. (See Figure 16.5.)

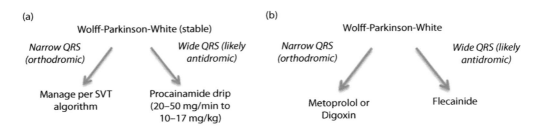

FIGURE 16.4   Management of Wolff-Parkinson-White syndrome in pregnancy.

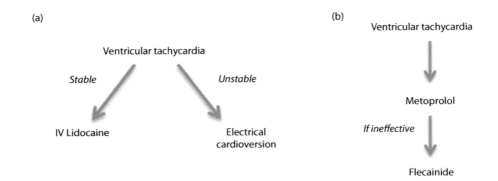

FIGURE 16.5   Management of ventricular tachycardia.

Genetic Syndromes

Brugada

In the acute setting of electrical storm, treatment includes *cardioversion* and *isoproterenol* (1-2 μg bolus intravenously followed by continuous infusion of 0.15–2.0 μg/min). Brugada mainstay is avoiding certain medications (listed previously) and *definitive treatment* in the at-risk group is *AICD placement*. However, *quinidine* can be used for *prophylaxis* [28,29].

Prolonged QT Syndrome

The specific interventions for acute arrhythmia in the setting of prolonged QT include intravenous *magnesium*, *beta-blockade*, and if needed, *defibrillation*. In some cases, temporary overdrive pacing is indicated. The risk of cardiac event and death is largely attenuated with use of beta-blockers [31]. Fetal safety of beta-blocker therapy within this group has been documented and the patient can be reassured [39]. If the patient has been on successful prophylaxis with a beta-blocker prior to pregnancy, she should continue the same beta-blocker that she has been on (possibly with exception of atenolol). This is one setting in pregnancy that *nonselective beta-blocker* may be preferred as there have been documented differences in efficacy among the beta-blockers [41,42].

Recurrence

Patients with prior history of some arrhythmias have been documented to have an increased recurrence rate. Those with a history of symptomatic SVT were found to have a recurrence rate of 22%–50% with further increased prevalence in those with structural heart disease [15,45]. More than 50% of patients with prior history of atrial fibrillation will have a symptomatic recurrence during pregnancy warranting prompt evaluation. The risk of recurrent ventricular tachycardia is nearly 30% during pregnancy [15].

Cardiac Procedures for Arrhythmias in Pregnancy

Electrical Cardioversion

Direct current cardioversion is used in the setting of hemodynamic instability and is considered safe for the fetus. There is no alteration in the defibrillation protocol recommended for the pregnant patient as compared to the nonpregnant patient. Anterolateral pad positioning is felt to be a reasonable default. Airway protection and management may be problematic, and therefore experienced personnel should be readily available [46].

Implantable Cardioverter-Defibrillator

In the limited reported literature available, the presence of an implantable cardioverter-defibrillator (ICD) does not seem to influence the outcomes of pregnancy nor does pregnancy negatively affect its function [47,48]. No ICD adjustment is necessary for vaginal delivery. There are various recommendations available regarding ICD management during surgery. Knowledge of the device and whether the patient is pacemaker dependent should be obtained from the last device clinic note. This allows surgical planning should delivery be done by cesarean section. It is important to consider electromagnetic interference of the pacemaker secondary to monopolar cautery. If monocautery must be used, it is recommended to use short bursts. The pacemaker can be programmed ahead of time to avoid inactivation, or a magnet can be used to convert the pacemaker to an asynchronous mode

[49]. Since cesarean section is below the umbilicus (>6 inches from the device), it is not required to deactivate the device preoperatively [50]. Placement of an ICD, if required during pregnancy, should be performed after the first 8 weeks to minimize risks of radiation [30]. Use of non-radiation-exposing techniques such as echocardiographic guidance is recommended. ICD placement using electroanatomic techniques and no fluoroscopy have been reported [51].

Life Vest

Also known as a wearable cardioverter-defibrillator (WCV), life vest has been utilized as a way of limiting risk of sudden death that may resolve with time. A good example is newly diagnosed peripartum cardiomyopathy with low ejection fraction felt to be at high risk for sudden death but with good odds of recovery. There is limited literature on this, but one series reported 12% of the patients with ventricular tachyarrhythmia, including one with partial recovery of ejection fraction. Additional possible uses include while awaiting placement of a permanent defibrillator due to inheritable arrhythmias diagnosed in pregnancy, while pending referral to a center with experience with non-radiation-based techniques in ICD placement, or even in cases where placement of permanent defibrillator is being delayed until after pregnancy [52,53].

Radiofrequency Catheter Ablation

Catheter ablation in pregnancy is considered safe and effective for both SVT and ventricular arrhythmias using electroanatomical mapping and catheter navigation systems. Although ablation in general should be deferred until postpartum, there has been reported ablation in pregnancy using low or no radiation techniques in patients with recalcitrant arrhythmias. Regardless, if necessary, procedure should be delayed until after the first trimester when most of organogenesis is complete [8,54]. However, it should be used as a last resort effort to control recalcitrant ventricular tachycardia and recalcitrant poorly tolerated SVT [30,55].

Antepartum Follow-Up

Cardiology Follow-Up

Cardiology follow-up is indicated for all patients with significant arrhythmia and/or structural heart disease. Stable arrhythmias without significant risk (i.e., SVT, AF) may see cardiology twice during pregnancy, whereas the higher risk arrhythmias (unstable SVT or VT, those with ICDs) and those with more potential adjustment of medications require closer cardiology follow-up, anywhere from every month to every trimester [30]. If the patient has a device in place, information about the device is made readily available and any special care is planned pre-delivery. In patients with a high burden of PVCs [19,20]:

- Burden of >5% but <10% may benefit from an additional visit late pregnancy in the 34–36 week range
- Burden of >10% may benefit from monthly cardiology visit with low threshold for checking a BNP and/or follow-up echo

- Burden of 20% or more should have follow-up echocardiograms every 4–8 weeks and clinic visit monthly with aggressive PVC suppression with first signs of LV dysfunction

Obstetrical Follow-Up

Obstetrical follow-up is largely determined by obstetrical indications; however, close tracking for growth may be indicated in patients on beta-blockers given their association with IUGR. SVT in pregnancy has an association with preterm delivery in one study [24], and quinidine can increase risk for preterm labor.

Commonly Used Medications on Labor and Delivery to Use with Caution or Avoid in a Patient with Arrhythmia

- Pitocin if used with a patient who has a congenital arrhythmia such as prolonged QT: Oxytocin, although potentially harmful and death reported with a high dose bolus, it is probably safe if given as a slow infusion [56]
- Magnesium sulfate
- Terbutaline
- Methergine
- Hemabate

Delivery Planning
Who Needs Telemetry?

In general, stable arrhythmias without significant risk do not need telemetry postpartum. In women with PVC burden greater than 5%, we recommend maternal telemetry peripartum. While if asymptomatic PVCs and low burden of arrhythmia, telemetry is not necessary [19,20]. For atrial fibrillation, telemetry may be useful postpartum but it is not absolutely necessary if rate is stable and controlled. If unable to achieve rate control, however, telemetry should be used, especially while loading medications used for rhythm control such as flecainide. Patients with congenital prolonged QT syndrome should remain on telemetry for the intrapartum and postpartum period.

Multidisciplinary Team Approach

In general, arrhythmias can safely be managed in a multidisciplinary manner with input from maternal-fetal medicine, anesthesia, and cardiology.

One Special Note about Congenital Prolonged QT Syndrome

All local anesthetics have been used successfully for regional anesthesia. Some drugs which are commonly used peripartum that should be avoided include many of the inhalation anesthetics, ketamine, and thiopental. Acceptable medications commonly used include etomidate, propofol, nitrous oxide, and methohexital. Fentanyl, morphine, and midazolam are all acceptable. Droperidol and ondansetron have been associated with prolonged QT [57].

Anticoagulation Considerations

See Chapter 9 for details.

Postpartum Follow-Up

Follow-up in the postpartum period is highly dependent on the type of arrhythmia. PVCs often improve in the postpartum period [3]. In cases of new-onset pregnancy-associated lone atrial fibrillation, it is reasonable to give a trial off of rate and/or rhythm control after 6–8 weeks postpartum. For patients on anticoagulation at that point, one may consider placing a 30-day monitor to exclude silent atrial fibrillation prior to discussion with patient about discontinuing anticoagulation. Patients who are potential candidates for catheter ablation therapy, such as those with SVTs and certain ventricular arrhythmias, should be evaluated in the postpartum period for potential intervention.

Conclusion

Palpitations are extremely common in pregnancy and the incidence of cardiac arrhythmias is higher during pregnancy, and highest in pregnant women with a history of heart disease. It can be challenging to manage symptoms of arrhythmia in pregnancy, such as palpitations and shortness of breath, as they often mimic normal pregnancy symptoms. Fortunately, most arrhythmias during pregnancy are benign and do not require therapy. However, all patients should be evaluated based on frequency and severity of symptoms, risk factors, and physical examination findings. The goal is not to miss potentially harmful arrhythmias that can be safely managed in pregnancy, ideally in a multidisciplinary manner with input from maternal-fetal medicine, anesthesia, and cardiology.

REFERENCES

1. Kroenke K, Arrington ME, Mangelsdorff AD. The prevalence of symptoms in medical outpatients and the adequacy of therapy. *Arch Intern Med.* 1990;150(8):1685–9.
2. Turner AS, Watson OF, Adey HS, Cottle LP, Spence R. The prevalence of disturbance of cardiac rhythm in randomly selected New Zealand adults. *N Z Med J.* 1981;93(682):253–5.
3. Shotan A, Ostrzega E, Mehra A, Johnson JV, Elkayam U. Incidence of arrhythmias in normal pregnancy and relation to palpitations, dizziness, and syncope. *Am J Cardiol.* 1997;79(8):1061–4.
4. Choi HS et al. Dyspnea and palpitation during pregnancy. *Korean J Intern Med.* 2001;16(4):247–9.
5. Raviele A et al. Management of patients with palpitations: A position paper from the European Heart Rhythm Association. *Europace.* 2011;13(7):920–34.
6. Mahendru AA, Everett TR, Wilkinson IB, Lees CC, McEniery CM. A longitudinal study of maternal cardiovascular function from preconception to the postpartum period. *J Hypertens.* 2014;32(4):849–56.
7. Li J-M, Nguyen C, Joglar JA, Hamdan MH, Page RL. Frequency and outcome of arrhythmias complicating admission during pregnancy: Experience from a high-volume and ethnically-diverse obstetric service. *Clin Cardiol.* 2008;31(11):538–41.
8. Page RL et al. 2015 ACC/AHA/HRS guideline for the management of adult patients with supraventricular tachycardia. *Heart Rhythm.* 2016;13(4).
9. Knotts RJ, Garan H. Cardiac arrhythmias in pregnancy. *Semin Perinatol.* 2014;38(5):285–8.
10. Fuster V et al. ACC/AHA/ESC 2006 guidelines for the management of patients with atrial fibrillation. *Europace.* 2006; 8(9):651–745.
11. Antonelli D, Bloch L, Rosenfeld T. Implantation of permanent dual chamber pacemaker in a pregnant woman by transesophageal echocardiographic guidance. *Pacing Clin Electrophysiol.* 1999;22(3):534–5.
12. Al-Yaseen E, Al-Na'ar A, Hassan M, Al-Ostad G, Ibrahim E. Palpitation in pregnancy: Experience in one major hospital in Kuwait. *Med J Islam Repub Iran.* 2013;27(1):31–4.
13. Drenthen W et al. Predictors of pregnancy complications in women with congenital heart disease. *Eur Heart J.* 2010;31(17):2124–32.
14. Sanghavi M, Rutherford JD. Cardiovascular physiology of pregnancy. *Circulation.* 130(12), 2014;1003–8.
15. Silversides CK et al. Pregnancy outcomes in women with heart disease. *J Am Coll Cardiol.* 2018;71(21):2419–30.
16. Lee AK, Deyell MW. Premature ventricular contraction-induced cardiomyopathy. *Curr Opin Cardiol.* 2016;31(1):1–10.
17. Weber BE, Kapoor WN. Evaluation and outcomes of patients with palpitations. *Am J Med.* 1996;100(2):138–48.
18. Mayou R, Sprigings D, Birkhead J, Price J. Characteristics of patients presenting to a cardiac clinic with palpitation. *QJM.* 2003;96(2):115–23.
19. Tong C et al. Impact of frequent premature ventricular contractions on pregnancy outcomes. *Heart.* 2018;104(16):1370–5.
20. Razvi S et al. Thyroid hormones and cardiovascular function and diseases. *J Am Coll Cardiol.* 2018;71(16):1781–96.
21. Salam AM et al. Atrial fibrillation or flutter during pregnancy in patients with structural heart disease. *JACC: Clin Electrophysiol.* 2015;1(4):284–92.
22. Lee MS et al. Atrial fibrillation and atrial flutter in pregnant women-a population based study. *J Am Heart Assoc.* 2016;5(4):e003182.
23. Renoux C, Coulombe J, Suissa S. Revisiting sex differences in outcomes in non-valvular atrial fibrillation: A population-based cohort study. *Eur Heart J.* 2017;May 14;38(19):1473–9.
24. Chang S-H et al. Outcomes associated with paroxysmal supraventricular tachycardia during pregnancy. *Circulation.* 2017;135(6):616–8.
25. Vaidya VR et al. Burden of arrhythmia in pregnancy. *Circulation.* 2017;135(6):619–21.
26. Ertekin E et al. Ventricular tachyarrhythmia during pregnancy in women with heart disease: Data from the ROPAC, a registry from the European Society of Cardiology. *Int J Cardiol.* 2016;220: 131–6.
27. Nakagawa M et al. Characteristics of new-onset ventricular arrhythmias in pregnancy. *J Electrocardiol.* 2004;37(1):47–53
28. Brugada Syndrome. www.brugada.org/. Brugada Foundation. 2018. Web. 24 Sept 2019.
29. Rodríguez-Mañero M et al. The clinical significance of pregnancy in Brugada syndrome. *Rev Esp Cardiol (Engl Ed).* 2014;67(3):176–80.

30. Regitz-Zagrosek V et al. 2018 ESC Guidelines for the management of cardiovascular diseases during pregnancy. *Eur Heart J.* 2018;39(34):3165–241.

31. Seth R et al. Long QT Syndrome and pregnancy. *J Am Coll Cardiol.* 2007;49(10):1092–8.

32. Walker N, Cobbe S, McGavigan A. Paroxysmal bidirectional ventricular tachycardia with tachycardiomyopathy in a pregnant woman. *Acta Cardiologica.* 2009;64(3):419–22.

33. Gandjbakhch E et al. Pregnancy and newborn outcomes in arrhythmogenic right ventricular cardiomyopathy/dysplasia. *Int J Cardiol.* 2018;258:172–8.

34. Hodes AR et al. Pregnancy course and outcomes in women with arrhythmogenic right ventricular cardiomyopathy. *Heart.* 2015;102(4):303–12.

35. Hidaka N et al. Short communication: Is intrapartum temporary pacing required for women with complete atrioventricular block? An analysis of seven cases. *BJOG.* 2006;113(5):605–7.

36. Thaman R et al. Cardiac outcome of pregnancy in women with a pacemaker and women with untreated atrioventricular conduction block. *Europace.* 2011;13(6):859–63.

37. Korzets Z et al. Bradycardia as a presenting feature of late postpartum eclampsia. *Nephrol Dial Transplant.* 1994;9(8):1174–5.

38. Wright JM et al. Antiarrhythmic drugs in pregnancy. *Expert Rev Cardiovasc Ther.* 2015;13(12):1433–44.

39. Ishibashi K et al. Arrhythmia risk and β-blocker therapy in pregnant women with long QT syndrome. *Heart.* 2017;103(17):1374–9.

40. Ersbøll A, Hedegaard M, Søndergaard L, Ersbøll M, Johansen M. Treatment with oral beta-blockers during pregnancy complicated by maternal heart disease increases the risk of fetal growth restriction. *BJOG.* 2014;121(5):618–26.

41. Abu-Zeitone A, Peterson DR, Polonsky B, Mcnitt S, Moss AJ. Efficacy of different beta-blockers in the treatment of long QT syndrome. *J Am Coll Cardiol.* 2014;64(13):1352–8.

42. Kim H. Not all beta-blockers are equal in the management of long QT syndrome types 1 and 2: Higher recurrence of events under metoprolol. *J Emerg Med.* 2013;44(3):732–3.

43. Wang YC, Chen CH, Su HY, Yu MH. The impact of maternal cardioversion on fetal haemodynamics. *Eur J Obstet Gynecol Reprod Biol.* 2006;126(2):268–9.

44. Alshawabkeh L, Economy KE, Valente AM. Anticoagulation during pregnancy. *J Am Coll Cardiol.* 2016;68(16):1804–13.

45. Lee SH et al. Effects of pregnancy on first onset and symptoms of paroxysmal supraventricular tachycardia. *Am J Cardiol.* 1995;76(10):675–8

46. Jeejeebhoy FM et al. Cardiac arrest in pregnancy. *Circulation.* 2015;132(18):1747–73.

47. Boule S et al. Pregnancy in women with an implantable cardioverter-defibrillator: Is it safe? *Europace.* 2014;16(11):1587–94.

48. Miyoshi T et al. Safety and efficacy of implantable cardioverter defibrillator during pregnancy and after delivery. *Cir J.* 2013;77(5):1166–70.

49. Neelankavil JP, Thompson A, Mahajan A. Managing cardiovascular implantable electronic devices (CIEDs) during perioperative care. *APSF Newsletter.* 2013;28(2):32–5.

50. Crossley GH et al. The Heart Rhythm Society (HRS)/American Society of Anesthesiologists (ASA) Expert Consensus Statement on the Perioperative Management of Patients with Implantable Defibrillators, Pacemakers and Arrhythmia Monitors: Facilities and Patient Management. *Heart Rhythm.* 2011;8(7):1114–54.

51. Quartieri F et al. Implantation of single lead cardioverter defibrillator with floating atrial sensing dipole in a pregnant patient without using fluoroscopy. *Indian Pacing Electrophysiol J.* 2016;16(2):70–2.

52. Piccini JP, Allen LA, Kudenchuk PJ, Page RL, Patel MR, Turakhia MP. Wearable cardioverter-defibrillator therapy for the prevention of sudden cardiac death. *Circulation.* 2016;133(17):1715–27.

53. Duncker D et al. Risk for life-threatening arrhythmia in newly diagnosed peripartum cardiomyopathy with low ejection fraction: A German multi-centre analysis. *Clin Res Cardiol.* 2017;106(8):582–9.

54. Kaspar G, Sanam K, Gundlapalli S, Shah D. Successful fluoroless radiofrequency catheter ablation of supraventricular tachycardia during pregnancy. *Clin Case Rep.* 2018;6(7):1334–7.

55. Chen G et al. Zero-fluoroscopy catheter ablation of severe drug-resistant arrhythmia guided by Ensite NavX system during pregnancy. *Medicine.* 2016;95(32).

56. Martillotti G, Talajic M, Rey E, Leduc L. Long QT syndrome in pregnancy: Are vaginal delivery and use of oxytocin permitted? A case report. *J Obstet Gynaecol Can.* 2012;34(11):1073–6.

57. Drake E, Preston R, Douglas J. Brief review: Anesthetic implications of long QT syndrome in pregnancy. *Can J Anesth.* 2007;54(7):561–72.

17

Thromboembolism and Amniotic Fluid Embolism

Arthur J. Vaught

KEY POINTS

- Pulmonary embolism accounts for 10% of maternal deaths
- The gold standard for diagnosis of pulmonary embolism in pregnancy is computed tomographic angiography of the pulmonary arteries
- Pulmonary embolism is considered massive (10%) if it is accompanied by systemic arterial hypotension resulting in shock

- Treatment considerations for massive pulmonary embolism include systemic thrombolytic therapy, catheter-directed thrombolysis, or emergent thrombectomy
- Amniotic fluid embolism occurs in 2–6 per 100,000 deliveries characterized by cardiovascular collapse, disseminated intravascular coagulopathy, and refractory hypoxemia resulting from acute respiratory distress syndrome

Pulmonary Embolism

Epidemiology

Both pulmonary embolism (PE) and deep venous thrombosis (DVT) occur more frequently in pregnancy. In a pooled meta-analysis, the overall prevalence of DVT and PE in pregnancy were 1.1% and 0.2%, respectively [1]. Although PE occurs less frequently, its associated morbidity and mortality is higher than DVT [2]. Despite the significant decrease in maternal mortality secondary to thromboembolic events, PE still remains a leader of maternal hospital cost, severe maternal morbidity, and prolonged hospital stay, and accounts for 10% of maternal deaths [3]. See Figure 17.1.

Risk Factors

Obesity, hypertensive disorders, postpartum hemorrhage, and inherited thrombophilia are all risk factors for PE in pregnancy [4]. In fact, the physiologic and anatomic changes of pregnancy further augment these risks by increasing clotting factors and compression of the inferior vena cava (IVC) causing decreased venous flow and stasis [4]. Although all of these factors increase the risk of a PE or thromboembolic event, the most important risk factor is a history of prior venous thromboembolic event (VTE). The risk of recurrent VTE during pregnancy increases by fourfold, and one-quarter of all VTEs in pregnancy are recurrences [5]. Many women with VTE do not get a diagnosis of thrombophilia during pregnancy; however, these mutations certainly increase the risk and likelihood of having a clot. Routine screening for thrombophilia is not recommended; however, it is reasonable to screen if there is history of multiple VTE in a given woman, a strong family history, or if the VTE was severe (i.e., massive pulmonary embolism) [6].

Diagnosis

Diagnosis of pulmonary embolism may be challenging in pregnancy, as shortness of breath and tachycardia are common features of normal pregnancy. (See Chapter 3 for more details of physiologic changes.)

Symptoms

Classic clinical signs and symptoms of PE include but are not limited to hypoxemia, tachypnea, changes in cardiac imaging studies, mild elevations of troponin levels, and tachyarrhythmia. Common presenting symptoms are listed in Table 17.1. It is important to note that symptoms of PE are neither sensitive nor specific, and therefore the obstetric practitioner should continue to have a wide differential when diagnosis of PE is being entertained.

Differential Diagnosis

Includes pneumonia, myocardial infarction, preeclampsia, cardiac failure, and non-cardiogenic pulmonary edema.

Diagnostic Testing

Oddly enough, significant hypoxemia was a rare finding in PE, with many patients with oxygenation >95% [7]. Cardiac arrhythmias are present in approximately 10% of patients diagnosed with a PE, usually a tachyarrhythmia. Although sinus tachycardia is the most common tachyarrhythmia, others can present with atrial fibrillation, atrial flutter, and multifocal atrial tachycardia [8].

Arterial blood gas is also clinically useful. Often blood gases will show a respiratory alkalosis and hypoxemia or normal oxygenation. Other lab parameters abnormally elevated in PE are

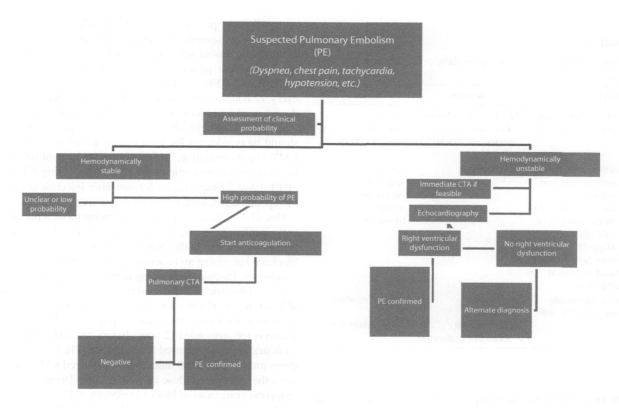

FIGURE 17.1 Management of suspected pulmonary embolism in pregnancy.

D-dimer, cardiac troponins, and brain natriuretic peptide (BNP) levels. It should be noted that D-dimer levels increase in pregnancy and are not considered reliable in diagnosing PE during pregnancy [4,7–10]. Likewise, false negative results for D-dimer have been reported, and therefore D-dimer test is not used as part of the workup for PE [11].

Although not used to diagnose PE, cardiac troponins and BNP can be helpful in the risk stratification of patients with PE. Overall, approximately 50% of patients with PE will have a "positive" or elevated cardiac troponins [12]. Further, approximately 30% of the patients exhibit right ventricular dysfunction that is associated with worsened short- and long-term mortality [13]. BNP has also been shown to help stratify patients with PE into lower and higher risk categories. In particular, nonpregnant patients with pro-BNP

TABLE 17.1

Clinical Features and Diagnostic Testing in Pulmonary Embolism

Signs and Symptoms	Diagnostic Testing
Dyspnea (73%)	Arterial blood gas
Tachypnea (54%)	Electrocardiography
Arrhythmia/Tachycardia (24%)	Chest CT angiography
Pleuritic chest pain (66%)	Ventilation/perfusion scan
Cough (37%)	Lower extremity Doppler
Hemoptysis (13%)	Echocardiography
Wheezing (21%)	Pro-brain natriuretic peptide
Fever (3%)	or B-type natriuretic peptide

levels >600 pg/mL were at increased risk of short-term mortality secondary to PE [14]. Therefore, it is reasonable to check cardiac troponins and BNP levels at diagnosis of PE. High levels can help stratify patients into low- and high-risk categories which could aid practitioners in obtaining additional imaging (i.e., echo), consultation (cardiology, hematology, cardiac surgery), and transfer to higher levels of care (critical care, hospital transfer).

Although practitioners can use physical exam and lab data to aid in the diagnosis of PE, *the gold standard for diagnosis is computed tomographic angiography (CTA) of the pulmonary arteries, even in pregnancy* [4]. In clinical practice, practitioners may argue against CTA for fear of radiation exposure to the fetus; however, this exposure is very low and rarely if at all causes fetal harm from just one CTA [4]. Further, the fetus can be shielded by placing the lead on the maternal abdomen if there is concern. In clinical scenarios of renal injury, failure, or severe contrast allergy, ventilation-perfusion scan is a reasonable alternative; however, this imaging modality also has radiation exposure [15]. *Fetal radiation exposure from CTA is lower than ventilation-perfusion scan (0.32–0.64 mGy vs. 0.003–0.1398 mGy); however, the maternal radiation exposure to the breast is lower with ventilation-perfusion scan* [16]. See Table 17.2.

After a PE is diagnosed it should be categorized appropriately to help delineate severity, treatment options, and reduce maternal morbidity.

Types of Pulmonary Embolism

The three types of PE are subsegmental, submassive, and massive. Many PEs experienced in obstetric practice are subsegmental and

TABLE 17.2

Risks and Benefits of Imaging Modalities in Pulmonary Embolism

Modality	Benefits	Risks
CT Pulmonary Arteries *Sensitivity of 90%–95%*	Detects other pulmonary abnormalities, i.e., pneumonia, fibrotic disease	Radiation exposure Contrast allergy
Ventilation/Perfusion *Sensitivity varies on probability* *Low: 4% risk of PE* *Intermediate: 15% risk of PE* *High: 16% risk of PE* *Scoring further changes based on clinical probability*	No contrast	Radiation exposure Intermediate results 1-hour test
Echocardiography *Sensitivity 30%–40%*	No contrast No radiation Diagnosis right ventricular dysfunction	Not gold standard Needs confirmatory test

can be treated with careful therapeutic anticoagulation. However, massive and submassive PE account for 5–10% and 20%–25% of cases, respectively, in the general population and carry an increase in morbidity and mortality [17–19]. A PE is considered massive if it is accompanied by systemic arterial hypotension resulting in shock [19]. A PE is considered submassive when systemic hemodynamics are preserved but there is evidence of right ventricular dysfunction on either electrocardiogram, echocardiography, or CTA. The 90-day mortality for a massive PE can reach as high as 50%, and up to 19% for submassive PE. Therefore, when a PE is diagnosed proper categorization should be undertaken.

Management of Pulmonary Embolism

Prevention

One could argue that the mainstay of treatment of PE in pregnancy is prevention. Ideally, personal or family history of thromboembolism should be reviewed for each and every pregnant patient to identify those at high risk of complications. Patients without current PE but with risk factors should be considered for prophylactic, intermediate, or adjusted dose low molecular weight heparin (LMWH) or unfractionated heparin (UFH) per ACOG guidelines [4]. When selecting an appropriate dose of LMWH or UFH for prevention, maternal weight, past medical history, severity of previous disease (i.e., massive PE), thrombophilia workup (high-risk thrombophilia vs. low-risk thrombophilia), and other hypercoagulable comorbidities (nephrotic syndrome, ulcerative colitis, antiphospholipid antibody) should be considered.

Anticoagulation

Women diagnosed with a PE should be treated with full anticoagulation for at least 3–6 months and for at least 6 weeks postpartum.

Although many practitioners will keep patients on full anticoagulation, it is reasonable to decrease this dose to intermediate or prophylactic dosing after the initial 3–6 months of therapy into the postpartum period [4]. Acceptable therapeutic dosing for LMWH and UFH are 1 mg/kg every 12 hours or 250 units/kg every 12 hours, respectively. Usually, patients receiving LMWH do not need anti-factor Xa levels tested. However, patients with renal injury, morbid obesity, and antithrombin III deficiency should be considered for level testing which is 4–6 hours after LMWH administration. An anti-factor Xa level of 0.6–1.0 u/mL is considered therapeutic range [20]. When using UFH, a goal aPTT 1.5–2.5 times control 6 hours after injection is considered therapeutic (see Chapter 9 for more details).

One of the central issues the obstetrician faces is managing full anticoagulation around the timing of delivery. Full anticoagulation is not a contraindication to vaginal delivery or neuroaxial blockade but timing and coordination with obstetric anesthesia is paramount. Decisions regarding delivery timing should be based on usual obstetric and maternal indication; however, it is reasonable to time an induction for coordination purposes after 39 weeks. In general, for women receiving prophylactic LMWH, discontinuation is recommended 12 hours before neuroaxial blockade and 24 hours before an adjusted dose regimen [21]. Concerning UFH, doses greater than 7500 units twice daily need a 12-hour interval from the most recent dose as well as coagulation studies before induction or neuroaxial blockade placement [21].

The optimal time to resume full anticoagulation therapy postpartum is unknown. Obstetricians must weigh severity of disease burden and risk of hemorrhage or bleeding. A reasonable approach to minimize bleeding is to resume therapy no sooner than 4–6 hours after vaginal delivery and 6–12 hours after cesarean section [4,22]. Although it is safe to use LMWH in the postpartum period, it is reasonable to use intravenous UFH protocol to avoid further hemorrhage.

Warfarin is a vitamin K antagonist that easily crosses the placenta. In the setting of acute VTE and PE in pregnancy, warfarin is seldom used secondary to increased fetal risks which include fetal embryopathy (nasal bone hypoplasia and stippled epiphyses), fetal bleeding (intracranial, intraabdominal hemorrhage), and fetal loss [23,24]. Although warfarin is shown to be teratogenic, it is dose dependent and a dose of less than 5 mg/daily is rarely associated with poor fetal outcome. Although warfarin is infrequently used antenatally, it can be used in the postpartum period as it safe in breastfeeding [25,26].

New oral anticoagulants (NOAC) have shown great promise in the nonpregnant populations. They are preferred over LMWH in the prevention and treatment of VTE and PE, as there is no transition therapy needed for many NOACs; they are also superior in reducing the recurrence in VTE and PE, and the risk of bleeding appears less when compared to warfarin [27,28]. Despite these advances, LMWH is still the preferred anticoagulant in pregnancy and postpartum. There are no randomized trials on NOAC versus LMWH in pregnancy or in the immediate postpartum period. Further, fetal effects are unknown, and the medication is in breast milk [28]. There are also treatment failures noted in case reports with use postpartum. The pharmacologic failure is thought to be secondary to a shared hypermetabolic renal and hepatic system in the pregnant and immediate postpartum woman [29].

Treatment of Massive and Submassive Pulmonary Embolism

As stated earlier, submassive and massive PE are associated with high mortality; this is increasingly complex and morbid in the setting of a third trimester pregnancy. Although systemic thrombolysis with tissue plasminogen activator (tPA) improves pulmonary perfusion and improves right-sided heart failure, it is not without risk [30]. In fact, systemic tPA use has a major bleeding risk of 10% and a 3%–5% risk of hemorrhagic stroke [31]. Therefore, use of systemic tPA is FDA approved for massive PE, but use for submassive PE remains controversial. In addition, tPA is "relatively" contraindicated in the setting of pregnancy and recent surgery (cesarean section) because of risk of urgent delivery and hemorrhage [32]. Therefore, other targeted options in the setting of pregnancy may be preferred if available.

In a systematic review of pregnant patients, 83 severe PE in pregnancy received systemic thrombolytic therapy; 61 were antenatal and 9 were treated with catheter-directed thrombolysis (CDT) or emergent thrombectomy. Of the cohort, 80% were massive PEs and 20% underwent cardiac arrest. Among all massive PEs, maternal survival was 93%, with 96% survival antepartum and 85% postpartum [33]. Systemic thrombolysis was efficacious in hemodynamic improvement, and the five women who died received thrombolysis during or after cardiac arrest [33]. Major maternal bleeding occurred in approximately 30% of pregnant cases treated with systemic thrombolysis, with the greatest risk in the immediate postpartum period. In antenatal massive PE, fetal and neonatal death was 12%, and spontaneous preterm labor occurred in 14% of pregnancies [33].

In the review, 36 pregnancies underwent surgical thrombectomy, of which 13 had cardiac arrest. In this cohort, maternal survival was 84%, and major bleeding was prevalent at 20%. When thrombectomy occurred in the antepartum period without combined delivery, fetal loss reached 20%.

CDT represents an alternative to systemic thrombolysis and surgical thrombectomy as it acutely preserves right ventricular function as well as immediate pulmonary perfusion [30]. CDT with thrombectomy is reported in the literature, with seven cases reported. In these seven cases, two had suboptimal results and required use of extracorporeal membranous oxygenation (ECMO) [33]. However, maternal survival in this group was 100%, with only one episode of major bleeding, or 20%; fetal loss was 25%.

In the setting of massive PE, practitioners should consider systemic thrombolysis, CDT thrombolysis, and thrombectomy as well as surgical thrombectomy and ECMO.

All of these therapeutic options carry high risk of major hemorrhage, stroke, and fetal loss. However, overall outcomes are promising, with survival reaching 90% in the pregnant population. The obstetric specialist must balance risk and benefits in these settings optimally with a multidisciplinary team, including intensivist, cardiac surgery, and skilled interventional radiologist if available.

Amniotic Fluid Embolism

Amniotic fluid embolism (AFE) is a rare and usually lethal condition characterized by cardiovascular collapse, disseminated intravascular coagulopathy (DIC), and refractory hypoxemia resulting from acute respiratory distress syndrome (ARDS). The exact incidence of AFE is unknown but is estimated to affect 2–6 women per 100,000 deliveries [34]. In the past, diagnostic criteria were lacking; however, the Society of Maternal Fetal Medicine and the Amniotic Fluid Embolism Foundation created criteria. The diagnostic criteria are intended for research purposes but can also aid in clinical diagnosis (Table 17.3) [35].

The true pathogenesis of AFE is still not clear; however, it is theorized that entry of amniotic fluid into the maternal circulation causes an anaphylactic and hyperimmune response leading to shock and other above-mentioned sequela [35].

The remainder of the chapter will focus on organ systems most affected by AFE, and the treatment of these systems: cardiovascular, pulmonary, and hematologic.

Cardiovascular Collapse

Cardiovascular collapse in AFE is unique to the disease. In AFE, there is transient acute pulmonary hypertension from pulmonary artery vasoconstriction, resulting in right ventricular dysfunction and eventually failure. There is also concomitant left ventricular function and failure [35,36]. Aside from profound cardiogenic shock, there is also distributive shock from the massive vasoplegia of the systemic circulatory system.

The harbinger of treatment of cardiovascular collapse relies on urgent, immediate delivery in the setting of current pregnancy and high-quality cardiopulmonary resuscitation per ACLS guidelines [35]. When return of spontaneous circulation (ROSC) is achieved, the cardiovascular system must be maintained. Resuscitative efforts are multidisciplinary and employ maternal-fetal medicine, intensive care, cardiac surgery, and pulmonary medicine. In the setting of acute right-sided failure, inotropic support with milrinone and dobutamine may be of great use. Both agents aid in right-sided cardiac contractility, and also milrinone has pulmonary artery vasodilatory effects which allows further optimization of preload in biventricular failure resulting

TABLE 17.3

Diagnostic Criteria for Amniotic Fluid Embolism

✓ Sudden onset of cardiorespiratory arrest or refractory hypotension

Overt disseminated intravascular coagulopathy (Score ≥3)

Platelet count		
	>100,000/mL	0 points
	<100,000/mL	1 point
	<50,000/mL	2 points
PT or INR		
	<25% increase	0 points
	25–50% increase	1 point
	>50% increase	2 points
Fibrinogen		
	>200 mg/L	0 points
	<200 mg/L	1 point

Clinical onset during labor or within 30 minutes of placental delivery

Absence of fever (38°C) during labor

in an increased cardiac output [37,38]. However, care must be taken with these medications because they can be arrhythmogenic and cause systemic hypotension, which is undesirable with the combined distributive shock of an AFE.

Concomitant pulmonary vasodilators (inhaled prostacyclin, inhaled nitric oxide, intravenous prostacyclin) can be useful, as the right-sided heart failure is usually transient and lasts for a few hours after initial presentation. These partially selective dilators can provide the patient with a decrease in pulmonary vasculature resistance in an effort to improve right ventricular systolic function [37,39,40].

Acute Respiratory Distress Syndrome

Patients experiencing AFE also have rapid and refractory hypoxemia. On imaging, patients usually have components of both cardiogenic and noncardiogenic pulmonary edema. For this reason, many of these patients are intubated and do not tolerate noninvasive ventilation strategies [35]. In this setting, urgent intubation is necessary and should be undertaken by the most skilled provider. In the setting of cardiac arrest, ventilation should be done per ACLS guidelines. When ROSC is obtained, if applicable, patients may benefit from lung protective ventilation per ARDSnet guidelines and systemic pharmacologic paralysis [41,42]. Although shown to change overall mortality, inhaled nitric oxide can be used with refractory hypoxemia to help patients get through the first 48 hours of ARDS from AFE [43].

Hemorrhage and Disseminated Intravascular Coagulation

Hemorrhage and disseminated intravascular coagulation (DIC) are present in the majority of cases of AFE, and usually in conjunction with severe hemorrhage. Hemorrhage is usually present in the forms of uterine atony, large-bore intravenous access sets, and needed incision or tears. Bleeding should be controlled with surgical and compressive maneuvers, and blood should be aggressively replaced with massive transfusion protocols [35]. Adjuncts to massive transfusion such as tranexamic acid, fibrinogen concentrate, and factor VIIa can also be used; however, these should be used in the setting of controlled bleeding and aggressive ongoing resuscitation [44].

Conclusion

PE and AFE can be rapidly progressing and highly morbid events. Obstetricians should be aware of not only standards of care for treatment but salvage therapies for both of the disease processes, which include thrombectomy and mechanical circulatory support. A multidisciplinary approach and transition to higher levels of care when appropriate reduce maternal morbidity and mortality.

REFERENCES

1. Meng K, Hu X, Peng X, Zhang Z. Incidence of venous thromboembolism during pregnancy and the puerperium: A systematic review and meta-analysis. *J Matern Fetal Neonatal Med.* 2015;28(3):245–53.

2. Jacobsen AF, Skjeldestad FE, Sandset PM. Incidence and risk patterns of venous thromboembolism in pregnancy and puerperium—A register-based case-control study. *Am J Obstet Gynecol.* 2008;198(2):233.e1–e7.

3. ACOG practice bulletin no. 197: Inherited thrombophilias in pregnancy. *Obstet Gynecol.* 2018;132(1):e18–34.

4. ACOG practice bulletin no. 196: Thromboembolism in pregnancy. *Obstet Gynecol.* 2018;132(1):e1–e17.

5. Pabinger I et al. Temporary increase in the risk for recurrence during pregnancy in women with a history of venous thromboembolism. *Blood.* 2002;100(3):1060–2.

6. Agnelli G, Becattini C. Acute pulmonary embolism. *N Engl J Med.* 2010;363(3):266–74.

7. Pollack CV et al. Clinical characteristics, management, and outcomes of patients diagnosed with acute pulmonary embolism in the emergency department: Initial report of EMPEROR (Multicenter Emergency Medicine Pulmonary Embolism in the Real World Registry). *J Am Coll Cardiol.* 2011;57(6):700–6.

8. Stein PD et al. Clinical, laboratory, roentgenographic, and electrocardiographic findings in patients with acute pulmonary embolism and no pre-existing cardiac or pulmonary disease. *Chest.* 1991;100(3):598–603.

9. Wan T, Skeith L, Karovitch A, Rodger M, Le Gal G. Guidance for the diagnosis of pulmonary embolism during pregnancy: Consensus and controversies. *Thromb Res.* 2017;157:23–8.

10. Righini M et al. Diagnosis of pulmonary embolism during pregnancy: A multicenter prospective management outcome study. *Ann Intern Med.* 2018;169(11):766–73.

11. Van der Pol LM, Mairuhu ATA, Tromeur C, Couturaud F, Huisman MV, Klok FA. Use of clinical prediction rules and D-dimer tests in the diagnostic management of pregnant patients with suspected acute pulmonary embolism. *Blood Rev.* 2017;31(2):31–6.

12. El-Menyar A, Asim M, Nabir S, Ahmed MN, Al-Thani H. Implications of elevated cardiac troponin in patients presenting with acute pulmonary embolism: An observational study. *J Thorac Dis.* 2019;11(8):3302–14.

13. El-Menyar A, Sathian B, Al-Thani H. Elevated serum cardiac troponin and mortality in acute pulmonary embolism: Systematic review and meta-analysis. *Respir Med.* 2019;157:26–35.

14. Lankeit M et al. Validation of N-terminal pro-brain natriuretic peptide cut-off values for risk stratification of pulmonary embolism. *Eur Respir J.* 2014;43(6):1669–77.

15. Chunilal SD, Bates SM. Venous thromboembolism in pregnancy: Diagnosis, management and prevention. *Thromb Haemost.* 2009;101(3):428–38.

16. Leung AN et al. American Thoracic Society documents: An official American Thoracic Society/Society of Thoracic Radiology Clinical Practice Guideline—Evaluation of Suspected Pulmonary Embolism in Pregnancy. *Radiology.* 2012;262(2):635–46.

17. Piazza G, Goldhaber SZ. Management of submassive pulmonary embolism. *Circulation.* 2010;122(11):1124–9.

18. Sadiq I, Goldhaber SZ, Liu P-Y, Piazza G, Submassive and Massive Pulmonary Embolism Treatment with Ultrasound AcceleraTed ThromboLysis ThErapy (SEATTLE II) Investigators. Risk factors for major bleeding in the SEATTLE II trial. *Vasc Med.* 2017;22(1):44–50.

19. Kucher N, Rossi E, De Rosa M, Goldhaber SZ. Massive pulmonary embolism. *Circulation.* 2006;113(4):577–82.

20. Bates SM, Greer IA, Middeldorp S, Veenstra DL, Prabulos A-M, Vandvik PO. VTE, thrombophilia, antithrombotic therapy, and pregnancy: Antithrombotic Therapy and Prevention of Thrombosis, 9th ed: American College of Chest Physicians Evidence-Based Clinical Practice Guidelines. *Chest* 2012;141(2 Suppl):e691S–736S.

21. Leffert L et al. The Society for Obstetric Anesthesia and Perinatology Consensus Statement on the anesthetic management of pregnant and postpartum women receiving thromboprophylaxis or higher dose anticoagulants. *Anesth Analg.* 2018;126(3):928–44.

22. Freedman RA, Bauer KA, Neuberg DS, Zwicker JI. Timing of postpartum enoxaparin administration and severe postpartum hemorrhage. *Blood Coagul Fibrinolysis.* 2008;19(1):55–9.

23. Yarrington CD, Valente AM, Economy KE. Cardiovascular management in pregnancy: Antithrombotic agents and antiplatelet agents. *Circulation.* 2015;132(14):1354–64.

24. Economy KE, Valente AM. Mechanical heart valves in pregnancy: A sticky business. *Circulation.* 2015;132(2):79–81.

25. Vitale N, De Feo M, De Santo LS, Pollice A, Tedesco N, Cotrufo M. Dose-dependent fetal complications of warfarin in pregnant women with mechanical heart valves. *J Am Coll Cardiol.* 1999;33(6):1637–41.

26. Khamooshi AJ, Kashfi F, Hoseini S, Tabatabaei MB, Javadpour H, Noohi F. Anticoagulation for prosthetic heart valves in pregnancy. Is there an answer? *Asian Cardiovasc Thorac Ann.* 2007;15(6):493–6.

27. Castellucci LA et al. Clinical and safety outcomes associated with treatment of acute venous thromboembolism: A systematic review and meta-analysis. *JAMA.* 2014;312(11):1122–35.

28. Kearon C et al. Antithrombotic therapy for VTE disease: CHEST Guideline and Expert Panel Report. *Chest.* 2016;149(2):315–52.

29. Rudd KM, Winans ARM, Panneerselvam N. Possible rivaroxaban failure during the postpartum period. *Pharmacotherapy.* 2015;35(11):e164–8.

30. Hennemeyer C, Khan A, McGregor H, Moffett C, Woodhead G. Outcomes of catheter-directed therapy plus anticoagulation versus anticoagulation alone for submassive and massive pulmonary embolism. *Am J Med.* 2019;132(2):240–6.

31. Konstantinides SV et al. Corrigendum to: 2014 ESC Guidelines on the diagnosis and management of acute pulmonary embolism. *Eur Heart J.* 2015;36(39):2642.

32. Martin C, Sobolewski K, Bridgeman P, Boutsikaris D. Systemic thrombolysis for pulmonary embolism: A review. *P T.* 2016;41(12):770–5.

33. Martillotti G, Boehlen F, Robert-Ebadi H, Jastrow N, Righini M, Blondon M. Treatment options for severe pulmonary embolism during pregnancy and the postpartum period: A systematic review. *J Thromb Haemost.* 2017; 15(10):1942–50.

34. Knight M et al. Amniotic fluid embolism incidence, risk factors and outcomes: A review and recommendations. *BMC Pregnancy Childbirth.* 2012;12:7.

35. Society for Maternal-Fetal Medicine (SMFM). Electronic address: pubs@smfm.org, Pacheco LD, Saade G, Hankins GDV, Clark SL. Amniotic fluid embolism: Diagnosis and management. *Am J Obstet Gynecol.* 2016;215(2):B16–24.

36. Balazic J, Rott T, Jancigaj T, Popović M, Zajfert-Slabe M, Svigelj V. Amniotic fluid embolism with involvement of the brain, lungs, adrenal glands, and heart. *Int J Legal Med.* 2003;117(3):165–9.

37. Konstam MA et al. Evaluation and management of right-sided heart failure: A scientific statement from the American Heart Association. *Circulation.* 2018;137(20):e578–622.

38. Colucci WS, Wright RF, Jaski BE, Fifer MA, Braunwald E. Milrinone and dobutamine in severe heart failure: Differing hemodynamic effects and individual patient responsiveness. *Circulation.* 1986;73(3 Pt 2):III175–83.

39. Wasson S, Govindarajan G, Reddy HK, Flaker G. The role of nitric oxide and vasopressin in refractory right heart failure. *J Cardiovasc Pharmacol Ther.* 2004;9(1):9–11.

40. McLaughlin VV, Genthner DE, Panella MM, Rich S. Reduction in pulmonary vascular resistance with long-term epoprostenol (prostacyclin) therapy in primary pulmonary hypertension. *N Engl J Med.* 1998;338(5):273–7.

41. Papazian L et al. Neuromuscular blockers in early acute respiratory distress syndrome. *N Engl J Med.* 2010; 363(12):1107–16.

42. Acute Respiratory Distress Syndrome Network, Brower RG et al. Ventilation with lower tidal volumes as compared with traditional tidal volumes for acute lung injury and the acute respiratory distress syndrome. *N Engl J Med.* 2000;342(18):1301–8.

43. Gebistorf F, Karam O, Wetterslev J, Afshari A. Inhaled nitric oxide for acute respiratory distress syndrome (ARDS) in children and adults. *Cochrane Database Syst Rev.* 2016;(6):CD002787.

44. Kogutt BK, Vaught AJ. Postpartum hemorrhage: Blood product management and massive transfusion. *Semin Perinatol.* 2019;43(1):44–50.

18

Endocarditis in Pregnancy

Ann K. Lal and Thaddeus P. Waters

KEY POINTS

- In pregnancy, the most common risk factors for infective endocarditis (IE) are intravenous drug use and congenital heart disease
- For early diagnosis and treatment, endocarditis should be considered in the differential diagnosis for any patient presenting with fever along with relevant risk factors
- Any compromise of the cardiac structure and/or function related to IE may accelerate maternal cardiovascular decompensation

- Endocarditis prophylaxis in pregnancy is indicated for the same non-obstetric procedures as nonpregnant patients in the highest risk patients (see Table 18.7)
- Prophylaxis for IE is not recommended at the time of delivery (either vaginal or cesarean) in the absence of infection

---

Introduction

Infective endocarditis (IE) is defined as an infection of a heart valve (native or prosthetic), the endocardial surface, or an indwelling cardiac device [1–4]. The yearly incidence of IE is estimated at 3-10/100,000 in the general population [4], similar to that reported in pregnancy [5–8] (see Figure 18.1). IE can be a life-threatening infection associated with significant morbidity and mortality. Hospitalization rates for IE in the United States have increased from 28,195 in 1998 to 43,419 in 2009 in keeping with the increasing comorbidities and aging in the general population. While the majority of cases of IE during pregnancy are identified antepartum, it can also present up to 6 weeks postpartum or after an abortion [9].

Pregnancy imposes significant challenges to the cardiovascular system. Any compromise of the cardiac structure and/or function related to IE may accelerate maternal cardiovascular decompensation [11] with an increased risk of both maternal and fetal mortality, i.e., 22.1% and 14.7%, respectively [10]. In addition, cardiac surgery, which may sometimes be required, may lead to significant maternal mortality between 1.5%–5%, and fetal mortality of 14%–38% [11–13].

Risk Factors

While the risk factors for IE have remained overall unchanged, the distribution has evolved over time (see Table 18.1), as is true for pregnant and nonpregnant adults. Previously, rheumatic heart disease was a major contributing factor for IE, the prevalence

of which has fallen significantly in developed countries and its contribution to IE is negligible. In pregnancy, the most common risk factors are intravenous (IV) drug use and congenital heart disease that constitute 14%–43% and 12%–38% of cases of IE, respectively [9,17].

Pathogens

The microbes causing IE have also changed over the last 20 years. Currently, 50% of IE is health care–associated, with 42.5% being community-acquired and 7.5% nosocomial [16]. The vast majority of cases of IE (80%–90%) are caused by gram-positive cocci, staphylococcus, streptococcus, or enterococcus, with 5% reported as no identifiable organism and less than 2% are polymicrobial [2,14]. *Staphylococcus aureus* (26%–38%) and *Streptococcus viridans* (19%–43%) are the most common organisms isolated in cases of IE in pregnancy [9,17] (see Table 18.2).

TABLE 18.1

Predisposing Risk Factors for Infective Endocarditis[a]

Prosthetic cardiac valve
Congenital heart disease
Immunosuppression
IV drug use
Diabetes
Rheumatic heart disease

[a] See further references [9,14,15].

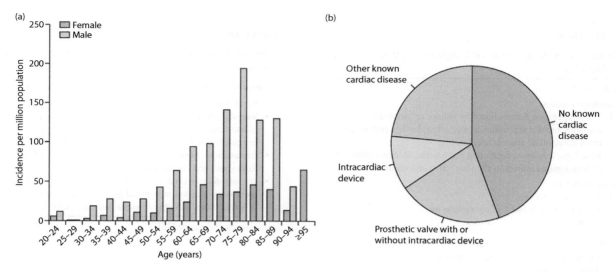

FIGURE 18.1 Epidemiology of infective endocarditis; incidence of infective endocarditis according to (a) age and sex, and (b) previous cardiac history, in a French cohort of 497 adults. The incidence peaks at 194 cases per million in men aged 75–79 years. (Adapted from Selton-Suty C et al. *Clin Infect Dis.* 2012;54:1230–9.)

TABLE 18.2

Organisms Associated with Infective Endocarditis[a]

Staphylococcus	Both *Staphylococcus aureus*, including methicillin-resistant strains, and coagulase-negative organisms (*S. epidermidis*, *S. lugdunensis*, *S. capitis*)
Streptococcus (oral, gastrointestinal tract, and genitourinary tract)	*Streptococcus mutans*, *S. salivarius*, *S. anginosus*, *S. mitis*, *S. sanguinis*
Enterococcus	*Enterococcus faecalis* is most common
HACEK	*Haemophilus*, *Aggregatibacter*, *Cardiobacterium*, *Eikenella corrodens*, *Kingella*
Fungus	*Candida* species
Other rare organisms	*Coxiella burnetii*, *Brucella*, *Bartonella*, *Chlamydia psittaci*, Enterobacteriaceae, *Propionibcaterium acnes*, *Lactobacillus*, *Acinetobacter*, *Pseudomonas aeruginosa*, *Legionella*, *Mycoplasma*, *Tropheryma whippelii*

[a] See further references [2,14,18,19].

Clinical Features of Endocarditis

The clinical features of IE are varied and nonspecific, causing a diagnostic challenge in most cases [20–22]. Nonspecific symptoms may include low-grade fever, chills, weight loss, poor appetite, or low-grade sepsis. Typical physical examination findings are a new-onset cardiac murmur, splinter hemorrhages, microscopic hematuria, embolic complications, or heart failure. Electrocardiogram may reveal new-onset conduction system abnormalities. Atypical presentation is more likely to occur in older and immunocompromised patients including pregnant population [23]. To avoid delays in diagnosis and treatment, IE should be in the differential diagnosis for any pregnant patient presenting with fever along with relevant risk factors.

Diagnosis

The diagnosis of IE is straightforward in patients with a consistent history and classic Oslerian manifestations, including sustained bacteremia or fungemia, evidence of acute valvulitis, peripheral emboli, and immunologic vascular phenomena [24]. However, as the majority of cases do not present with these classic signs and symptoms, initial evaluation of suspected IE includes both expeditious cardiac imaging and laboratory assessment, including:

1. Three sets of blood cultures should be taken from different venipuncture sights, with the first and last samples drawn at least 1 hour apart.
2. Echocardiogram is the main diagnostic test for the diagnosis of IE.
   a. Transthoracic echocardiogram (TTE) should be done initially in all suspected IE cases.
   b. Transesophageal echocardiogram (TEE) is recommended for cases with poor visualization on TTE or in patients with negative TTE, but high suspicion for IE [24].

The majority of cases in pregnancy involve a left-sided, either mitral or aortic valve, abnormality [9]. Duke criteria for IE were proposed in 1994 to aid both clinicians and researchers to make this challenging diagnosis [25]. Modified Duke criteria were subsequently published in 2000 in an attempt to decrease the number of patients classified as possible IE; these criteria are still used today [26] (see Tables 18.3 through 18.5).

A recent systematic review summarized maternal and fetal outcomes of pregnant or postpartum women with IE [9]. In total, 72 articles were identified with 90 cases of IE (56.7% (n = 51) pregnant versus 43.3% (n = 39) postpartum. The modified Duke criteria [26] were applied to all cases included in the publication. IV drug use was the most common identified risk factor for IE (n = 13), followed by congenital heart disease (n = 11) and rheumatic heart disease (n = 11). These observed frequencies were

TABLE 18.3

Modified Duke Criteria for the Diagnosis of Infective Endocarditis[a]

Definitive IE

Pathologic criteria

1. Microorganisms demonstrated by culture or histologic examination of a vegetation, a vegetation that has embolized, or an intracardiac abscess specimen
2. Pathologic lesions; vegetation or intracardiac abscess confirmed by histologic examination showing active endocarditis

Clinical criteria

1. 2 major criteria or
2. 1 major criterion and 3 minor criteria or
3. 5 minor criteria

Possible IE

1. 1 major criterion and 1 minor criterion
2. 3 minor criteria

Rejected IE

1. Firm alternate diagnosis explaining evidence of infective endocarditis or
2. Resolution of infective endocarditis syndrome with antibiotic therapy for ≤4 days or
3. No pathologic evidence of infective endocarditis at surgery or autopsy, with antibiotic therapy for ≤4 days or
4. Does not meet criteria for possible infective endocarditis, as above

[a] See further reference [26].

TABLE 18.4

Modified Major Duke Criteria for the Diagnosis of Infective Endocarditis[a]

Blood culture positive for IE

- Typical microorganisms consistent with IE from 2 separate blood cultures
  - *Viridans streptococci, Streptococcus bovis,* HACEK group, *Staphylococcus aureus,* or community-acquired enterococci, in the absence of a primary focus; or
  - Microorganisms consistent with IE from persistently positive blood cultures, defined as follows: At least 2 positive cultures of blood samples drawn 112 h apart; or all of 3; or a majority of >4 separate cultures of blood (with first and last sample drawn at least 1 h apart)
  - Single positive blood culture for *Coxiella burnetii* or antiphase I IgG antibody titer 1:800

Evidence of endocardial involvement

Echocardiogram positive for IE (TEE recommended in patients with prosthetic valves, rated at least "possible IE" by clinical criteria, or complicated IE [paravalvular abscess]; TTE as first test in other patients), defined as follows

- Oscillating intracardiac mass on valve or supporting structures, in the path of regurgitant jets, or on implanted material in the absence of an alternative anatomic explanation; or
- Abscess; or
- New partial dehiscence of prosthetic valve

New valvular regurgitation (worsening or changing of preexisting murmur not sufficient)

[a] See further reference [26].

TABLE 18.5

Modified Minor Duke Criteria for the Diagnosis of Infective Endocarditis[a]

Predisposition, predisposing heart condition, or injection drug use

- Fever, temperature >38°C
- Vascular phenomena, major arterial emboli, septic pulmonary infarcts, mycotic aneurysm, intracranial hemorrhage, conjunctival hemorrhages, and Janeway lesions
- *Immunologic phenomena:* Glomerulonephritis, Osler nodes, Roth spots, and rheumatoid factor
- *Microbiological evidence:* Positive blood culture but does not meet a major criterion as noted above or serological evidence of active infection with organism consistent with IE

[a] See further reference [26].

slightly lower than reported previously in pregnancy [17]; however, IV drug use and congenital heart disease were the most frequent identifiable causes in both studies on IE in pregnancy. The most commonly identified pathogens were streptococcal (n = 39) and staphylococcal species (n = 23), with 8 patients being culture-negative (8.9%). Other identified pathogens included *Neisseria* species (n = 4), gram stain-positive cocci (n = 3), *Escherichia coli* (n = 3), *Listeria* species (n = 2), *Pseudomonas* species (n = 2), *Salmonella* species (n = 1), *Rickettsia* species (n = 1), *Enterobacter* species (n = 1), *Enterococcus* species (n = 1), and *Haemophilus* species (n = 1) with 4 not reported and 3 being polymicrobial. Surgical interventions were performed in 48 cases, with 7 of these occurring during pregnancy. Maternal mortality was 11% overall (n = 10) with a relative equal distribution of deaths antepartum or postpartum (11.5 vs. 10.5%). Mortality was highest for the 16 non-staphylococcal and non-streptococcal cases (25%) with no observed deaths in the culture-negative group. Other complications included septic pulmonary emboli for 21 patients (23.3%), CNS emboli in 11 (12.2%), and other embolic complications in 7 women (7.8%). For the 51 pregnant women, IE involved native valves in 98% (n = 50) with the mitral valve being the most commonly affected (n = 21). Seven fetal deaths were observed (13.7%) with 41 deliveries with survival to discharge (80.4%), with the remaining 3 pregnancies lost to follow up (n = 2) and 1 termination of pregnancy.

See further Figure 18.2.

What Is the Rationale for Infective Endocarditis Prophylaxis?

Due to the morbidity and mortality of IE, significant efforts have been focused on prevention of IE particularly with antibiotic prophylaxis. Healthy cardiac tissue is resistant to bacteremia. However, after endothelial injury, bacterial adherence can occur, resulting in IE [27]. Endocarditis usually occurs in three steps [14]:

1. *Endothelial damage:* Bacteremia, from a multitude of sources, including oral (chewing, toothbrushing), gastrointestinal (GI), or genitourinary (GU), is the

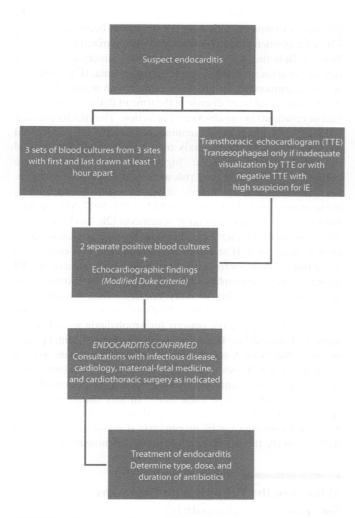

FIGURE 18.2 Endocarditis algorithm.

initial inciting event [15]. Bacteria are able to adhere to damaged endothelium, which can be caused by valve sclerosis, rheumatic valvulitis, or direct bacterial activity [15].

2. *Colonization*: After adhesion, colonization occurs, followed by endothelial injury, thrombosis formation, and inflammation, which lead to an infected vegetation, IE.

3. *Biofilm*: Biofilm development, which is seen with several of the common IE organisms, including staphylococci, streptococci, and enterococci, is an important part of the pathophysiology of IE. Biofilms are a multilayer of bacteria within a matrix, which provides resistance from host defenses and reduces antimicrobial effectiveness, thereby facilitating "bacterial persistence." [14–15]

However, despite the appreciated pathophysiology of IE, guidelines aimed at reducing IE from interventions such as prophylaxis have not demonstrated clear benefit. As such, several revisions have been made over time to the American Heart Association (AHA) guidelines for IE prophylaxis. In general, these revisions have conveyed a lack of clear evidence for IE prophylaxis and have limited the situations where prophylaxis is recommended (Table 18.6) [28].

TABLE 18.6

Primary Reasons for Revision of the Infective Endocarditis Prophylaxis Guidelines

IE is much more likely to result from frequent exposure to random bacteria associated with daily activities than from bacteremia caused by dental, GI tract, or GU tract procedure

Prophylaxis may prevent an exceedingly small number of cases of IE, if any, in individuals who undergo a dental, GI tract, or GU tract procedure

The risk of antibiotic-associated adverse events exceeds the benefit, if any, from prophylactic antibiotic therapy

Maintenance of optimal oral health and hygiene may reduce the incidence of bacteremia from daily activities and is more important than prophylactic antibiotics for dental procedure to reduce the risk of IE

Source: Wilson W et al. *Circulation* 2007 October 9;116(15):1736–54. With permission.

What Cardiac Conditions Need Infective Endocarditis Prophylaxis?

The list of cardiac conditions that require endocarditis prophylaxis has evolved over time, with the most recent AHA guidelines published in 2007 [28]. Since the first released AHA guidelines in 1955, there have been 10 revisions [28–37]. The goal of the 2007 publication is to use IE prophylaxis only in patients with the greatest chance of developing IE and the highest risk of adverse outcomes (Table 18.7) [28].

The British Society for Antimicrobial Chemotherapy has also published guidelines on prevention of IE. While acknowledging that evidence is limited regarding the benefit of antibiotic prophylaxis for the prevention of IE and that prevention should not be based on antibiotics alone, a list of conditions for which

TABLE 18.7

Cardiac Conditions Associated with the Highest Risk of Adverse Outcome from Endocarditis for Which Prophylaxis with Dental Procedures Is Reasonable

I	Prosthetic cardiac valve or prosthetic material used for cardiac valve repair
II	Previous infective endocarditis
III	Congenital heart disease (CHD)
	Unrepaired cyanotic CHD, including palliative shunts and conduits
	Completely repaired congenital heart defect with prosthetic material or device, whether placed by surgery or by catheter intervention, during the first 6 months after the procedure
	Repaired CHD with residual defects at the site or adjacent site to the site of a prosthetic patch or prosthetic device (which inhibit endothelialization)
IV	Cardiac transplantation recipients who develop cardiac valvulopathy

Source: Wilson W et al. *Circulation* 2007 October 9;116(15):1736–54. With permission.

antibiotic prophylaxis is recommended was proposed, including previous IE, prosthetic cardiac valves, and surgically constructed shunts and/or conduits [38]. The National Institute for Health and Care Excellence (NICE) currently does not recommend any antibiotic prophylaxis for the prevention of IE [39].

What Procedures during Pregnancy Require Endocarditis Prophylaxis?

Current recommendations for endocarditis prophylaxis during pregnancy are, in general, similar to those for nonpregnant patients. The 2007 AHA guidelines for the prevention of IE recommend that high-risk pregnant women (summarized in Table 18.7) receive prophylaxis. Procedures include:

1. Dental procedures with involvement of the gingival tissue or the periapical region of teeth or perforation of the oral mucosa [28]. However, this recommendation was also accompanied by a statement reiterating the lack of clear data establishing the efficacy of this approach.

2. Invasive respiratory tract procedures with incision or biopsy of respiratory mucosa or undergoing an invasive procedure to treat an established infection. For these situations, the authors recommended antibiotic coverage should include *Viridans* group streptococci. Prophylaxis was also recommended to include coverage for *Staphylococcus aureus* when suspected.

3. When surgical procedures for infected skin, skin structure, or musculoskeletal tissues is performed, it is reasonable to include antibiotics that would target staphylococcus and streptococcus. Limitations of these recommendations include a lack of a clear consensus for which patients are truly at increased risk for IE, as well as conflicting recommendations from different organizations regarding which patients should receive antibiotic prophylaxis, and for which procedures [40]. As majority of the cases of IE related to seeding from the oral microflora is likely from random bacteremia caused by routine daily activities, emphasis should be placed on optimal dental hygiene and good oral health.

4. For GI or GU procedures, including vaginal delivery and cesarean section, antibiotic prophylaxis is not recommended. While other procedures such as cerclage, amniocentesis, chorionic villous sampling, D&C, or D&E are not addressed in the currently published guidelines, IE prophylaxis would not be indicated for these procedures in the absence of infection. The 2007 AHA guidelines suggest antibiotics should include coverage of enterococci for the situation of a GI or GU procedure with a suspected enterococcus infection, but no studies specifically address if this will prevent enterococcal IE.

5. IE prophylaxis was also not recommended for the majority of skin or non-infected surgical procedures.

The 2007 AHA guidelines did not address specific issues of IE prophylaxis or treatment in pregnancy but these were addressed in the 2017 AHA scientific statement on the management of pregnancy in women with complex congenital heart disease [41]. These recommendations were recently summarized in an ACOG Practice Bulletin [42]. As neither a vaginal delivery nor cesarean delivery is associated with significant bacteremia, IE prophylaxis is not recommended for pregnant women with acquired or congenital structural heart disease at the time of delivery (either vaginal or cesarean) in the absence of infection. The ACOG practice bulletin supplements these recommendations with the additional suggestion that IE prophylaxis may be of benefit for vaginal delivery in patients with the "highest risk" of adverse cardiac outcomes. Women at highest risk were defined as those with cyanotic cardiac disease, prosthetic valves, or both [42]. Importantly, these recommendations were not within the 2007 AHA guidelines or the 2017 AHA scientific statements [28,40,41]; however, the use of antibiotics for these situations based solely upon expert opinion was noted. If antibiotic prophylaxis for IE is considered at the time of delivery for this subset of high-risk patients, ACOG suggests antibiotic prophylaxis can be given 30–60 minutes prior to the anticipated vaginal delivery. For this subset of highest risk women not already receiving antibiotics that would provide coverage for IE prophylaxis, options for prophylaxis would be the same as those used for IE prophylaxis at the time of dental procedures (Table 18.8). A separate circumstance is pregnant women at high risk for IE (see Key Points) with a concomitant infection (such as chorioamnionitis, endometritis, or pyelonephritis, etc.) that could result in bacteremia. In this situation, ACOG suggested the underlying infection should be treated without additional coverage for IE prophylaxis if adequate coverage is included in the treatment regimen already administered.

What Are the Prophylactic Regimens for Infective Endocarditis?

If prophylaxis is warranted, antibiotic choice should be governed by clinical factors including the patient's relevant allergies and current medication and antibiotic use. Prophylaxis should be given as a single dose 30–60 minutes prior to the anticipated procedure but may be given up to 2 hours after a procedure if needed (Wilson). Current recommended antibiotic prophylaxis regiments are summarized below (Table 18.8). If the patient is already receiving antibiotics intrapartum for another indication, coverage for IE is often provided by the antibiotic(s) administered for the obstetric indication.

Management of Endocarditis in Pregnancy

Current recommendations for both the diagnosis and treatment of pregnant women with IE do not vary from nonpregnant adults. The complete summary of the approach to IE is beyond the scope of this chapter and can be found in the AHA Scientific Statement regarding the diagnosis, treatment, and management of adults with IE [24].

As no randomized controlled data exist for pregnant women with IE, management continues to rely on current evidence-based guidelines for nonpregnant adults with a multidisciplinary approach including involvement of maternal-fetal medicine, infectious disease, cardiology, and cardiovascular surgery. As noted earlier, the

TABLE 18.8

Infective Endocarditis Antibiotic Prophylaxis Regiments for High-Risk Women

Treatment	Antibiotics	Regimen
Intravenous therapy	Ampicillin or	2 g intravenously
	Cefazolin or	1 g intravenously
	Ceftriaxone	1 g intravenously
Intravenous therapy with allergy to penicillin or ampicillin	Cefazolin[a] or	1 g intravenously
	Ceftriaxone[a] or	1 g intravenously
	Clindamycin	600 mg intravenously
Oral therapy	Amoxicillin	2 g
Oral therapy with allergy to penicillin or ampicillin	Cephalexin[a] or	2 g
	Clindamycin or	600 mg
	Azithromycin or clarithromycin	500 mg

Source: Adapted from Wilson W et al. *Circulation.* 2007 October 9;116(15):1736–54.

[a] Cephalosporin should not be used for penicillin- or ampicillin-allergic patients with a history of anaphylaxis, angioedema, or urticaria with penicillin, ampicillin, or an allergy to cephalosporin.

recommendations and protocols for the evaluation, treatment, and management of IE in nonpregnant adults is the current recommended care for the pregnant patient with IE. While variation from these established protocols are not endorsed based upon pregnancy status, this view needs to be balanced with limited information during pregnancy. This may particularly apply to the risks of appropriate interventions for the nonpregnant adult, including surgery, which likely carries a different risk-to-benefit tradeoff for the pregnant patient when including both maternal and fetal risks.

In general, the basic principles once the diagnosis of IE is established include the following.

1. Bactericidal antibiotics are preferred that target specific pathogens identified.
2. The dose and duration of parenteral antibiotics use is based on the identified pathogen and the site of infection.
3. Most patients require 6 weeks of parenteral antibiotics.
4. Patients with complications related to IE may require surgical intervention, and therefore a multidisciplinary team approach is mandatory.

The specific role of cardiovascular surgery in the treatment of IE during pregnancy poses particular challenges given the controversial role of surgery for IE, the risks of cardiac surgery during pregnancy, and the paucity of data regarding cardiac surgery for pregnant women with IE. Surgical intervention may be indicated for select cases in pregnancy [24]. The 2018 ESC Guidelines recommend urgent surgery for cardiogenic shock or refractory heart failure due to acute regurgitation [43]. Other scenarios where an individualized approach is advisable include need for valve surgery, uncontrolled infection, and prevention of embolism [43]. Considerations include the current gestational age prior to surgery and the consequential risks due to prematurity if intervention is urgent versus the option of expectant care which may impose an increased maternal risk. As in most complex obstetric situations, the "best" plan of care is individualized to the specific patient needs, balancing all of the above.

Conclusion

Infective endocarditis, although rare, is a serious cardiac complication that may lead to significant maternal and fetal morbidity and mortality. Predominant risk factors for the development of IE in pregnancy are IV drug use and a preexisting cardiac abnormality. Similar to nonpregnant patients, the majority of pregnant women with IE do not present in a clear and straightforward manner. Therefore, the diagnosis can be elusive and requires a high degree of clinical suspicion. The modified Duke criteria is the most commonly used and is the recommended tool to assist with the diagnosis. Once diagnosed, the management in pregnancy is similar to the nonpregnant patient with a multidisciplinary approach including maternal-fetal medicine, infectious disease, cardiology, and cardiovascular surgery.

REFERENCES

1. Murdoch DR et al. International Collaboration on Endocarditis-Prospective Cohort Study (ICE-PCS) Investigators. Clinical presentation, etiology, and outcome of infective endocarditis in the 21st century: The International Collaboration on Endocarditis-Prospective Cohort Study. *Arch Intern Med.* 2009;169:463–73.
2. Selton-Suty C et al. AEPEI Study Group. Preeminence of *Staphylococcus aureus* in infective endocarditis: A 1-year population-based survey. *Clin Infect Dis.* 2012;54:1230–9.
3. Pant S et al. Trends in infective endocarditis incidence, microbiology, and valve replacement in the United States from 2000 to 2011. *J Am Coll Cardiol.* 2015;65:2070–6.
4. Bor DH et al. Infective endocarditis in the U.S., 1998–2009: A nationwide study. *PLOS ONE.* 2013;8:e60033.
5. Nazarian M, McCullough GH, Fielder DL. Bacterial endocarditis in pregnancy: Successful surgical correction. *J Thorac Cardiovasc Surg.* 1976 Jun;71(6):880–3.
6. Montoya ME, Karnath BM, Ahmad M. Endocarditis during pregnancy. *South Med J.* 2003;96:1156–7.

7. Shah M, Patnaik S, Wongrakpanich S, Alhamshari Y, Alnabelsi T. Infective endocarditis due to *Bacillus cereus* in a pregnant female: A case report and literature review. *IDCases*. 2015 Oct 17;2(4):120–3.

8. Cox SM, Hankins GD, Leveno KJ, Cunningham FG. Bacterial endocarditis. A serious pregnancy complication. *J Reprod Med*. 1988 Jul;33(7):671–4.

9. Kebed KY, Bishu K, Al Adham RI, Baddour LM, Connolly HM, Sohail MR, Steckelberg JM, Wilson WR, Murad MH, Anavekar NS. Pregnancy and postpartum infective endocarditis: A systematic review. *Mayo Clin Proc*. 2014 Aug;89(8):1143–52.

10. Campuzano K, Roqué H, Bolnick A, Leo MV, Campbell WA. Bacterial endocarditis complicating pregnancy: Case report and systematic review of the literature. *Arch Gynecol Obstet*. 2003 Oct;268(4):251–5.

11. Sepehripour AH et al. Can pregnant women be safely placed on cardiopulmonary bypass? *Interact Cardiovascular Thorac Surg*. 2012;15:1063–70.

12. Pomini F et al. Cardiopulmonary bypass in pregnancy. *Ann Thorac Surg*. 1996;61:259–68.

13. Weiss BM et al. Outcome of cardiovascular surgery and pregnancy: A systematic review of the period 1984–1996. *Am J Obstet Gynecol*. 1998;179(Pt 1):1643–53.

14. Cahill TJ, Baddour LM, Habib G, Hoen B, Salaun E, Pettersson GB, Schäfers HJ, Prendergast BD. Challenges in infective endocarditis. *J Am Coll Cardiol*. 2017;69(3):325–44.

15. Cahill TJ, Prendergast BD. Infective endocarditis *Lancet*. 2016;387:882–93.

16. Correa de Sa D et al. Epidemiological trends of infective endocarditis: A population-based study in Olmsted County, Minnesota. *Mayo Clin Proc*. 2010 May;85(5):422–6.

17. Yuan SM. Infective endocarditis during pregnancy. *J Coll Physicians Surg Pak*. 2015 Feb;25(2):134–9.

18. Das M, Badley AD, Cockerill FR, Steckelberg JM, Wilson WR. Infective endocarditis caused by HACEK microorganisms. *Annu Rev Med*. 1997;48:25–33.

19. Brouqui P, Raoult D. Endocarditis due to rare and fastidious bacteria. *Clin Microbiol Rev*. 2001;14:177–207.

20. Dickerman SA et al. ICE Investigators. The relationship between the initiation of antimicrobial therapy and the incidence of stroke in infective endocarditis: An analysis from the ICE Prospective Cohort Study (ICE-PCS). *Am Heart J*. 2007;154:1086–94.

21. Nihoyannopoulos P et al. Duration of symptoms and the effects of a more aggressive surgical policy: Two factors affecting prognosis of infective endocarditis. *Eur Heart J*. 1985;6:380–90.

22. Lodise TP et al. Outcomes analysis of delayed antibiotic treatment for hospital-acquired *Staphylococcus aureus* bacteremia. *Clin Infect Dis*. 2003;36:1418–23.

23. Perez de Isla L, Zamorano J, Lennie V, Vazquez J, Ribera JM, Macaya C. Negative blood culture infective endocarditis in the elderly: Long-term follow-up. *Gerontology*. 2007;53:245–9.

24. Baddour LM et al. American Heart Association Committee on Rheumatic Fever, Endocarditis, and Kawasaki Disease of the Council on Cardiovascular Disease in the Young, Council on Clinical Cardiology, Council on Cardiovascular Surgery and Anesthesia, and Stroke Council. Infective endocarditis in adults: Diagnosis, Antimicrobial Therapy, and Management of Complications: A Scientific Statement for Healthcare Professionals from the American Heart Association. *Circulation*. 2015 Oct 13;132(15):1435–86.

25. Durack DT, Lukes AS, Bright DK, Duke Endocarditis Service. New criteria for diagnosis of infective endocarditis: Utilization of specific echocardiographic findings. *Am J Med*. 1994;96:200–9.

26. Li JS, Sexton DJ, Mick N, Nettles R, Fowler VG Jr, Ryan T, Bashore T, Corey GR. Proposed modifications to the duke criteria for the diagnosis of infective endocarditis. *Clin Infect Dis*. 2000;30:633–8.

27. Lockhart PB, Brennan MT, Sasser HC, Fox PC, Paster BJ, Bahrani-Mougeot FK. Bacteremia associated with tooth-brushing and dental extraction. *Circulation*. 2008 Jun 17;117(24):3118–25.

28. Wilson W et al. Prevention of infective endocarditis. *Circulation*. 2007 October 9;116(15):1736–54.

29. Jones TD, Baumgartner L, Bellows MT, Breese BB, Kuttner AG, McCarty M, Rammelkamp CH (Committee on Prevention of Rheumatic Fever and Bacterial Endocarditis, American Heart Association). Prevention of rheumatic fever and bacterial endocarditis through control of streptococcal infections. *Circulation*. 1955;11:317–20.

30. Rammelkamp CH Jr, Breese BB, Griffeath HI, Houser HB, Kaplan MH, Kuttner AG, McCarty M, Stollerman GH, Wannamaker LW (Committee on Prevention of Rheumatic Fever and Bacterial Endocarditis, American Heart Association). Prevention of rheumatic fever and bacterial endocarditis through control of streptococcal infections. *Circulation*. 1957; 15:154 –8.

31. Committee on Prevention of Rheumatic Fever and Bacterial Endocarditis, American Heart Association. Prevention of rheumatic fever and bacterial endocarditis through control of streptococcal infections. *Circulation*. 1960;21:151–5.

32. Wannamaker LW et al. (Committee on Prevention of Rheumatic Fever and Bacterial Endocarditis, American Heart Association). Prevention of bacterial endocarditis. *Circulation*. 1965;31:953–4.

33. Rheumatic Fever Committee and the Committee on Congenital Cardiac Defects, American Heart Association. Prevention of bacterial endocarditis. *Circulation*. 1972;46: S3–6.

34. Kaplan EL et al. (Committee on Rheumatic Fever and Bacterial Endocarditis, American Heart Association). Prevention of bacterial endocarditis. *Circulation*. 1977;56:139A–43A.

35. Shulman ST et al. (Committee on Rheumatic Fever and Infective Endocarditis, American Heart Association). Prevention of bacterial endocarditis: A statement for health professionals by the Committee on Rheumatic Fever and Infective Endocarditis of the Council on Cardiovascular Disease in the Young. *Circulation*. 1984;70:1123A–7A.

36. Dajani AS et al. Prevention of bacterial endocarditis: Recommendations by the American Heart Association. *JAMA*. 1990;264:2919–22.

37. Dajani AS et al. Prevention of bacterial endocarditis: Recommendations by the American Heart Association. *Clin Infect Dis*. 1997 Dec;25(6):1448–58.

38. Gould FK, Elliott TS, Foweraker J, Fulford M, Perry JD, Roberts GJ, Sandoe JA, Watkin RW, Working Party of the British Society for Antimicrobial Chemotherapy. Guidelines for the prevention of endocarditis: Report of the Working Party of the British Society for Antimicrobial Chemotherapy. *J Antimicrob Chemother*. 2006 Jun;57(6):1035–42.

39. National Institute for Health and Care Excellence (NICE). *Prophylaxis Against Infective Endocarditis*. National Institute for Health and Clinical Excellence, 2008. (with 2016 update). http://www.nice.org.uk/CG64

40. Nishimura RA et al. 2017AHA/ACC focused update of the 2014 AHA/ACC guidelines for the management of patients with valvular heart disease: A report of the American College of Cardiology/American Heart Association Task Force on Clinical Practice Guidelines. *Circulation*. 2017;135:e1159–95.

41. Canobbio MM et al. Management of pregnancy inpatients with complex congenital heart disease: A scientific statement for healthcare professionals from the American Heart Association. *Circulation*. 2017;135:e50–87.

42. American College of Obstetricians and Gynecologists. ACOG Practice Bulletin No. 199. Use of prophylactic antibiotics in labor and delivery. *Obstet Gynecol*. 2018;132:e103–19.

43. Neumann FJ et al. 2018 ESC/EACTS guidelines on myocardial revascularization. *Eur Heart J*. 2019;40(2):87–165.

19

Cardiac Surgery in Pregnancy

Kathryn Lindley

KEY POINTS

- Multidisciplinary planning is essential for optimal maternal and fetal care
- Maternal mortality is comparable to the nonpregnant setting, unless surgery is emergent
- Fetal loss is ~33% and increases with earlier gestational age, emergent surgery, deep hypothermia, and prolonged cardiopulmonary bypass time

- Beyond 28 weeks' gestation, cesarean delivery followed by cardiopulmonary bypass is typically preferred
- Continued postoperative fetal monitoring is important to identify sustained contractions and preterm labor

---

Introduction

Cardiopulmonary bypass during pregnancy carries similar risk to the mother as their nonpregnant counterparts; however, fetal mortality remains high [1]. Fortunately, the need for cardiac surgery during pregnancy is relatively rare. However, with a growing number of women of childbearing age with congenital heart disease and underlying cardiovascular risk factors such as hypertension and diabetes, these numbers may increase in the future [2]. While most cardiovascular conditions can be adequately temporized with medical therapy throughout the pregnancy, there are a variety of conditions which may necessitate urgent or emergent surgery in a pregnant or immediately postpartum woman.

Cardiac Surgery during Pregnancy

Cardiac surgery during pregnancy carries the risk of morbidity and mortality for both the mother and the fetus. In the current era, maternal perioperative mortality is comparable to that in the nonpregnant women unless the surgery occurs in an emergent setting [3]. *Though prior studies reported mortality between 3%–15%, current estimates of maternal mortality are approximately 5%–9% [4–6].* For women who undergo cardiac surgery immediately following cesarean delivery, additional blood products are often required during surgery, but excessive uterine bleeding is not typically reported [5]. Some of the common indications for cardiac surgery in pregnancy are reviewed in Table 19.1.

TABLE 19.1

Indications for Cardiac Surgery during Pregnancy

	Surgical Indications
Valvular lesions	• Severe symptomatic aortic stenosis • Severe symptomatic mitral stenosis • Mechanical valve thrombosis • Valvular endocarditis
Aortopathies	• Acute aortic dissection • Expanding aortic aneurysm • Severely dilated aortic aneurysm
CABG coronary dissection	• Myocardial infarction with cardiogenic shock

Valve Disease

While regurgitant valvular heart conditions are generally well tolerated during pregnancy, severe left-sided stenotic lesions may become symptomatic as the hemodynamic load of pregnancy increases throughout the second and third trimester. This is most commonly related to congenital heart defects such as bicuspid aortic valve or Shone complex, or rheumatic heart disease [7]. Severe prosthetic valve dysfunction may also present in this manner [8].

If the patient cannot be temporized with medical therapy or percutaneous interventions, surgery may be required to relieve symptomatic heart failure during pregnancy or the immediate postpartum period [7,9]. Mechanical heart valves require meticulous care throughout pregnancy to avoid thrombotic and bleeding complications. In the setting of mechanical valve thrombosis, emergent valve replacement may be required:

- If the patient is too unstable for or otherwise deemed not a candidate for thrombolysis [9]

Valvular endocarditis may also require surgical intervention during pregnancy in the setting of

- Large, mobile vegetations
- Recurrent embolic phenomena
- Severe valvular destruction causing heart failure
- Highly resistant organisms
- Abscess formation [9]

Aortopathies

Aortic enlargement, particularly in the setting of underlying connective tissue disorders such as Marfan syndrome, Loeys-Dietz syndrome, Ehlers-Danlos IV, Turner syndrome, coarctation of the aorta, and bicuspid aortic valve, can be associated with significant maternal morbidity and mortality [10]. *These risks are further elevated among women with additional risk factors such as a family history of aortic dissection, hypertension, prior personal history of aortic dissection, and tobacco use.* Patients with underlying aortopathy may require emergent aortic repair or replacement in the setting of an aortic dissection during pregnancy [10]. Semi-elective aortic root replacement may be undertaken in women with severely dilated aortic root discovered during pregnancy if termination is declined, or if progressive dilatation occurs during pregnancy [10].

Coronary Artery Bypass Grafting

Coronary artery dissection is the most common cause of myocardial infarction in pregnant and postpartum women [11]. This is most commonly managed conservatively [11]. However, in the setting of cardiogenic shock, such as in the setting of left main coronary artery dissection or mechanical complications of myocardial infarction, or after technical failure or complication of attempted percutaneous intervention, coronary artery bypass grafting may be elected [11].

While atherosclerotic coronary disease is less common among women of childbearing age, it may occur in women with risk factors such as diabetes, familial hyperlipidemia, hypertension, obesity, or tobacco use [12,13]. In the setting of coronary ischemia with severe three-vessel disease or high-risk features for percutaneous intervention, such as left main disease, surgical revascularization may be selected during pregnancy or immediately following delivery in select patients [12,14].

Surgery Timing

Preconception

Ideally, cardiovascular evaluation including imaging will occur prior to conception, and surgery may be considered at that time to potentially reduce the risk of cardiovascular complications of pregnancy [7]. This approach also reduces the potential risks of exposure to cardiopulmonary bypass to the fetus during pregnancy. However, prophylactic preconceptual surgery must be weighed against the intrinsic risks of the surgical procedure itself and the long-term sequelae of the surgery. For example, it is reasonable for preconceptual patients with asymptomatic severe aortic stenosis with aortic velocity ≥4.0 m/s or mean pressure gradient ≥40 mmHg to undergo prophylactic aortic valve replacement [9]. However, if a bioprosthetic valve is placed, the patient will inevitably require a repeat valve surgery in the future. If a mechanical valve is placed, the pregnancy will be complicated by anticoagulation management and the risk for warfarin embryopathy [7,10]. Preconceptual surgical intervention should be performed for symptomatic severe aortic or mitral stenosis [9].

Pre-pregnancy surgical intervention is also recommended for patients with aortopathy and Marfan or related disorders with ascending aorta size ≥45 mm [10]. For other patients, such as those with a bicuspid aorta, surgery should be performed when the aorta size is ≥50 mm [10]. For patients with Turner syndrome or an otherwise small body surface area, surgery should be done prior to pregnancy when the aorta exceeds ≥27 mm/m^2 [10].

Pregnancy

If the patient is already pregnant and surgery is being contemplated, optimal timing of surgery presents challenges for both the mother and the fetus. Shared decision making in a multidisciplinary manner is preferred. Surgical decisions must be tailored to the specific needs of the patient based on the underlying lesion, maternal status, and the gestational age of the fetus. The best time period for cardiac surgery in pregnancy is between 13–28 weeks.

Role of the Multidisciplinary Team

The decision for cardiac surgery in pregnancy should always be made in the context of an experienced multidisciplinary team, including maternal-fetal medicine specialists, cardiologists, obstetric and cardiac anesthesiologists, cardiac surgeons, and neonatologists.

Timing of Surgery

The ideal surgical timing depends partially on the urgency of the procedure.

i. In the setting of life-threatening conditions requiring urgent surgical intervention, such as aortic dissection or mechanical valve thrombosis, surgery should be undertaken as soon as possible.

ii. For less urgent procedures, the procedure may be delayed for fetal benefit, as it has been shown that fetal mortality declines as gestational age progresses [15].

iii. Prior to fetal viability around 24 weeks' gestation, preterm labor or delivery would lead to demise of the fetus, thus delay until closer to viability may be of some benefit for fetal survival. Subsequent to fetal viability, preterm labor or fetal distress requiring delivery will be associated with increased infant morbidity and mortality proportionate to degree of prematurity [16]. Thus, consequences of very premature birth must be considered in women undergoing cardiac surgery in the late second trimester.

iv. For patients in the third trimester, cesarean delivery immediately followed by initiation of cardiopulmonary bypass for cardiac surgery is usually the preferred strategy, as the fetus is typically developed well enough for reasonably good survival after delivery [5].

Maternal and Fetal Complications of Cardiac Surgery

Maternal complications are reported in 15% of patients, with persistent heart failure (6%), cardiac arrhythmia (2%), and postoperative bleeding (2%) being most common [4]. Maternal complications are higher in women undergoing urgent or emergent cardiac surgeries [4]. Fetal complications are reported in 12%, with respiratory distress syndrome (5%) and developmental delay (3%) being most common [4].

Risk of fetal demise related to cardiac surgery has been reported as between 14% and 33% [3–6]. The risk appears to be higher if there are additional maternal risk factors for fetal loss, or if the surgery occurs in an emergent setting or at an early gestational age [5]. Most of this risk is related to cardiopulmonary bypass, and not the anesthesia itself [5].

Cardiopulmonary Bypass in Pregnancy

Physiologic changes during cardiopulmonary bypass:

i. During cardiopulmonary bypass, there is a decrease in mean arterial blood pressure and flow pulsatility, which tends to decrease uteroplacental perfusion and may lead to onset of uterine contractions [5]. Uterine blood flow is not auto regulated, but depends entirely on maternal blood pressure and uterine vascular resistance [3]. Animal studies demonstrate that nonpulsatile flow leads to significant placental dysfunction due to severe vasoconstriction [3].

ii. Hypothermia increases the risk of fetal arrhythmias and acid–base imbalance [3].

iii. Both cooling and warming during cardiopulmonary bypass are also associated with sustained contractions [3]. The deeper the hypothermia, the greater the risk of fetal death [3].

Sustained contractions are the most common cause of fetal demise, which may occur after the conclusion of cardiopulmonary bypass and cardiac surgery [3,5]. Stillbirth and fetal demise have been reported to occur up to several days after surgery [5]. Sustained contractions lead to a reduction in uteroplacental blood flow, causing fetal hypoxia and subsequent fetal demise [3]. One proposed mechanism for this is dilution of progesterone in the setting of cardiopulmonary bypass, and post-cardiopulmonary bypass progesterone administration has been used to stop premature labor [3]. Reports of successful tocolysis with magnesium have also been reported [5].

Optimizing Fetal Outcomes during Cardiopulmonary Bypass

When possible, if surgery is not urgent, it should be delayed until the second trimester for women with early gestation pregnancies. For all pregnant women undergoing cardiac surgery, the following recommendations can help optimize fetal outcomes (Table 19.2). Maintenance of normothermia reduces fetal loss [3,5,17,18]. Attempts should be made to minimize blood loss and maintain normokalemia (<5 mmol/L) [5]. Avoid maternal hypoxemia and hypoglycemia to reduce the risk of fetal bradycardia [5,19,20]. Attempts should be made to minimize cardiopulmonary bypass times and maintain pulsatile flow, a high flow rate (>2.5 L/min/m^2), and a mean arterial pressure >70–75 mmHg [5]. Blood pressure should ideally be managed via flow rates of cardiopulmonary bypass rather than through sympathomimetic drugs, though these can be used if needed, preferably phenylephrine

TABLE 19.2

Measures to Optimize Outcomes in Pregnant Women Undergoing Cardiopulmonary Bypass

	How to Optimize Outcomes?
Maternal	*Avoid emergent surgery if possible*
Heart failure	• Monitor volume status • Judicious fluid use • Diuresis to attain a euvolemia
Arrhythmia	• Monitor and replete electrolytes as needed • Use beta-blockers and antiarrhythmic drugs as needed
Bleeding	• Vertical skin incision for cesarean delivery • Ensure obstetric incision hemostasis before proceeding with cardiopulmonary bypass • Uterotonic medications as needed
Fetal	*Delay cardiac surgery to later gestational age if possible* *Avoid emergent surgery if possible*
Fetal demise	• Avoid hypothermia • Maintain normal potassium levels • Avoid hypoxemia • Minimize blood loss • Avoid hypoglycemia • Minimize cardiopulmonary bypass time • Maintain high flow rate (>2.5 L/min/m^2) and pulsatile flow • Fetal heart rate monitoring intraoperatively (goal 110–160 bpm) • Post-operative progesterone administration • Magnesium administration in select cases
Preterm birth	• Avoid hypothermia • Pulsatile flow to the uterus • Maintain adequate mean arterial pressure (70–75 mmHg) • Minimize cardiopulmonary bypass time • Postoperative progesterone administration and magnesium administration have been proposed with limited data
RDS	Preoperative administration of steroids for fetal benefit

Abbreviation: RDS, respiratory distress syndrome.

and ephedrine [3,5]. Pregnancy is intrinsically a hypercoagulable state, so antifibrinolytic agents such as tranexamic acid should be limited to patients with concern for ongoing bleeding [5]. For women beyond 20 weeks' gestational age, uterine displacement by placement in the left lateral recumbent position is recommended [5]. For women beyond 24 weeks gestational age, it is reasonable to administer preoperative steroid for fetal lung maturation [3]. Fetal heart rate monitoring is recommended, with adjustment in hemodynamics for a goal fetal heart rate of 110–160 bpm. Following surgery, continuous and frequent fetal monitoring is recommended due to the high risk of fetal demise in the early postoperative period [3]. Preoperative neonatology consultation is also advised, in the event of premature delivery.

Clinical Scenarios That May Benefit by a Combined Cesarean Delivery and Cardiopulmonary Bypass Surgical Procedure

There are times when a combined cesarean delivery and cardiac surgery is the most appropriate management plan for the patient. *This typically involves a cesarean delivery in the cardiac operating room, with immediate institution of cardiopulmonary bypass following closure of the uterine incision and packing of the abdominal wound* [5]. After completion of the cardiac procedure and chest closure, the abdominal wound is inspected and closed after hemostasis is established [5]. This combined procedure should be considered when the patient requires an emergent surgical intervention in the setting of a viable fetus.

- *Viability*: If the fetus is viable (more than 24 weeks' gestation), one must balance the risk of exposing the fetus to cardiopulmonary bypass (undelivered) versus proceeding with preterm delivery immediately prior to cardiac surgery.
- *Gestational age*: If the fetus is more than 28 weeks' gestation, it is typically lower risk for the baby to deliver immediately prior to initiation of cardiopulmonary bypass than to proceed with surgery while the patient is still pregnant. This reduces the exposure of the baby to cardiopulmonary bypass.
- *Risk versus benefit*: A combined procedure reduces fetal exposure to cardiopulmonary bypass, though additional blood products may be required during surgery. Overall this strategy has been reported as safe for mother and baby [5].

Anesthesia Considerations

The rate of failed intubation in pregnant patients is higher in the pregnant patient than in the general population due to physiologic and anatomic change associated with pregnancy [21]. Cricoid pressure is often applied during airway intubation, and assistance of videolaryngoscopy may be useful [21]. Pregnant women are also at higher risk of aspiration and have reduced functional capacity, increased minute ventilation, and the potential for rapid

---

BOX 19.1 CHECKLIST FOR PREGNANT WOMEN UNDERGOING CARDIAC SURGERY

PREOPERATIVE

☐ Multidisciplinary consultation
  - Maternal-fetal medicine
  - Cardiology
  - Cardiac surgery
  - Obstetric anesthesia
  - Cardiac anesthesia
  - Neonatology
  - Nursing
☐ Fetal steroid administration (if >24 weeks' gestation)
☐ Fetal magnesium sulfate administration (if <32 weeks' gestation)

OPERATIVE

☐ Airway: Videolaryngoscopy
☐ Positioning: Left uterine displacement
☐ Fetal heart monitoring
☐ Cesarean delivery tray available
☐ Obstetrician available

POSTOPERATIVE

☐ Continuous fetal monitoring

---

desaturation [21]. Pregnant women undoing general anesthesia are generally preoxygenated, and an induction agent such as propofol or ketamine is administered in addition to a muscle relaxant such as succinylcholine or rocuronium [21]. Due to lipid solubility, all inhaled and most intravenous anesthetic agents cross the placenta [1]. Volatile anesthetics also may reduce placental blood flow and cause uterine relaxation [1].

Multidisciplinary team planning plays a crucial role in successful outcome of the mother and the fetus, as shown in the checklist in Box 19.1.

Conclusion

Cardiac surgery can be safely performed in pregnant women, however, it should be reserved for cardiac conditions refractory to medical therapy, without an option for an interventional procedure in a mother whose life is at stake. Maternal risks are comparable to surgical risks in the nonpregnant state unless surgery is emergent. Fetal risks are optimized through careful multidisciplinary planning, management of cardiopulmonary bypass, and intraoperative fetal heart rate monitoring. Gestational age must be taken into account when determining the timing of cardiac surgery and the need for cesarean delivery, as fetal outcomes are undoubtedly better at later gestational ages. In these situations, preterm delivery may be a safer option for the baby prior to proceeding with cardiac surgery for the mother.

REFERENCES

1. Kapoor MC. Cardiopulmonary bypass in pregnancy. *Ann Card Anaesth*. 2014;17:33–9.
2. ACOG Practice Bulletin no. 212: Pregnancy and heart disease. *Obstet Gynecol*. 2019;133:e320–56.
3. Patel A, Asopa S, Tang AT, Ohri SK. Cardiac surgery during pregnancy. *Tex Heart Inst J*. 2008;35:307–12.
4. Jha N, Jha AK, Chand Chauhan R, Chauhan NS. Maternal and fetal outcome after cardiac operations during pregnancy: A meta-analysis. *Ann Thorac Surg*. 2018;106:618–26.
5. John AS, Gurley F, Schaff HV, Warnes CA, Phillips SD, Arendt KW, Abel MD, Rose CH, Connolly HM. Cardiopulmonary bypass during pregnancy. *Ann Thorac Surg*. 2011;91:1191–6.
6. Chambers CE, Clark SL. Cardiac surgery during pregnancy. *Clin Obstet Gynecol*. 1994;37:316–23.
7. Canobbio MM, Warnes CA, Aboulhosn J, Connolly HM, Khanna A, Koos BJ, Mital S, Rose C, Silversides C, Stout K. Management of pregnancy in patients with complex congenital heart disease: A scientific statement for healthcare professionals from the American Heart Association. *Circulation*. 2017;135(8):e50–e87.
8. O'Sullivan CJ, Buhlmann Lerjen E, Pellegrini D, Eberli FR. Sudden cardiac arrest during emergency caesarean delivery in a 31-year-old woman, due to accelerated structural valve degeneration of an aortic valve bioprosthesis. *BMJ Case Rep*. 2015;2015.
9. Nishimura RA et al. 2014 AHA/ACC guideline for the management of patients with valvular heart disease. Executive summary: A report of the American College of Cardiology/American Heart Association Task Force on Practice Guidelines. *Circulation*. 2014;129(23):2440–92.
10. Regitz-Zagrosek V et al. ESC guidelines on the management of cardiovascular diseases during pregnancy: The task force on the management of cardiovascular diseases during pregnancy of the European Society of Cardiology (ESC). *Eur Heart J*. 2011;32:3147–97.
11. Hayes SN et al. Spontaneous coronary artery dissection: Current state of the science: A scientific statement from the American Heart Association. *Circulation* 2018;137:e523–57.
12. Lameijer H, Burchill LJ, Baris L, Ruys TP, Roos-Hesselink JW, Mulder BJM, Silversides CK, van Veldhuisen DJ, Pieper PG. Pregnancy in women with pre-existent ischaemic heart disease: A systematic review with individualised patient data. *Heart*. 2019;105(11):873–880.
13. Leifheit-Limson EC, D'Onofrio G, Daneshvar M, Geda M, Bueno H, Spertus JA, Krumholz HM, Lichtman JH. Sex differences in cardiac risk factors, perceived risk, and health care provider discussion of risk and risk modification among young patients with acute myocardial infarction: The VIRGO study. *J Am Coll Cardiol*. 2015;66:1949–57.
14. Hillis LD et al. 2011 ACCF/AHA guideline for coronary artery bypass graft surgery: A report of the American College of Cardiology Foundation/American Heart Association task force on practice guidelines. *Circulation*. 2011;124:e652–735.
15. Weiss BM, Zemp L, Seifert B, Hess OM. Outcome of pulmonary vascular disease in pregnancy: A systematic overview from 1978 through 1996. *J Am Coll Cardiol*. 1998;31:1650–7.
16. Callaghan WM, MacDorman MF, Rasmussen SA, Qin C, Lackritz EM. The contribution of preterm birth to infant mortality rates in the United States. *Pediatrics*. 2006;118:1566–73.
17. Pomini F, Mercogliano D, Cavalletti C, Caruso A, Pomini P. Cardiopulmonary bypass in pregnancy. *Ann Thorac Surg*. 1996;61:259–68.
18. Hawkins JA, Paape KL, Adkins TP, Shaddy RE, Gay WA Jr. Extracorporeal circulation in the fetal lamb. Effects of hypothermia and perfusion rate. *J Cardiovasc Surg (Torino)*. 1991;32:295–300.
19. Parry AJ, Westaby S. Cardiopulmonary bypass during pregnancy. *Ann Thorac Surg*. 1996;61:1865–9.
20. Kole SD, Jain SM, Walia A, Sharma M. Cardiopulmonary bypass in pregnancy. *Ann Thorac Surg*. 1997;63(3):915–6.
21. ACOG Practice Bulletin no. 209: Obstetric analgesia and anesthesia. *Obstet Gynecol*. 2019;133:e208–25.

20

Cardiovascular Medications in Pregnancy

Alice Chan and Ali N. Zaidi

KEY POINTS

- Pharmacokinetics of the cardiovascular medications are affected in pregnancy due to physiologic changes that affect metabolism and efficacy of various drugs
- Hydralazine and nitrates can be substituted for ACE inhibitors in treatment of heart failure in pregnancy

- Beta-blockers are the most commonly used cardiac medication in pregnancy
- Drugs that easily cross the blood–brain barrier usually enter breast milk more readily
- Nifedipine and propranolol have similar drug concentrations in the breast milk as in the maternal plasma

---

Introduction

Cardiovascular disease (CVD) is currently one of the leading causes of mortality in pregnant women [1–4], affecting 1%–2% of pregnancies [5]. Having a good understanding of the use of cardiac medications during this time is important to ensure appropriate management of these patients. However, pharmacological therapy for CVD during pregnancy can be challenging because the effects of the medications often change throughout gestation. The pharmacokinetics of the cardiovascular medications is affected by the physiological changes in pregnant women; the metabolism and the efficacy of the medications are usually altered [4]. Most cardiac conditions require use of medications. According to the Registry of Pregnancy and Cardiac Disease (ROPAC), up to one-third of women with CVD use cardiac medications during pregnancy, and this use was associated with increased fetal risk such as intrauterine fetal growth restriction (IUGR) [6]. The majority of data on the safety of medication use during pregnancy rely on observational studies and expert opinion. It should be kept in mind that drug use in pregnancy affects both the mother and the fetus, and therefore pharmacologic agents are chosen to address those concerns.

Drug Risk Categorization

The U.S. Food and Drug Administration (FDA) previously used pregnancy risk categories A, B, C, D, and X, with most cardiovascular drugs categorized as B (no animal studies have shown risk/no controlled studies in humans) or C (animal studies have shown adverse effect/no controlled studies in humans). In 2015, the FDA introduced new risk guidelines for various medications in pregnancy and lactation [7]. This new categorization provides narrative sections for pregnancy and lactation, an overall

risk based on known data, and the effects on women and men of reproductive potential. However, implementation of these guidelines will occur in stages over a 5-year period. Even though most providers continue to use the U.S. FDA-approved pregnancy risk categories as outlined above [4], the new system should be followed as much as possible, as it is a more detailed description of effects of drugs on pregnancy and lactation.

Pharmacokinetics in Pregnancy

The physiological changes in pregnancy affect many body organs, including the cardiac, hepatic, and renal systems (Table 20.1). Important changes include:

1. Delayed gastric emptying and motility
2. Prolonged small bowel transit time
3. Gastroesophageal reflux
4. Increased plasma volume and fat accumulation
5. Increased volume of distribution
6. Decreased albumin and plasma binding proteins
7. Increased minute ventilation
8. Increased hepatic clearance
9. Increased renal clearance
10. Hypercoagulability

All of these changes may affect drug distribution and clearance [5]. For instance, the glomerular filtration rate (GFR) increases by 25% during pregnancy leading to an increase in the clearance rate on medications that are primarily excreted by the kidneys [5,8]. The increase in the amount of body fat and plasma volume can also affect the medication's concentrations [4]. These factors

TABLE 20.1

Pharmacology and Hemodynamic Changes in Pregnancy

Renal	Circulation	Hematology
Increased reabsorption	Hemodilution	Increase in fibrinogen
Decreased urinary motility	Decreased in binding proteins	Increased von Willebrand factor
Increased glomerular filtration rate	Increased in volume of distribution	Decreased fibrinolysis
Increased secretion	Increased tissue fat	Increased coagulation
Increased renal clearance	Increased plasma	Decreased protein C
	Increased red blood cells	Decrease in protein S
		Increased clotting factors
Gastrointestinal	**Hepatic**	**Pulmonary**
Increase in gastric pH	Increased hepatic clearance	Decreased total lung capacity
Decreased absorption	Increased hepatic perfusion	Hyperventilation
Decreased bowel motility	Increased enzymatic activity	Increased minute ventilation

TABLE 20.2

Medications Contraindicated in Pregnancy

Medication Classification	FDA Category	Safety in Pregnancy	Safety in Lactation
Aldosterone antagonists	Variable	Contraindicated	Contraindicated
Statin	X	Contraindicated	Contraindicated
DOACs	Variable	Contraindicated	Contraindicated
ERAs	X	Contraindicated	Contraindicated
ACEI[a]	D	Contraindicated	Use with caution
ARB	D	Contraindicated	Unknown

Abbreviation: DOACs, direct oral anticoagulants; ERAs, endothelin receptor antagonists; ACEI, angiotensin converting enzyme inhibitor; ARB, angiotensin receptor blocker.

[a] Some ACEI medications such as enalapril, captopril, and benazepril are safe in lactation.

are important to keep in mind when prescribing medications to women during their pregnancy. The hormonal influences during pregnancy on the liver increase or decrease metabolism of some drugs without clear patterns. It should also be kept in mind that pregnancy is a hypercoagulable state associated with increased risk of thromboembolism.

The dynamic physiological changes of pregnancy clearly affect the pharmacokinetic processes. Increased activity of liver enzyme systems, GFR, plasma volume, protein binding changes, and decreased serum albumin levels contribute to changes in the pharmacokinetics of many medications [9,10]. The hormonally induced alterations in receptor and transport expression may affect drug activity at receptor sites, and therefore pregnancy introduces unpredictability to the body's handling of medications.

Absorption

Increased progesterone levels can delay intestinal motility in the small bowel while nausea and emesis can inhibit the absorption of medications. Many changes in medication absorption during pregnancy remain mostly theoretical and not proven.

Volume of Distribution (Vd)

There is an ~50% increase in plasma volume and total body water during pregnancy, increasing the Vd of hydrophilic and lipophilic substances. As Vd rises throughout pregnancy, the concentrations of a drug may decrease, requiring an increase in drug dosage. The concentration of drugs during pregnancy depends not only on the Vd but also on the clearance of the drug by the different organ systems (i.e., lungs, kidneys, and liver). Vd is also affected by the amount of drug bound to plasma proteins (e.g., albumin). Therefore, the net exposure of a drug during pregnancy depends on the interplay between Vd, degree of binding to serum proteins, extraction ratio, and clearance [11].

Hepatic Clearance

Hepatic extraction ratio refers to the fraction of drug removed from the circulation by the liver. Some drugs like propranolol, verapamil, and nitroglycerin are rapidly taken up into hepatocytes, and their clearance depends on the rate of blood flow to the liver. In pregnancy, perfusion to the liver stays stable or increases, causing some drugs to be metabolized faster, which in turn may require an increase in drug dosing. Clearance of those drugs that are not affected by hepatic clearance, such as warfarin, depends on the intrinsic hepatic activity as well as on the unbound fraction of the drug in plasma [12].

Renal Clearance

Effective renal plasma flow increases as much as 50%–85% in pregnancy [8]. GFR increases by 45%–50% by the end of the first trimester [8] and continues to rise until term, with a possible downtrend in the last few weeks. The tubular function remains variable [13].

Medications in Pregnancy

Some cardiovascular medications may be continued in pregnancy, but others are teratogenic and will need to be changed during pregnancy. Medications such as beta blockers, digoxin, and furosemide are safe in pregnancy [4], whereas angiotensin-converting enzyme inhibitors (ACEIs) and angiotensin receptor blockers (ARBs) are contraindicated in pregnancy (Table 20.2). Patients on ACEI or ARB for treatment of heart failure and/or hypertension would need to switch these medications to a safer alternative because of their teratogenic potential once pregnancy is confirmed, or ideally, prior to anticipated pregnancy [1,4]. Table 20.3 lists commonly used cardiovascular medications.

Hypertension

Hypertension is one of the most common comorbidities seen in pregnant women, affecting approximately 5%–10% of

TABLE 20.3

Common Cardiac Medications in Pregnancy

Medication	FDA	Teratogenicity	Fetal Effects	Safety in Lactation
Antiarrhythmic				
Amiodarone	D	No	Fetal thyroid toxicity	Contraindicated
Procainamide	C	No	Use with caution	Use with caution
Sotalol	B	No	Human data suggests risk	Possibly hazardous
Lidocaine	B	No	Safe	Safe
Flecainide	C	No	Limited human information	Use with caution
Phenytoin	C	No	Hemorrhagic disease of newborn	Safe
Atrioventricular nodal blocking drugs				
Adenosine	C	No information	Safe	Use with caution
Digoxin	C	No	Safe	Safe
Beta-blockers				
Metoprolol	C	No	Potential growth restriction	Use with caution
Atenolol	D	No	Potential growth restriction	Use with caution
Esmolol		No	Beta blockade in the fetus	Unknown
Labetalol	C	No	Safe	Use with caution
Carvedilol	C	Limited information	Potential growth restriction	Unknown
Propranolol	C	No	Safe	Use with caution
Calcium channel blockers				
Nifedipine	C	No	Safe	Safe
Amlodipine	C	No	Use with caution	Use with caution
Diltiazem	C	No	Safe	Use with caution
Verapamil	C	No	Safe	Safe
Inotropic drugs				
Dopamine	C	No	Safe	May inhibit prolactin release
Dobutamine	B	No	Safe	Unknown
Norepinephrine	C	No	Safe	Unknown
Vasodilators				
Hydralazine	C	No	Safe	Safe
Ephedrine sulfate	C	No	Safe	Caution with chronic use
Nitroglycerin	C	No	Use with caution	Unknown
Isosorbide dinitrate	C	No	Use with caution	Unknown
Nitroprusside	C	No	Potential fetal cyanide toxicity with high doses	Use with caution
Antiplatelet				
Aspirin	C	No	Use with caution	Use with caution
Clopidogrel	B	No	Use with caution	Use with caution
Ticagrelor	C	Limited information	Use with caution	Unknown
Anticoagulation				
Heparin	C	No	Safe	Safe
Enoxaparin	B	No	Safe	Safe
Warfarin	D	Limb defects, nasal hypoplasia	Fetal hemorrhage	Safe
Argatroban	B	No	Use with caution	Unknown
Direct factor Xa inhibitors (rivaroxaban or apixaban)		No	Crosses placenta, bleeding risk	No information
Alpha blockers				
Alpha-methyldopa	B	No	Safe	Safe
Clonidine	C	No	Use with caution	Unknown

(Continued)

TABLE 20.3 (*Continued*)

Common Cardiac Medications in Pregnancy

Medication	FDA	Teratogenicity	Fetal Effects	Safety in Lactation
Diuretics				
Furosemide	C	No	Safe	Caution
Hydrochlorothiazide	B	No	Use with caution	Safe
Metolazone	B	No	Use with caution	Unknown
Torsemide	B	No	Use with caution	Unknown
Pulmonary hypertension drugs				
Sildenafil	B	No	Use with caution	Use with caution
Treprostinil	C	No	Unknown	Unknown
Epoprotenol	B	No	Use with caution	Unknown

Source: Data derived from Halpern DG et al. *J Am Coll Cardiol*. 2019;73(4):457; ACOG Practice Bulletin #212 2019; https://chemm.nlm.nih.gov/pregnancycategories.htm.

FDA Categories: (A) Well-controlled studies have not shown fetal risk. (B) Animal studies have not shown fetal risk. (C) Animal studies have shown side effects on the fetus. (D) Human studies have shown side effects on the fetus. However, use of the medications may be warranted if there are potential benefits. (X) Human and animal studies have shown fetal risk or abnormalities, which outweigh potential benefits.

Abbreviation: FDA, Food and Drug Administration.

pregnancies globally [1,5]. In the United States, high blood pressure (BP) during pregnancy is a serious concern since it contributes to maternal and fetal morbidity and mortality [14]. Maternal complications can include strokes, organ failure, and placental abruption [1,14,15]. The fetal complications can include preterm delivery, growth restriction or retardation, and fetal death [1,14].

Pharmacological management is needed for hypertensive pregnant patients, but the medication used will depend on the patient's condition and its effect on the fetus [1]. Studies show labetalol, methyldopa, and nifedipine can safely be used during pregnancy [1,5,15,16]. Although frequently used in nonpregnant patients, treatment with diuretics for hypertensive disorders in pregnancy requires balancing BP control with adequate placental perfusion. There is a theoretical risk of decreased uterine blood flow and fetal growth restriction due to decreased blood volume when starting hydrochlorothiazide, so initiation during pregnancy is generally not advised [14]. A review of 11 randomized controlled trials on thiazide diuretics in the treatment of hypertension during pregnancy showed an overall reduction in risk of progression to preeclampsia and proteinuria (RR 0.66, $p = 0.001$, and 0.86, $p < 0.005$) without a statistically significant change in fetal mortality or stillbirths. In addition, women taking hydrochlorothiazide before pregnancy were not found to have changes in maternal or fetal outcomes compared with those who were not on the medication [17].

Beta blockers are an additional option for BP control. Although literature notes that fetal exposure to beta blockers may be associated with low birthweight, labetalol is a pregnancy class-C alpha- and beta-adrenergic antagonist that has traditionally been a first-line agent against hypertensive disorders in pregnancy. Labetalol has been shown to effectively reduce maternal BP and decrease both maternal and fetal morbidity and mortality in mild to moderate hypertension [18]. Metoprolol succinate is a beta-selective adrenergic antagonist in pregnancy class C. An open controlled trial for its use in moderate hypertension in pregnancy showed significantly better BP control than placebo without increases in preterm labor or maternal and fetal complications [19]. Carvedilol is dependent on renal elimination, which

can lead to greater amounts of drug excretion and thus higher doses during pregnancy given increases in GFR. Atenolol is a pregnancy class-D beta-adrenergic antagonist, which should be avoided in pregnancy, especially in the first trimester [20,21].

Methyldopa is a pregnancy class-B alpha-2 receptor agonist traditionally used in hypertensive pregnant women. Its use shows no observed differences in fetal morbidity and mortality compared with placebo and similar maternal BP control and outcomes to labetalol. Methyldopa use against hypertension in pregnancy is thus both safe and effective [22].

Nifedipine is also a dihydropyridine calcium channel antagonist in pregnancy class C, available in long- and short-acting formulations [23]. Diltiazem and verapamil are non-dihydropyridine calcium channel antagonists, and also fall into pregnancy category C [24].

Nitroglycerin is the drug of choice for women who have preeclampsia with pulmonary edema [1]. Hydralazine has been used in pregnancy for maintenance therapy as well as for the treatment of hypertensive emergencies [16]. An increased risk of fetal cyanide poisoning has been shown with sodium nitroprusside so it should be avoided when possible. In general, according to the American College of Cardiology/American Heart Association Task Force clinical practice guideline recommendations on the management of pregnant patients with high BP, women should be switched over to nifedipine, methyldopa, or labetalol if they are currently pregnant or plan to become pregnant in the near future [25].

ACEIs are a mainstay of hypertension and heart failure treatment in nonpregnant populations. In pregnant women, they have been associated with complications, including renal dysplasia, pulmonary hypoplasia, and growth restriction [26]. As approximately 50% of pregnancies are unplanned, ACEIs should be avoided not only in pregnant women but also in all women of childbearing age using no contraception, given their severe side effects [22]. ARBs such as losartan and valsartan, also commonly used to treat hypertension and heart failure, are classed pregnancy category D due to congenital abnormalities similar to those for ACEI use [26].

Heart Failure

One of the causes of morbidity and mortality in pregnant women and their fetus is heart failure. However, due to its nonspecific symptoms, it is sometimes difficult to diagnose. Women experience swelling to their lower extremities, dyspnea on exertion, and fatigue, but all of these symptoms can be considered normal in pregnancy [4]. Patient complaints need to be assessed carefully based on the heart failure guidelines. Once it is diagnosed, the management is not significantly different from patients who are not pregnant, except teratogenic medications need to be avoided. The goal of managing heart failure is improving prognosis and symptoms. Heart failure should be treated according to guidelines on acute and chronic heart failure. During pregnancy, ACE inhibitors, ARBs, and renin inhibitors are contraindicated because of fetotoxicity.

Medications with proven mortality benefit include beta-blockers, ACEIs, ARBs, and aldosterone antagonists [27]. These medications include mineralocorticoid receptor antagonists, angiotensin receptor neprilysin, ACEI, ARB, and atenolol [1]. Diuretics can be used if needed for pulmonary congestion, but since it can decrease cardiac output and placental blood flow, avoiding them would be preferable [1,5].

Heart failure with pulmonary congestion is treated with loop diuretics and thiazides if required; however, diuretics should be avoided in the absence of pulmonary congestion, due to the potential reduction in placental blood flow [28]. Hydralazine and nitrates can be used instead of ACEIs/ARBs for afterload reduction. Dopamine and levosimendan can be used if inotropic drugs are needed. Beta blockers can also be used in pregnancy but should be prescribed with careful titration to the tolerated dose [1]. Beta-blocker treatment is indicated for all patients with congestive heart failure if it is tolerated, with the preference of using B1-selective drugs (i.e., metoprolol). Atenolol should not be used. Diuretics should only be used if pulmonary congestion is present since they may decrease blood flow over the placenta [29]. Furosemide and hydrochlorothiazide are the two most frequently used. Aldosterone antagonists such as spironolactone should also be avoided since it can be associated with antiandrogenic effects in the first trimester. Data for eplerenone are lacking [30].

Management of acute heart failure and cardiogenic shock in pregnancy is based on current heart failure guidelines. Diuretics such as furosemide, bumetanide, and hydrochlorothiazide are used for symptomatic pulmonary edema and, as mentioned before, hold the risk of decreasing placental perfusion and causing an electrolyte imbalance in the fetus. For afterload reduction, hydralazine plus nitrates are used in place of ACE inhibitors and ARBs. After initial stabilization, beta blockers should be initiated, and digoxin can be considered. Postpartum, neurohormonal blockade can be restarted [1]. Paucity of data and lack of guidelines exist in regard to inotrope and vasopressor use for the critically ill pregnant patient. For inotrope support, dopamine and dobutamine have been safely used in pregnancy (119). Levosimendan, a calcium sensitizer, is recommended in the setting of postpartum cardiomyopathy, as dobutamine may be associated with heart failure progression in these patients [31].

Digoxin is a pregnancy class-C sodium/potassium ATPase inhibitor and direct suppressor of atrioventricular nodal conduction. It crosses the placenta readily during later pregnancy, but no adverse effects have been observed to the mother or fetus. Digoxin is generally used in pregnant women with persistent heart failure symptoms on beta-blockers, nitrate/hydralazine, and diuretic therapy [32].

Overall, review of the literature showed that when beta blockade is indicated, metoprolol is the most effective and safest option of beta-blockers studied. Furosemide is effective for volume control in heart failure, but with limited outcome data for mothers and fetuses, its use should be sparing and carefully monitored. Digoxin is safe for patients with persistent symptoms despite beta blockade, nitrate/hydralazine therapy, BP control, and fluid status optimization. ACEIs, ARBs, aldosterone antagonists, and newer agents such as sacubitril should be avoided.

Medication Safety during Lactation

All medications can enter breast milk, but how readily the drug passes into mature milk depends on several factors including:

1. Drug molecular weight
2. Lipid solubility
3. Protein binding
4. Volume of distribution
5. Half-life
6. Acid dissociation constant (pKa)

Generally, agents that easily cross the blood–brain barrier usually enter breast milk more readily [1,33]. Many women need to continue with their medications postpartum for the management of cardiomyopathies and hypertension so it is important for providers to consider the effects these medications may have on breastfeeding [4].

Patients on medications during lactation should be informed that their cardiac medications can be passed on to their breast milk, but fortunately, the small quantity that enter the breast milk are usually insignificant. Medications that are categorized as safe have a relative infant dose of less than 10%, and a majority of the cardiac medications have a relative infant dose of less than 1% [4]. The two antihypertensive medications that have similar drug concentrations in the breast milk as maternal plasma are nifedipine and propranolol. Most of the other antihypertensives have very low drug concentrations when they reach the breast milk [1].

It is also important to note the possible adverse effects associated with each of the different classification of medications. Diuretics can reduce the amount of milk produced in lactating women, which can lead to dehydration and lethargy in their infants. For women taking calcium channel blockers or beta-blockers, their infants should be assessed for drowsiness, pallor, weight gain, and poor feeding, as well as lethargy. The use of ACEIs such as enalapril appears to be safe in women who are lactating and breastfeeding, as long as the fetal weight is monitored routinely (every 4 weeks). ARB use during lactation, however, is not well described and their use postpartum is not advised with breastfeeding since little data is known about its effects [4,33].

Conclusion

Patients with cardiovascular disease who have higher-risk pregnancies should be followed with a multidisciplinary team that includes maternal-fetal medicine, obstetrics, cardiologists, anesthesia, primary care providers, and pharmacology experts [4,34–36]. Certain hypertension and heart failure medications are safe during pregnancy and play an important role in the management of high-risk patients, mitigating the rise in maternal mortality. Nevertheless, continued research evaluating safety and efficacy profiles of other cardiac medications in pregnancy is critical to reversing the trend of increasing maternal mortality in the United States.

REFERENCES

1. Regitz-Zagrosek V et al. 2018 ESC Guidelines for the management of cardiovascular diseases during pregnancy. *Eur Heart J.* 2018;39(34):3165–3241.
2. van Hagen IM et al. Global cardiac risk assessment in the registry of pregnancy and cardiac disease: Results of a registry from the European Society of Cardiology. *Eur J Heart Fail.* 2016;18(5):523–33.
3. Elkayam U et al. High-risk cardiac disease in pregnancy: Part II. *J Am Coll Cardiol.* 2016;68(5):502–516.
4. Kaye AB et al. Review of cardiovascular drugs in pregnancy. *J Womens Health (Larchmt).* 2019;28(5):686–697.
5. Halpern DG et al. Use of medication for cardiovascular disease during pregnancy: JACC State-of-the-Art review. *J Am Coll Cardiol.* 2019;73(4):457–476.
6. Ruys TP et al. Cardiac medication during pregnancy, data from the ROPAC. *Int J Cardiol.* 2014;177(1):124–8.
7. Pernia S, DeMaagd G. The new pregnancy and lactation labeling rule. *P T* 2016;41(11):713–715.
8. Costantine MM. Physiologic and pharmacokinetic changes in pregnancy. *Front Pharmacol.* 2014;5:65.
9. Pieper PG. Use of medication for cardiovascular disease during pregnancy. *Nat Rev Cardiol.* 2015;12(12):718–29.
10. Pieper PG et al. Uteroplacental blood flow, cardiac function, and pregnancy outcome in women with congenital heart disease. *Circulation.* 2013;128(23):2478–87.
11. Anderson GD. Using pharmacokinetics to predict the effects of pregnancy and maternal-infant transfer of drugs during lactation. *Expert Opin Drug Metab Toxicol.* 2006;2(6):947–60.
12. Feghali M, Venkataramanan R, Caritis S. Pharmacokinetics of drugs in pregnancy. *Semin Perinatol.* 2015;39(7):512–9.
13. Cheung KL, Lafayette RA. Renal physiology of pregnancy. *Adv Chronic Kidney Dis.* 2013;20(3):209–14.
14. Hypertension in pregnancy. Report of the American College of Obstetricians and Gynecologists' Task Force on Hypertension in Pregnancy. *Obstet Gynecol.* 2013;122(5):1122–31.
15. Firoz T et al. Oral antihypertensive therapy for severe hypertension in pregnancy and postpartum: A systematic review. *BJOG.* 2014;121(10):1210–8; discussion 1220.
16. Frishman WH, Elkayam U, Aronow WS. Cardiovascular drugs in pregnancy. *Cardiol Clin.* 2012;30(3):463–91.
17. Collins R, Yusuf S, Peto R. Overview of randomised trials of diuretics in pregnancy. *Br Med J (Clin Res Ed).* 1985;290(6461):17–23.
18. Molvi SN et al. Role of antihypertensive therapy in mild to moderate pregnancy-induced hypertension: A prospective randomized study comparing labetalol with alpha methyldopa. *Arch Gynecol Obstet.* 2012;285(6):1553–62.
19. Hogstedt S et al. A prospective controlled trial of metoprolol-hydralazine treatment in hypertension during pregnancy. *Acta Obstet Gynecol Scand.* 1985;64(6):505–10.
20. Lydakis C et al. Atenolol and fetal growth in pregnancies complicated by hypertension. *Am J Hypertens.* 1999;12(6):541–7.
21. Cruickshank DJ, Campbell DM. Atenolol in essential hypertension during pregnancy. *BMJ.* 1990;301(6760):1103.
22. Cockburn J et al. Final report of study on hypertension during pregnancy: The effects of specific treatment on the growth and development of the children. *Lancet.* 1982;1(8273):647–9.
23. Manninen AK, Juhakoski A. Nifedipine concentrations in maternal and umbilical serum, amniotic fluid, breast milk and urine of mothers and offspring. *Int J Clin Pharmacol Res.* 1991;11(5):231–6.
24. Lubbe WF. Use of diltiazem during pregnancy. *N Z Med J.* 1987;100(818):121.
25. Whelton PK et al. 2017 ACC/AHA/AAPA/ABC/ACPM/AGS/APhA/ASH/ASPC/NMA/PCNA Guideline for the prevention, detection, evaluation, and management of high blood pressure in adults: Executive Summary: A Report of the American College of Cardiology/American Heart Association Task Force on Clinical Practice Guidelines. *Circulation* 2018;138(17):e426–e483.
26. Schaefer C. Angiotensin II-receptor-antagonists: Further evidence of fetotoxicity but not teratogenicity. *Birth Defects Res A Clin Mol Teratol.* 2003;67(8):591–4.
27. Yancy CW et al. 2013 ACCF/AHA guideline for the management of heart failure: A report of the American College of Cardiology Foundation/American Heart Association Task Force on Practice Guidelines. *J Am Coll Cardiol.* 2013;62(16):e147–239.
28. Hilfiker-Kleiner D et al. A management algorithm for acute heart failure in pregnancy. The Hannover experience. *Eur Heart J.* 2015;36(13):769–70.
29. Sliwa K, Fett J, Elkayam U. Peripartum cardiomyopathy. *Lancet.* 2006;368(9536):687–93.
30. Mirshahi M et al. The blockade of mineralocorticoid hormone signaling provokes dramatic teratogenesis in cultured rat embryos. *Int J Toxicol.* 2002;21(3):191–9.
31. Bauersachs J et al. Current management of patients with severe acute peripartum cardiomyopathy: Practical guidance from the Heart Failure Association of the European Society of Cardiology Study Group on peripartum cardiomyopathy. *Eur J Heart Fail.* 2016;18(9):1096–105.
32. Widerhorn J et al. Cardiovascular drugs in pregnancy. *Cardiol Clin.* 1987;5(4):651–74.
33. Newton ER, Hale TW. Drugs in breast milk. *Clin Obstet Gynecol.* 2015;58(4):868–84.
34. Khairy P et al. Pregnancy outcomes in women with congenital heart disease. *Circulation.* 2006;113(4):517–24.
35. Earing MG, Webb GD. Congenital heart disease and pregnancy: Maternal and fetal risks. *Clin Perinatol.* 2005;32(4):913–9, viii–ix.
36. Swan L. Congenital heart disease in pregnancy. *Best Prac Res Clin Obstet Gynaecol.* 2014;28(4):495–506.

21

Cardiopulmonary Resuscitation in Pregnancy

Lauren A. Plante

KEY POINTS

- Maternal cardiac arrest occurs in 8–8.5 per 100,000 delivery hospitalizations
- Manual chest compressions with rescue breaths is inherently inefficient with respect to generating adequate cardiac output
- Additional differential diagnosis of maternal cardiac arrest includes amniotic fluid embolism, magnesium toxicity, and local anesthetic systemic toxicity

- In most cases of maternal cardiac arrest, the initial rhythm is not shockable
- Preparations for early resuscitative cesarean delivery should occur in parallel to maternal resuscitation to affect delivery within 5 minutes of maternal cardiac arrest

Incidence

The incidence of cardiac arrest in pregnancy is between 1:12,000 and 1:36,000 pregnancies. Population-based estimates *of the incidence of maternal cardiac arrest show about 8–8.5 cases per 100,000 delivery hospitalizations in North America* [1,2]; however, these data do not distinguish between antepartum, intrapartum, and postpartum cardiac arrests. Similar rates have been reported in the United Kingdom, i.e., 6.3 per 100,000 (1:16,000).

Etiology

Maternal cardiac arrest may result from any of the factors associated with adult cardiac arrest. *Pregnancy-specific etiologies must be included in the differential, such as amniotic fluid embolism, magnesium toxicity, and local anesthetic systemic toxicity.*

Survival Rates

Analysis of 56 million U.S. delivery hospitalizations between 1998 and 2011, containing 4843 cases of maternal cardiopulmonary arrest [1], showed that overall survival to hospital discharge was 59%, which is about three times higher than the cardiac arrest survival of women of childbearing age who are not pregnant (19%) [4]. Survival varies with the etiology of cardiac arrest, with highest rates (86%) noted in arrest due to magnesium toxicity and 82% due to anesthesia-related causes. Maternal survival after cardiac arrest due to anesthetic complications from the UK was reported excellent (100%), while lower in etiologies [3]. Furthermore, survival was much lower when the arrest occurred at home or in an ambulance rather than in the hospital (summarized in Box 21.1).

A direct comparison of women who received CPR in-hospital, drawn from the U.S. National Inpatient Sample, showed that

BOX 21.1 ETIOLOGY AND SURVIVAL OF MATERNAL CARDIAC ARREST[c]

Cause	Proportion of Maternal Cardiac Arrests (% of total)	Survival to Hospital Discharge (%)
Obstetric hemorrhage	45–60	43–73
Heart failure	13–32	71–74
Amniotic fluid embolism	12–13	52–67
Sepsis	9–11	47–60
Anesthesia complication	8–13	82–100
Venous embolism[a]	6–14	12–53
Eclampsia	6–7	76–85
Cerebrovascular disorder	4–5	0–40
Trauma	2–3	23–56
Pulmonary edema	2–5	71–77
Myocardial infarction	1–3	33–56
Magnesium toxicity[b]	1	86
Asthma	1–2	0–54
Anaphylaxis	<1–2	100
Aortic aneurysm, dissection, or rupture	<1–2	0–25 (this 25% represents 1 of 4 reported)
Hypoxia[b]	7	100
Hypovolemia[b]	22	62
Cardiac cause[b]	12	86

Note: Rounded to nearest integer; may not sum to 1 because differentially partitioned in different datasets.

[a] Category as "obstetric embolism" in [2], where it includes both venous and air embolism.
[b] Category appears in only one reference.
[c] Compiled from references [1–3].

pregnant women who received CPR were more likely to survive than nonpregnant women in the same age cohort (71% vs. 49%) [5]. There was no survival advantage to pregnancy when the arrest was due to trauma or traumatic injuries [6]. In a separate analysis of the American Heart Association's voluntary registry, survival for in-hospital maternal cardiac arrest was 41% [7].

Out-of-Hospital Cardiac Arrest

Limited information is available specifically on out-of-hospital cardiac arrest (OHCA) in pregnancy. In a Toronto database of OHCA between 2010 and 2014, there were six maternal OHCAs, all in the third trimester, out of a total of 1085 reproductive age women [8]. Only one woman (17%) and two newborns (33%) survived to hospital discharge, even though return of spontaneous circulation (ROSC) was achieved in 50% of pregnant women, a rate three times higher than in nonpregnant counterparts. A retrospective study identified two survivors among 16 pregnant women who sustained OHCA between 2009 and 2014; both women were in their first trimester who had arrested due to a cardiac cause with ROSC prior to arrival at the hospital [9]. The sole fetal survivor was born at term to one of these women. These small studies suggest that the outcome for OHCA in pregnancy is poor for both mother and baby. Nonpregnant young adults who experience OHCA also have a poor prognosis, with 6%–10% probability of survival [10,48].

Etiology and Risk Factors for Maternal Cardiac Arrest

Leading causes of maternal cardiac arrest are summarized in Box 21.2 [11,12].

- In most cases of maternal cardiac arrest, the initial rhythm is non-shockable, with 50% being pulseless electrical activity and 25% being asystole [7].
- African American women are overrepresented, comprising 25%–35% of cases of maternal cardiac arrest despite being about 10% of the population in the United States [1,7].
- Preexisting medical conditions are associated with higher odds of maternal cardiac arrest [1].
- The majority of cases of maternal cardiac arrest are preceded by respiratory insufficiency and/or hypotension [7].

Challenges in Performing CPR Pregnancy

Conventional cardiopulmonary resuscitation (CPR) is inherently inefficient with respect to generating cardiac output [13], and that is without the additional challenges imposed by pregnancy. In addition, there may be legal, sociologic, or cultural factors at play when a pregnant woman suffers a cardiac arrest [14].

Physiology

Normal pregnancy requires maternal physiologic adaption in all organ systems. The growing uterus, fetus, and placenta impose

---

BOX 21.2   ETIOLOGIES OF MATERNAL CARDIAC ARREST

A	Anesthesia-related	Airway loss
		Aspiration
		Local anesthetic systemic injury
		High spinal
	Accidents	Trauma
		Drowning
		Suicide
B	Bleeding	Placental abruption
		Uterine rupture
		Placenta previa/accreta
		Uterine atony
		Retained placenta
C	Cardiovascular	Arrhythmia
		Aortic dissection or rupture
		Myocardial infarction
		Cardiomyopathy
		Congenital heart disease
D	Drugs	Licit (oxytocin, magnesium, insulin, opioids)
		Illicit (opioids, others)
		Anaphylaxis
		Drug error
E	Embolism	Amniotic fluid embolism
		Pulmonary embolism
		Venous air embolism
		Cerebral embolism
F	Fever	Infection
G	General H's & T's	Hypovolemia
		Hypoxia
		Hypothermia
		Hydrogen ion (acidosis)
		Hypo/hyperkalemia
		Toxins
		Tamponade
		Tension pneumothorax
		Thrombosis (coronary or pulmonary)
H	Hypertension	Preeclampsia/eclampsia
		HELLP syndrome (hemolysis, elevated liver enzymes, low platelets)
		Stroke

Source: Jeejeebhoy FM et al. *Circulation.* 2015;132:1747–73; Zelop CM et al. *Am J Obstet Gynecol.* 2018;219(1):52–61.

---

mechanical and metabolic demands, which have the potential to complicate critical situations such as cardiac arrest and resuscitation. An understanding of pregnancy anatomy and physiology is crucial in recognizing and responding to critical situations (see Box 21.3).

A key point in pregnancy physiology is the decrease in cardiac output (CO) in the supine position past mid-pregnancy because of compression of the IVC by the enlarged uterus, which has been known for over 50 years [15]. More recently, cardiac magnetic resonance imaging (MRI) studies demonstrate an incremental effect of pregnancy-induced IVC compression in later gestation and the variation in cardiac output from supine to left lateral position. There is an increase in ejection fraction by 11%, left ventricular end diastolic volume by 21%, stroke volume by 35%, left atrial volume by 41%, and cardiac output by 24% by shifting the patient from supine to left lateral position [16]. MRI

BOX 21.3 PREGNANCY PHYSIOLOGY THAT AFFECTS MATERNAL RESUSCITATION[a]

	Physiologic Changes	Clinical Implications
Cardiovascular	Total cardiac output increases by 30%–50% with 20% of this directed to the uterus	Following delivery, this portion of cardiac output is redirected away from the uterus into maternal circulation that potentially may contribute to maternal resuscitation
	Increased venous capacitance and vasodilation leading to decrease in systemic vascular resistance	Decrease in blood pressure and contributing to dependent edema
	Decreased sensitivity to both endogenous and exogenous vasopressor substances	May affect response to vasopressors
Respiratory	Increased anteroposterior diameter of the chest	May affect efficacy of chest compressions
	Increased airway edema and mucosal capillary fragility	Difficult intubation
	Increased minute ventilation and oxygen consumption, and decreased functional residual capacity	Increased oxygen demand and quick desaturation when oxygenation is interrupted
	Decreased thoracic compliance due to elevation of diaphragm and mammary growth during pregnancy	May affect efficacy of chest compressions
	Compensated respiratory alkalosis with decrease in carbon dioxide, serum bicarbonate, and buffering capacity	May affect acid–base balance during resuscitation
Gastrointestinal	Relaxation of the lower esophageal sphincter and slowed transit time through the stomach and intestine	Increased risk of aspiration
	Decreased production of binding proteins	Increase in free concentration of protein-bound drugs
Renal	Increased renal blood flow and glomerular filtration rate	Drug clearance may be affected
	Decreased tubular absorption of protein and glucose	Protein and glucose spills in the urine at lower thresholds
	Relaxation of ureteric smooth muscle, compression of ureters at the pelvic brim by enlarging uterus	Urinary stasis
Hematologic	Hemodilution	Decreased colloid oncotic pressure and decrease in hematocrit
Neurologic	Increased sensitivity to local anesthetics	Dose adjustment may be necessary

[a] Compiled from references [11,70,109–112].

shows the inferior vena cava is almost completely occluded in the supine position when a pregnancy is at term [17], which can be remedied by lateral tilt positioning to a minimum of 30 degrees or more [16–18], a position which tends to see patients sliding off the underlying surface. Indirect methods also show a modest variation in CO [19]; however, these methods have not been validated for use in pregnancy [20,21].

CPR in a tilted position results in inefficient compressions [22], whereas CO is compromised in the supine position. Proposed solutions range from the Cardiff wooden wedge [22], preformed foam wedge [23], and the "human wedge" in which the patient is supported on the thighs of a kneeling rescuer [24]. The American Heart Association (AHA) and European Resuscitation Council (ERC) recommend that an additional rescuer manually displace the uterus, either pulling it from the left or pushing it from the right, with upward and lateral pressure [11,25,26] (see Figures 21.1 and 21.2). The International Consensus on Cardiopulmonary Resuscitation (ILCOR) guidelines, however, differ from most others, stating that there is inadequate evidence to make a recommendation about left lateral tilt or uterine displacement during CPR in a pregnant patient [27].

Fetoplacental Perfusion and Oxygenation

In humans, the uterine arteries dilate during pregnancy and increase in diameter by nearly fivefold [28], which makes placental perfusion largely dependent on a pressure head, with very limited or absent vasoreactivity. Oxygen (O_2) and carbon dioxide

(CO_2) transfer across the placenta along the pressure gradient between maternal intervillous blood and the fetal blood in villous capillaries [29]. As CO_2 diffuses into maternal blood, its decreasing pH favors release of O_2 and enhances O_2 transfer to the fetus. Fetal hemoglobin has inherently higher O_2 affinity, further favoring uptake.

The fetal response to impaired perfusion and asphyxia manifests by bradycardia and redistribution of blood flow [30], which are compensatory responses to allow defense against moderate hypoxia. The preterm fetus has a less robust cardiovascular response to interruption of blood flow, however, and may be able to survive longer primarily due to greater cardiac glycogen reserve compared to the term fetus [30]. Human studies are not feasible, but fetal lambs show a failure of compensatory responses by about 12 minutes following complete umbilical cord occlusion [30]. The fetus is clearly at risk of injury and/or death when uteroplacental blood flow is interrupted; however, maternal CPR takes precedence and delivery is advisable as a resuscitative measure for the mother.

Approach to Cardiac Arrest in the Pregnant Patient

ILCOR and AHA guidelines were revised in 2010 to emphasize circulation (rather than airway or breathing) as the initial step in resuscitation after cardiac arrest [31], and the most recent guidelines in 2015 [32] reiterate this focus. After verifying the scene

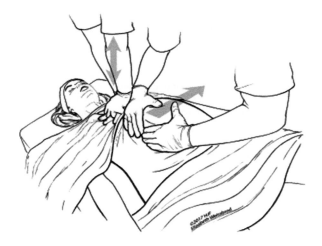

FIGURE 21.1 A method of manual left uterine displacement from the patient's left side. (From Kikuchi J, Deering S. *Semin Perinatol.* 2018;42:33–8. With permission [113].)

is *safe* and the patient is *unresponsive*, the health care provider should call for *help, activate* the emergency response team, and either get the *AED* or send someone else to do so. The *uterus should be displaced* manually as soon as a second rescuer is available [11], but another method of uterine displacement is needed when there is only one rescuer.

If the patient has no pulse and respiratory effort is absent or gasping, the immediate intervention is to begin CPR, cycling 30 compressions and 2 breaths. A firm underlying surface is required, such as a backboard. The AHA considers that actions in the basic life support (BLS) sequence should be simultaneous rather than sequential in maternal cardiac arrest [11], so the order of ventilation versus defibrillation is unclear in this population. In adults generally, immediate defibrillation is indicated if the rhythm is shockable [32,33]. Ventilations are delivered by bag-valve-mask with F_1O_2 of 1.0 at an O_2 flow rate of $\geq$15 L/min, at a rate of 2 ventilations to every 30 compressions; or an advanced airway is inserted (endotracheal or supraglottic device) and ventilations are delivered at a rate of 10 per minute, without coordinating or interrupting chest compressions (see Figure 21.3).

Old iterations of BLS suggested an A-B-C (Airway-Breathing-Circulation) order of tasks, but since 2010 the recommendation has been *C-A-B (Circulation-Airway-Breathing)* [34,35]. When the arrest victim is pregnant, experts have suggested C-A-B-U (Circulation-Airway-Breathing-Uterine displacement) [11] or C-A-B-D (Circulation-Airway-Breathing-Delivery). A shockable rhythm should always be defibrillated.

How Should CPR Be Modified in Pregnancy?

There are no randomized trials focused on cardiac arrest care modifications for pregnancy. A 2011 systematic review of cardiac arrest in pregnancy only addressed maternal physiology as it pertains to resuscitation [36]. They identified five pertinent articles: two on perimortem CS [37,38], two on the effect of lateral tilt on chest compressions [22,24], and one on thoracic impedance during pregnancy [39], from which they concluded that defibrillation energy requirements should not be altered in pregnancy.

Basic Life Support

Chest Compressions

The importance of high-quality chest compressions remains the utmost priority in national and international guidelines [32,49,50], as survival rates are directly linked to good-quality chest compressions.

The Society for Obstetric Anesthesia and Perinatology [35] and the European Resuscitation Council [26] had previously suggested hand placement higher on the sternum in pregnancy because of the elevation of the diaphragm. The current 2015 AHA guidelines [11,25] do not recommend higher hand placement on the sternum, nor do the ILCOR guidelines [27]. Cardiac MRI demonstrates no difference in cardiac position in a woman's third trimester compared to 3 months postpartum [52].

Chest compressions should be performed at a rate of 100–120 times per minute, with a compression depth 5–6 min, and recoil

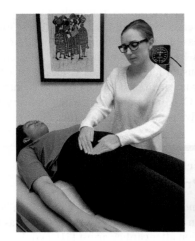
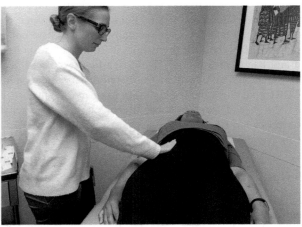

FIGURE 21.2 Method of manual left uterine displacement, performed from the patient's left (a) and right (b).

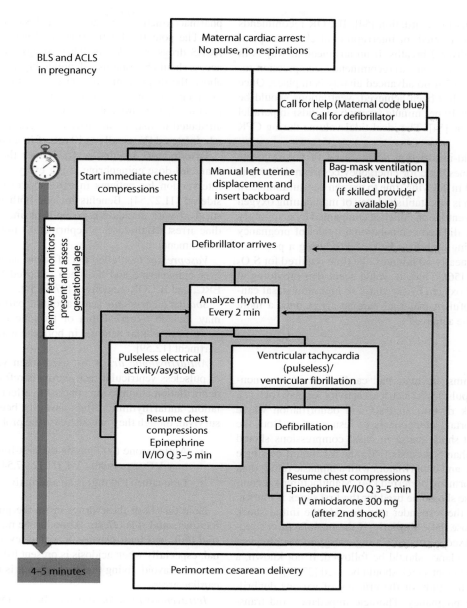

FIGURE 21.3 Suggested algorithm for maternal resuscitation following cardiac arrest. (From Zelop CM et al. *Am J Obstet Gynecol.* 2018;219(1):52–61. With permission.)

of the chest wall should be allowed between compressions, which means the rescuer cannot lean his/her weight on the chest [32,49,50]: *inadequate recoil interferes with right heart filling and coronary perfusion* [50]. *These recommendations are not altered in pregnancy.*

Ventilation and Oxygenation

The airway must be kept open during CPR either with head-tilt chin-lift, or jaw-thrust maneuver, or with the use of an oral airway; nasal airways are avoided in pregnancy because of edema and friability of nasal mucosa.

Hypoventilation or apnea causes hypoxemia faster in a pregnant woman, because of increased oxygen demand and reduced functional residual capacity. It takes only about 4 minutes of apnea for S_aO_2 to drop below 90% (compared to more than 7 minutes in a nonpregnant adult) when neither preoxygenation nor passive oxygen insufflation is provided [53]. Options for oxygenation and ventilation are listed below.

- Bag-valve-mask ventilation does not protect the airway, and therefore there is risk of aspiration in pregnancy.
- Endotracheal intubation is more difficult in a pregnant woman because of anatomic alterations and airway edema, and therefore it must be undertaken by the most experienced provider. Cricoid pressure is neither required nor recommended for intubation [11].
- Supraglottic airway devices (e.g., laryngeal mask airway) should be considered if intubation cannot be easily accomplished.

Excessive attention to ventilation may compromise high-quality CPR, and therefore chest compressions should continue without interruptions for ventilation [54]. ILCOR recommends that <10 seconds be allotted for interruption of chest compressions in order to deliver 2 breaths, if no advanced airway is in place [50]. Guidelines continue to recommend a compression-to-ventilation ratio of 30:2 if no advanced airway is in place. Once an advanced airway has been achieved, ventilations should be delivered at a rate of 10 per minute (every 6 seconds) in parallel to chest compressions [54]. The ideal tidal volume during CPR is unknown.

A high-flow rapid-insufflation device used to preoxygenate prior to a general anesthetic for emergency cesarean delivery is thought to be useful in delaying time to oxygen desaturation [55]. Apneic oxygenation is an established way of maintaining oxygen saturation without ventilation, albeit accompanied by respiratory acidosis, and in a validated computational model of pregnancy physiology, delivering high-flow F_1O_2 of 1.0 during a period of apnea increased to nearly 60 minutes, the time required for S_aO_2 to fall below 90% [56]. Thus, it would seem that providing at least a high flow of oxygen by facemask or high-flow nasal cannula might be helpful in maternal cardiac arrest until a more secure airway can be achieved.

Defibrillation

Most initial rhythms in maternal cardiac arrest are non-shockable, either pulseless electrical activity or asystole [7]. Nevertheless, quick rhythm analysis and defibrillation where indicated are important components of resuscitation. Both the pre-shock and post-shock pause in chest compressions should be limited to less than 5 seconds [35]. Shocks should be single rather than stacked, and defibrillators with a biphasic rather than monophasic waveform are preferred [54]. Manufacturer's recommended energy dose should be used for the first shock if known; if it is not known, the responder may provide the initial shock at the maximum dose [54]. Similarly, if the manufacturer's recommendation for fixed versus escalating energy in a subsequent shock is known, guidance should be followed; if not known, a higher-energy subsequent shock should be used [27,54].

There has been no study of the efficacy of various defibrillation strategies in pregnancy. Thoracic impedance and transmyocardial current delivered is unchanged in pregnancy [11,39]. The fibrillation threshold of the fetal heart is unknown [57], and it is unlikely that much of a transthoracic current delivered to the mother would be transmitted to the uterus.

Electronic fetal monitors if already in place should not be removed for the purpose of electrical safety in defibrillation [11,51]. Either the standard hospital defibrillator or an automated external defibrillator (AED) may be used with pads or paddles placed in the anterolateral position, with care taken to ensure the lateral pad is placed under the left breast [11].

Advanced Cardiac Life Support

In addition to BLS interventions (chest compressions, defibrillation, ventilation), advanced cardiac life support (ACLS) involves additional monitoring (such as capnography), endotracheal intubation, and pharmacologic therapies. Despite known alterations in volume of distribution, protein binding, and other pharmacokinetics of pregnancy, ACLS drug doses are no different. The potential for transplacental passage or fetal effects of ACLS drugs is irrelevant. These drugs are given IV, so venous access should be established, preferably large-bore venous access above the diaphragm. Any drugs that may have contributed to or precipitated maternal cardiac arrest such as oxytocin or magnesium should immediately be discontinued. If the arrest is attributed to magnesium toxicity, 1 gram of calcium should be administered IV, usually as 10 mL of 10% calcium gluconate [12].

Vasopressors require central rather than peripheral access. Standard-dose epinephrine (1 mg every 3–5 min) is a common intervention for patients in cardiac arrest and should be considered [11,27,54]. Benefits include both ROSC and improved survival with standard-dose epinephrine [54,59] in adult cardiac arrest. High-dose epinephrine (0.1 mg/kg and above) is not recommended.

Vasopressin has fallen out of favor, as it provides no benefit over epinephrine and has been removed from the 2015 AHA, ERC, and ILCOR guidelines [27,54,59].

Sodium bicarbonate is not a routine part of ACLS. Indications may include hyperkalemia or tricyclic overdose [59]. It may cause intracellular acidosis in both the maternal and fetal compartment [12,59].

Antiarrhythmic drugs are used when ventricular fibrillation or pulseless ventricular tachycardia is refractory to one or more defibrillation attempts. In contrast to effective CPR and defibrillation, antiarrhythmic drugs have not been shown to increase survival, though they may increase the probability of ROSC [54].

- Amiodarone (300 mg) is the first-line agent for refractory VF or pulseless VT [11,12,27,54,59]
- Lidocaine (100 mg) is an alternative [59]

Note that both these drugs cross the placenta with potential fetal/neonatal side effects. Amiodarone may affect the fetal thyroid [60], and fetal plasma lidocaine levels may exceed maternal, especially when acidosis is present [61]. Neither of these is a reason to avoid giving the drug when it is indicated in maternal cardiac arrest.

Intravenous lipid therapy may be used when cardiac arrest is attributed to local anesthetic systemic toxicity (LAST), though there are neither experimental nor observational studies in humans [27], let alone in pregnancy. The Society for Obstetric Anesthesia and Perinatology recommends lipid emulsion as adjunctive therapy in the case of local anesthetic-induced maternal cardiac arrest [35], dosed as a bolus of 1.5 mL/kg 20% lipid emulsion (Intralipid®), followed by 0.25–0.5 mL/kg/min infusion [12]. The majority of maternity units in both the United Kingdom and the United States keep lipid emulsion in stock for this indication [62,63] recommended by both the Association of Anesthetists' of Great Britain and Ireland [64] and the American Society of Regional Anesthesia and Pain Medicine [65]. Successful resuscitation from LAST-induced cardiac arrest may take 1 hour or more. Lidocaine must be avoided as an antiarrhythmic when LAST is suspected.

Opioid overdose, either from prescribed or illicit use, may precipitate maternal cardiac arrest. Several cases have been reported in association with remifentanil patient-controlled analgesia (PCA) in labor [66,67].

Fetal Assessment

Not Recommended

The primary focus of resuscitation is the pregnant woman, not the fetus. Fetal monitoring is irrelevant in the setting of maternal arrest as it will not contribute to maternal resuscitation and may well distract the team from proper resuscitation performance [35].

Perimortem Cesarean Delivery (Resuscitative Hysterotomy) and the 5-Minute "Rule"

- AHA recommends consideration of perimortem cesarean delivery or resuscitative hysterotomy [73] if the initial maternal resuscitative measures are unsuccessful in the presence of uterine size greater than or equal to 20 weeks.

- Guidelines for resuscitation in pregnancy commonly refer to a 5-minute rule or a 4-minute rule: after 4 (or 5) minutes of CPR without return of spontaneous circulation, perform perimortem cesarean (PMCD) with the goal of effecting delivery in the next minute [68].

Perimortem cesarean, or more precisely "resuscitative delivery," is primarily performed as a last-ditch attempt to resuscitate the mother. Decompressing the IVC by emptying the uterus has the potential to return CPR to its baseline effectiveness, which may be enough for return of spontaneous circulation and maternal survival. In addition, extraction of the fetus and placenta lowers maternal oxygen demand, increases functional residual capacity and chest wall compliance, and shifts that portion of circulating volume previously diverted to the uterus back into the central circulation. As a way of emphasizing the maternal effects of the procedure, some authors describe it as "resuscitative hysterotomy." [41,43,45,72–74]

- *Maternal survival* is clearly better when the interval from cardiac arrest to delivery is shorter. A systematic review of cases in English and German found that maternal survival was inversely correlated with time from arrest to delivery, in a gradual stepwise fashion [70] but there was no specific breakpoint; the time which marked 50% injury-free survival was 25 minutes. Even after 4 minutes (or more) of CPR without ROSC, there still appears to be maternal benefit in PMCD. The role of contemporary post-arrest care in improving injury-free survival after maternal cardiac arrest remains unexplored.

- PMCD may be associated with *survival of the newborn*. In a recent review, overall neonatal survival was 76%, and intact survival 57% [70]. Neonatal survival after maternal cardiac arrest is affected by the time elapsed between arrest and PMCD: in the UKOSS CAPS study [3], 96% of infants survived when PMCD was performed within 5 min, while 70% survived when PMCD was performed at later than 5 min. Infant survivors have, however, been reported when PMCD was performed as late as 30 [75,76] and even 43 [77] minutes after maternal cardiac arrest. In the 2016 review, just as for maternal survival, there was no sharp drop in newborn survival at 4 or 5 minutes after maternal arrest: the threshold for 50% injury-free neonatal survival was almost the same as the mothers at 26 min [70].

- PMCD should be performed at the *site of arrest*, because transport reduces success [3]. Transport to hospital is, of course, indicated when the arrest has occurred out of hospital. Little information is available about performing PMCS out of hospital [39,41], and no recommendation can be made here. The technique of PMCD is simple [11,78,79] (see Figure 21.4). If an obstetrician is not available, a general surgeon, family medicine physician, or emergency medicine physician may have the required surgical skills. Speed is of the essence. Though a cesarean tray with instruments should be used if one is at the site, no time should be wasted waiting for one: the operator may proceed with nothing more than a scalpel.

- *Antiseptic preparation* of the abdomen should be abbreviated or eliminated altogether ("splash and crash"). Either a vertical midline incision or a Pfannenstiel incision may be used at the operator's preference; the uterus may be opened vertically or via a transverse lower segment incision; ideally, delivery will be effected within 1 minute of abdominal incision. The cord may be clamped in one location or two so the infant can be handed off. Manual uterine displacement is released once the infant is delivered. A neonatal resuscitation team or provider should take charge of the newborn. Little or no maternal bleeding is expected in the absence of effective circulation. If circulation is restored, however, bleeding may be brisk. In some cases, the successfully resuscitated patient will require transport to an operating room for closure and hemorrhage control [12].

Extracorporeal Life Support

Extracorporeal life support (ECLS) during CPR is a way of supporting perfusion while reversible etiologies of cardiac arrest are being corrected. Analysis of data from an international registry showed that utilization of extracorporeal CPR (ECPR) increased between 2003 and 2014, but there was no improvement in survival (27%–30%) during those years [80]. Recent national and international guidelines on CPR are cautious in recommending ECPR but allow that there may be a place for it as a rescue therapy in selected patients with a reversible cause of cardiac arrest [27,54,59]. A few cases of postpartum ECPR have been reported [81–84], largely third trimester presentations of respiratory distress due to pulmonary embolus, in which the maternal arrest occurred in the operating room after cesarean delivery. The duration of CPR in these cases was surprisingly long (45 to 65 min) before ECPR was instituted. Maternal complications included coagulopathy with massive transfusion in all three, relaparotomy in two, compartment syndrome in two, renal insufficiency, hepatic insufficiency, and sepsis. Of the three cases in which the fetus was alive at the time, two newborns and all three mothers survived. Although ECLS in maternal arrest is possible, current experience is inadequate to make conclusive recommendations.

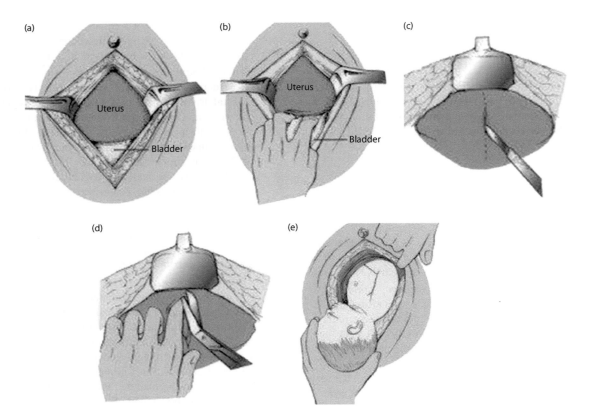

FIGURE 21.4 Technique of perimortem cesarean delivery, performed via vertical abdominal and uterine incision. (a) Vertical incision through the abdominal wall from the level of the uterine fundus to the symphysis pubis. (b) Retraction to expose the anterior surface of the uterus and retract the bladder inferiorly. (c) Small vertical incision through the lower uterine segment. (d) Extension of the incision superiorly to the fundus by bandage scissors. (e) Delivery of the fetus (suction the nose and mouth; clamp and cut the cord). (From Healy M et al. *J Emerg Med*. 2016;51:172−7. With permission.)

Post-Arrest Care

Survival is not the only outcome of interest after cardiac arrest, as survivors may experience significant morbidity. The post-cardiac arrest syndrome includes:

- Post-arrest brain injury
- Myocardial dysfunction
- Ischemia-reperfusion response manifested as inflammation
- Impaired vascular regulation
- Altered coagulation
- Temperature dysregulation
- Hemodynamic instability
- Hyperglycemia
- Immune dysfunction
- Multi-organ failure [33]

Treatment strategies for post-cardiac arrest syndrome can reduce morbidity and improve quality of life. Current [85] recommendations are:

1. Avoid/correct hypotension
2. Targeted temperature management (therapeutic hypothermia) followed by active measures to prevent fever

3. Detect and treat seizures
4. Maintain P_aCO_2 in the physiologic range
5. Maintain peripheral oxygen saturation $\geq 94\%$ while avoiding hyperoxia

In the majority of cases of maternal cardiac arrest, underlying etiology is typically ameliorated by delivery, e.g., obstetric hemorrhage, eclampsia, and amniotic fluid embolism, and therefore there is less contribution to the post-cardiac arrest syndrome.

Limited data are available on outcome for survivors of maternal cardiac arrest. The UKOSS CAPS study reported on 38 survivors, of whom 42% suffered additional morbidity during their hospital stay: 16% neurologic, 18% hemorrhage or coagulopathy, 5% renal, and 3% cardiac [3]. Unfortunately, no information was available on these survivors after hospital discharge; some have gone to term and been normal [9], others appeared to do well at the time of maternal resuscitation, only to be delivered weeks later with evidence of hypoxic ischemic encephalopathy [86].

The AHA 2015 guidelines explicitly state, "There are essentially no patients for whom temperature control somewhere in the range between 32°C and 36°C is contraindicated," and recommends targeted temperature management (TTM) for at least 24 hours following return of spontaneous circulation after cardiac arrest [85]. Data specific to TTM in pregnancy remain limited to case reports [87–92], but there have been some successful maternal outcomes. Information on the perinatal outcome with post-arrest TTM use in an ongoing pregnancy is more limited. Fetal heart rate monitoring may show fetal bradycardia in response to maternal hypothermia [91], but this is likely to resolve as rewarming occurs.

Pregnancy is no contraindication to implantable cardioverter defibrillator (ICD) implantation or continuation [11]. Limited case reports and case series [93–96] show ICDs to be safe during pregnancy. The majority of reports describe devices implanted prior to pregnancy, but implantation during pregnancy imposes no particular challenge, nor does the required fluoroscopy [97]; general principles of diagnostic imaging in pregnancy apply [98].

Maternal Prognosis and Long-Term Outcome after Cardiac Arrest

Long-term outcome after maternal cardiac arrest is unclear. In general, adults who have survived cardiac arrest often display a degree of cognitive impairment, post-traumatic stress disorder, and possibly anxiety and depression [99]. Risk score and a nomogram has been developed to predict the probability of survival with good neurological status after adult in-hospital cardiac arrest [100]. Although it has not been validated in pregnancy, the more favorable outcomes associated with younger age and absence of preexisting conditions suggest that pregnant patients who survive a cardiac arrest in hospital are not likely to do worse than other adults.

Neonatal Outcomes after Maternal Cardiac Arrest and Factors Influencing Infant Survival

Placental perfusion requires adequate maternal cardiac output and therefore it is not surprising that fetal bradycardia or even asystole commonly follows maternal cardiac arrest and during CPR [71].

When resuscitative cesarean delivery is performed, infant survival is inversely related to time elapsed from maternal arrest to delivery. In only a minority of cases has PMCD been effected within the 4 or 5 minutes commonly recommended, but a 50% probability of intact survival has been calculated even at 22 minutes [70], and neonatal survival has been reported with arrest-to-PMCD intervals as long as 30 [75,76] and 43 [77] minutes.

Neonatal survival is also highly predicated on gestational age at birth and the availability of neonatal resuscitation and intensive care services, which makes it difficult to incorporate cases from older literature or under-resourced areas. The largest datasets on maternal cardiac arrest seldom have information on neonatal outcomes. The UKOSS CAPS study provided information on 58 babies born to 66 women who had suffered cardiac arrest [3]. Of these 58, 12 were stillborn, and 5 of those born alive nevertheless died in the neonatal period, for a perinatal mortality rate of 29%. The survivors had much higher birthweights, indicating a more advanced gestational age. Neurologic, respiratory, and infectious complications are reported among 32% of the liveborn babies, but no further analysis was offered, and no information was provided about outcomes after discharge from the neonatal intensive care unit.

Institutional Planning

Hospitals that treat adults should have plans in place for maternal cardiopulmonary arrest and resuscitation. At the minimum, staff should know how to activate a team to respond to a maternal cardiac arrest, how to access the algorithms, and have the requisite equipment available [11]. (See Box 21.4 for a sample checklist.)

Simulation and Drills

Team training is mandatory to improve team performance in response to obstetrical emergencies. In a review of obstetric team performance during simulation of maternal cardiac arrest, authors from Stanford showed significant deficiencies in the performance of important tasks: not one of the teams performed all the recommended interventions properly, despite all team members being current in ACLS certification [101]. Teams were more likely to fail at the basics of adult resuscitation (firm surface, defibrillation, correct ventilation, and compression rate) and succeed at swift delivery of the fetus. Surprisingly, fewer than half the teams implemented left uterine displacement during CPR.

Early Warning and Rapid Response Systems

Women with preexisting disease or comorbidities including mental health issues are at increased risk of maternal death. Indirect

---

BOX 21.4   CHECKLIST (PERSONNEL AND EQUIPMENT) WHEN A RISK OF CARDIAC ARREST IS IDENTIFIED IN A PREGNANT PATIENT

Personnel

☐ Anesthesiologist

☐ Obstetrician   OB team

☐ Labor & delivery nurse

☐ Internist, intensivist, or ED physician: code leader

☐ Additional physician(s)

☐ Nurses: ED or critical care   Arrest team

☐ Respiratory therapist

☐ Recorder

☐ Neonatologist or pediatrician   Pediatric team

☐ Nurse with neonatology expertise

Equipment

☐ Posted algorithms (maternal and neonatal resuscitation)

☐ Airway management supplies

☐ Defibrillator or AED

☐ Crash cart with emergency drugs

☐ Cesarean tray

☐ Infant warmer

☐ Neonatal resuscitation supplies

maternal deaths (conditions aggravated by pregnancy-related physiologic changes) now constitute about two-thirds of all maternal deaths in the UK, with cardiac disease and sepsis being the most prevalent [102]. A review of maternal deaths in the United States identified 63% as being preventable. Common themes are:

- Missed or delayed diagnosis
- Delays in care or ineffective treatment
- Failure to seek specialty consultation
- Inadequate training of personnel/health care providers
- Lack of existing policies to identify or triage pregnant/ postpartum women
- Lack of coordination and/or communication between health care providers [103]

Regardless of underlying condition, all women are at risk of an acute event during pregnancy, birth, and the postpartum period. Analysis of 462 cases of in-hospital maternal cardiac arrest showed that 36% exhibited respiratory insufficiency and 33% signs of hypotension or hypoperfusion prior to the event [7]. The majority of adults who suffer in-hospital cardiac arrest demonstrate one or more abnormal vital signs in the preceding 1–4 hours, which underscores the utility of clinical warning signs [104]. The Royal College of Obstetricians & Gynecologists recommends that a obstetric early warning score be routinely used for all pregnant/postpartum women [69]. The National Partnership for Maternal Safety has made a similar recommendation in the United States [105]. Their proposed maternal early warning criteria include:

- Hypotension (systolic BP <90 mmHg)
- Hypertension (systolic BP >160 mmHg or diastolic BP >100 mmHg)
- Abnormal heart rate (<50/beats per minute or >120 beats per minute)
- Abnormal respiratory rate (<10/min or >30/min)
- Oxygen desaturation (<95% on room air)
- Oliguria
- Altered mental status

To date, maternal early warning systems have not been validated to prevent maternal cardiac arrest or to improve survival.

Rapid response teams or medical emergency teams are meant to respond to the patient's bedside if a patient exhibits clinical deterioration short of cardiac arrest [106]. There are several published reports on "obstetric emergency teams" but most of these seem to focus on obstetric emergencies [107,108]; only 2%–3% of team activations came from maternal cardiac or respiratory instability. The AHA endorses "bundling" of teams [11] by simultaneous activation of maternal (obstetric and acute care medical team) and neonatal resuscitation teams when maternal cardiac arrest is diagnosed.

Conclusion

Maternal cardiac arrest, though fortunately rare, is an emergency that threatens two lives, and therefore both the hospital and prehospital services must be prepared. A few modifications of basic and advanced life support are required to optimize maternal resuscitation such as manual displacement of the uterus, and early resuscitative hysterotomy or perimortem cesarean delivery; however, the sequence of defibrillation and drugs does not differ. Airway management may be challenging. Algorithms and checklists are likely to be helpful. Simulation drills and team-based training are crucial in maintaining knowledge and skills in a low-frequency, high-stakes situation such as maternal cardiac arrest. The role of early warning systems and rapid response teams as a means of preventing maternal cardiac arrest needs further investigation.

REFERENCES

1. Mhyre JM, Tsen LC, Einav S, Kuklina EV, Leffert LR, Bateman BT. Cardiac arrest during hospitalization for delivery in the United States, 1998–2011. *Anesthesiology.* 2014;120(4):810–81.
2. Balki M, Liu S, Leon JA, Baghirzada L. Epidemiology of cardiac arrest during hospitalization for delivery in Canada: A nationwide study. *Anesth Analg.* 2017;124:890–7.
3. Beckett VA, Knight M, Sharpe P. The CAPS Study: Incidence, management and outcomes of cardiac arrest in pregnant women in the UK: A prospective, descriptive study. *BJOG.* 2017;124:1374–81.
4. Topjian AA et al., for the American Heart Association National Registry of Cardiopulmonary Resuscitation Investigators. Women of child-bearing age have better in-hospital cardiac arrest survival outcomes than equal aged men. *Crit Care Med.* 2010;38:1254–60.
5. Mogos MF, Salemia JL, Spooner KK, McFarlin BL, Salihu HM, Differences in mortality between pregnant and non-pregnant women after cardiopulmonary resuscitation. *Obstet Gynecol.* 2016;128:880–8.
6. Lavecchia M, Abenhaim HA. Cardiopulmonary resuscitation of pregnant women in the emergency department. *Resuscitation.* 2015;91:104–7.
7. Zelop CM et al. Characteristics and outcomes of maternal cardiac arrest: A descriptive analysis of Get with the guidelines data. *Resuscitation.* 2018;132:17–20.
8. Lipowicz AA et al., on behalf of the Rescu Investigators. Incidence, outcomes and guideline compliance of out-of-hospital maternal cardiac arrest resuscitations: A population-based cohort study. *Resuscitation.* 2018;132:127–32.
9. Maurin O et al. Maternal out-of-hospital cardiac arrest: A retrospective observational study. *Resuscitation.* 2019;135: 205–11.
10. McNally B et al., Centers for Disease Control and Prevention. Out-of-hospital cardiac arrest surveillance—Cardiac Arrest Registry to Enhance Survival (CARES), United States, October 1, 2005 – December 31, 2010. *Morbid Mortal Weekly Rep.* 2011;60(8):1–25.
11. Jeejeebhoy FM et al., on behalf of the American Heart Association Emergency Cardiovascular Care Committee, Council on Cardiopulmonary, Critical Care, Perioperative and Resuscitation, Council on Cardiovascular Diseases in the Young, and Council on Clinical Cardiology. Cardiac arrest in pregnancy: A scientific statement from the American Heart Association. *Circulation.* 2015;132:1747–73.

12. Zelop CM, Einav S, Mhyre JM, Martin S. Cardiac arrest during pregnancy: Ongoing clinical conundrum. *Am J Obstet Gynecol.* 2018;219(1):52–61.

13. Brooks SC et al. Part 6: Alternative techniques and ancillary devices for cardiopulmonary resuscitation: 2015 American Heart Association guidelines update for cardiopulmonary resuscitation and emergency cardiovascular care. *Circulation.* 2015;132(suppl 2):S436–43

14. Burkle CM, Tessmer-Tuck J, Wijdicks EF. Medical, legal, and ethical challenges associated with pregnancy and catastrophic brain injury. *Int J Gynecol Obstet.* 2015;129:276–80.

15. Kerr MG, Scott DB, Samuel E. Studies of the inferior vena cava in late pregnancy. *Brit Med J.* 1964;1:532–3.

16. Rossi A et al. Quantitative cardiovascular magnetic resonance in pregnant women: Cross-sectional analysis of physiologic parameters throughout pregnancy and the impact of the supine position. *J Cardiovasc Magnetic Resonance.* 2011;13:31.

17. Higuchi H, Takagi S, Zhang K, Furui I, Ozaki M. Effect of lateral tilt angle on the volume of the abdominal aorta and inferior vena cava in pregnant and nonpregnant women determined by magnetic resonance imaging. *Anesthesiology.* 2015;122:286–93.

18. Lee AJ, Landau R. Aortocaval compression syndrome: Time to revisit certain dogmas. *Anesth Analg.* 2017;125:1979–85.

19. Lee SWY, Khaw KS, Ngan Jee WD, Leung TY, Critchley LAH. Haemodynamic effects from aortocaval compression at different angles of lateral tilt in non-labouring term pregnant women. *Br J Anaesth.* 2012;109:950–6.

20. McNamara H, Barclay P, Sharma V. Accuracy and precision of the ultrasound cardiac output monitor (USCOM 1A) in pregnancy: Comparison with three-dimensional transthoracic echocardiography. *Br J Anaesth.* 2014;113:669–76.

21. Mangos JG, Pettit F, Preece R, Harris K, Brown MA. Repeatability of USCOM®-measured cardiac output in normotensive nonpregnant and pregnant women. *Pregnancy Hypertens.* 2018;12:71–4.

22. Rees GA, Willis BA. Resuscitation in late pregnancy. *Anaesthesia.* 1988;43:347–9.

23. Butcher M, Ip J, Bushby D, Yentis SM. Efficacy of cardiopulmonary resuscitation with manual displacement of the uterus vs lateral tilt using a firm wedge: A manikin study. *Anaesthetsia.* 2014;69:868–71.

24. Goodwin AP, Pearce AJ. The human wedge. A manoeuvre to relive aortocaval compression during resuscitation in late pregnancy. *Anaesthesia.* 1992;47:433–4.

25. Lavonas EJ et al. Part 10: Special circumstances of resuscitation. 2015 American Heart Association guidelines update for cardiopulmonary resuscitation and emergency cardiovascular care. *Circulation.* 2015;132(suppl 2):S501–18.

26. Truhlaf A et al., on behalf of the cardiac arrest in special circumstances collaborators. European Resuscitation Council Guidelines for Resuscitation 2015. Section 4. Cardiac arrest in special circumstances. *Resuscitation.* 2015;95:148–201.

27. Soar J et al.; Advanced Life Support Chapter Collaborators. Part 4: Advanced life support. 2015 International Consensus on cardiopulmonary resuscitation and emergency cardiovascular care science with treatment recommendations. *Resuscitation.* 2015;95:e71–20.

28. Burton GJ, Fowden AL. The placenta: A multifaceted, transient organ. *Phil Trans R Soc B.* 2015;370(1663):20140066.

29. Nye GA et al. Human placental oxygenation in late gestation: Experimental and theoretical approaches. *J Physiol.* 2018;596:5523–34.

30. Bennet L. Sex, drugs and rock and roll: Tales from preterm fetal life. *J Physiol.* 2017;195:1865–81.

31. Berg RA et al. Part 5: Adult basic life support: American Heart Association guidelines for cardiopulmonary resuscitation and emergency cardiovascular care. *Circulation.* 2010;122(suppl 3):S685–705.

32. Kleinman ME et al. Part 5: Adult basic life support and cardiopulmonary resuscitation quality: 2015 American Heart Association guidelines update for cardiopulmonary resuscitation and emergency cardiovascular care. *Circulation.* 2015;132(suppl 2):S414–35.

33. Nolan JP et al. Post-cardiac arrest syndrome: Epidemiology, pathophysiology, treatment, and prognostication. A scientific statement from the International Liaison Committee on Resuscitation; the American Heart Association emergency cardiovascular care committee; the council on cardiovascular surgery and anesthesia; the Council on Cardiopulmonary, Perioperative, and Critical Care; the Council on Clinical Cardiology; the Council on Stroke. *Resuscitation.* 2008;79:350–79.

34. Field JM et al. Part 1: Executive summary: 2010 American Heart Association guidelines for cardiopulmonary resuscitation and emergency cardiovascular care. *Circulation.* 2010;122(suppl 3):S640–56.

35. Lipman S et al. The Society for Obstetric Anesthesia and Perinatology consensus statement on the management of cardiac arrest in pregnancy. *Anesth Analg.* 2014;118:1003–16.

36. Jeejeebhoy FM et al. Management of cardiac arrest in pregnancy: A systematic review. *Resuscitation.* 2011;82:801–9.

37. Katz V, Balderston K, DeFreeze M. Perimortem cesarean delivery: Were our assumptions correct? *Am J Obstet Gynecol.* 2005;192:1916–20.

38. Dijman A et al. Cardiac arrest in pregnancy: Increasing use of perimortem caesarean section due to emergency skills training? *BJOG.* 2010;117:282–7.

39. Nanson J, Elcock D, Williams M, Deakin CD. Do physiological changes in pregnancy change defibrillation energy requirements? *Br J Anaesth.* 2001;87:237–9.

40. Kupas DF, Harter SC, Vosk A. Out-of-hospital perimortem cesarean section. *Prehosp Emerg Care.* 1998;2(3):206–8.

41. Bloomer R, Reid C, Wheatley R. Prehospital resuscitative hysterotomy. *Eur J Emerg Med.* 2011;18:241–2.

42. Bowers W, Wagner C. Field perimortem cesarean section. *Air Medical J.* 2001;20(4):10–1.

43. Gatti F et al. Out-of-hospital perimortem cesarean section as resuscitative hysterotomy in maternal posttraumatic cardiac arrest. *Case Rep Emergency Med.* 2014;2014:121562.

44. Lenz H, Stenseth LB, Meidell N, Heimdal HJ. Out-of-hospital perimortem cesarean delivery performed in a woman at 32 weeks of gestation: A case report. *A A Case Rep.* 2017;8:72–4.

45. Tommila M, Pystynen M, Soukka H, Aydin F, Rantanen M. Two cases of low birthweight infant survival by prehospital emergency hysterotomy. *Scan J Trauma Resusc Emerg Med.* 2017;25:62.

46. Grasner JT et al., on behalf of EuReCa ONE Collaborators. EuReCa ONE—27 Nations, ONE Europe, ONE Registry. A prospective one month analysis of out-of-hospital cardiac arrest outcomes in 27 countries in Europe. *Ressuscitation.* 2016;105:188–95.

47. Girotra S et al., and collaboration with CARES Surveillance Group and the HeartRescue Project. Regional variation in out-of-hospital cardiac arrest survival in the United States. *Circulation.* 2016;133(2):2159–68.

48. Herlitz J et al. Characteristics and outcome amongst young adults suffering from out-of-hospital cardiac arrest in whom cardiopulmonary resuscitation is attempted. *J Intern Med.* 2006;260:435–41.

49. Perkins GD et al., on behalf of the Adult basic life support and automated external defibrillation section Collaborators. European Resuscitation Guidelines for Resuscitation 2015. Section 2. Adult basic life support and automated external defibrillation. *Resuscitation.* 2015;95:81–99.

50. Perkins GD et al., on behalf of the Basic Life Support Chapter Collaborators. Part 3: Adult basic life support and automated external defibrillation. 2015 International Consensus on cardiopulmonary resuscitation and emergency cardiovascular care science with treatment recommendations. *Resuscitation.* 2015;95:e3–e69.

51. Vanden Hoek TL et al. Part 12: Cardiac arrest in special situations: 2010 American Heart Association guidelines for cardiopulmonary resuscitation and emergency cardiovascular care. *Circulation.* 2010;122:S829–61.

52. Holmes S, Kirkpatrick IDC, Zelop CM, Jassal DS. MRI evaluation of maternal cardiac displacement in pregnancy: Implications for cardiopulmonary resuscitation. *Am J Obstet Gynecol.* 2015;213:401.e1–5.

53. McClelland SH, Bogod DG, Hardman JG. Apnoea in pregnancy: An investigation using physiological modeling. *Anaesthesia.* 2008;63:264–9.

54. Link MS et al. Part 7: Adult advanced cardiovascular life support: 2015 American Heart Association guidelines update for cardiopulmonary resuscitation and emergency cardiovascular care. *Circulation.* 2015;132(suppl 2):S444–64.

55. Hengen M et al. Transnasal humidified rapid-insufflation ventilator exchange for preoxygenation before cesarean delivery under general anesthesia: A case report. *A A Case Rep.* 2017;9:216–8.

56. Pillai A, Chikhani M, Hardman JG. Apnoeic oxygenation in pregnancy: A modeling investigation. *Anaesthesia.* 2016;71:1077–80.

57. Brown O, Davidson N, Palmer J. Cardioversion in the third trimester of pregnancy. *Aust NZ J Obstet Gynaecol.* 2001;41:241–2.

58. Kronick SL et al. Part 4: Systems of care and continuous quality improvement. 2015 American Heart Association guidelines update for cardiopulmonary resuscitation and emergency cardiovascular care. *Circulation.* 2015;132(suppl 2):S397–415.

59. Soar J et al., on behalf of the Adult advanced life support Collaborators, European Resuscitation Council Guidelines for Resuscitation 2015. Section 3. Adult advanced life support. *Resuscitation.* 2015;95:100–47.

60. Bartalena L, Bogazzi F, Braverman LE, Martino E. Effects of amiodarone administration on neonatal thyroid function and subsequent neurodevelopment. *J Endocrin Invest.* 2001;24:116–30.

61. Mitani GM, Steinberg E, Lien EJ, Harrison EC, Elkayam U. The pharmacokinetics of antiarrhythmic agents in pregnancy and lactation. *Clin Pharmacokinet.* 1987;12:253–91.

62. Williamson RM, Haines J. Availability of lipid emulsion in obstetric anaesthesia in the UK: A national questionnaire survey. *Anaesthesia.* 2008;63:385–8.

63. Toledo P et al. Availability of lipid emulsion in United States obstetric units. *Anesth Analg.* 2013;116:406–8.

64. Association of Anaesthetists of Great Britain & Ireland. London, 2010. AAGBI Safety Guideline. Management of severe local anaesthetic toxicity. https://www.aagbi.org/sites/default/files/la_toxicity_2010_0.pdf. Accessed 1/25/19.

65. American Society of Regional Anesthesia and Pain Medicine (ASRA). Pittsburgh, PA, 2011 Checklist for treatment of local anesthetic systemic toxicity. https://www.asra.com/content/documents/asra_last_checklist.2011.pdf. Accessed 1/25/19.

66. Kinney MA et al. Emergency bedside cesarean delivery: Lessons learned in teamwork and patient safety. *BMC Res Notes.* 2012 Aug 6;5:412.

67. Marr R, Myams J, Bythell V. Cardiac arrest in an obstetric patient using remifentanil patient-controlled analgesia. *Anaesthesia.* 2013;68:283–7.

68. Katz VL, Dotters DJ, Droegemueller W. Perimortem cesarean delivery. *Obstet Gynecol.* 1986;68:571–6.

69. Royal College of Obstetricians and Gynaecologists. *Maternal Collapse in Pregnancy and the Puerperium.* Green-top Guideline no. 56. RCOG; London UK; January 2011. https://www.rcog.org.uk/globalassets/documents/guidelines/gtg_56.pdf. Accessed 1/4/19

70. Benson MD, Padovano A, Bourjeily G, Zhou Y. Maternal collapse: Challenging the four-minute rule. *EBioMedicine.* 2016;6:253–7.

71. Einav S, Kaufman N, Sela HY. Maternal cardiac arrest and perimortem caesarean delivery: Evidence or expert-based? *Resuscitation.* 2012;83:1191–200.

72. Kamei H et al. Resuscitative hysterotomy in a patient with peripartum cardiomyopathy. *J Obstet Gynaecol Res.* 2018;45(3):724–8.

73. Rose CH et al. Challenging the 4- to 5-minute rule: From perimortem cesarean to resuscitative hysterotomy. *Am J Obstet Gynecol.* 2015;213:653–6.

74. Battaloglu E, Porter K. Management of pregnancy and obstetric complications in pre-hospital trauma care: Pre-hospital resuscitative hysterotomy/perimortem caesarean section. *Emerg Med J.* 2017;34:326–30.

75. Kazandi M et al. Post-mortem Caesarean section performed 30 minutes after maternal cardiopulmonary arrest. *Aust NZ J Obstet Gynaecol.* 2004;44:351–3.

76. Capobianco G et al. Perimortem cesarean delivery 30 minutes after a laboring patient jumped from a fourth-floor window: Baby survives and is normal at age 4 years. *Am J Obstet Gynecol.* 2008;198:e15–6.

77. Wu SH, Li RS, Hwu YM. Live birth after perimortem cesarean delivery in a 36-year-old out-of-hospital cardiac arrest nulliparous woman. *Taiwan J Obstet Gynecol.* 2019;58:43–5.

78. Drukker L et al. Perimortem cesarean section for maternal and fetal salvage: Concise review and protocol. *Acta Obstet Gynecol Scand.* 2014;93:965–72.

79. Healy M et al. Care of the critically ill pregnant patient and perimortem cesarean delivery in the emergency department. *J Emerg Med.* 2016;51:172–7.

80. Richardson AC, Schmidt M, Bailey M, Pellegrino VA, Rycus PT, Pilcher DV. ECMO cardiopulmonary resuscitation

(ECPR), trends in survival from an international multicentre cohort study over 12 years. *Resuscitation.* 2017;112:34–40.

81. Takacs ME, Damisch KE. Extracorporeal life support as salvage therapy for massive pulmonary embolus and cardiac arrest in pregnancy. *J Emerg Med.* 2018;55:121–4.

82. Leeper WR, Valdis M, Arntfield R, Guo LR. Extracorporeal membrane oxygenation in the acute treatment of cardiovascular collapse immediately post-partum. *Interact Cardiovasc Thorac Surg.* 2013;17:898–9.

83. Fernandes P, Allen P, Valdis M, Guo L. Successful use of extracorporeal membrane oxygenation for pulmonary embolism, prolonged cardiac arrest, post-partum: A cannulation dilemma. *Perfusion.* 2015;30:106–10.

84. McDonald C, Laurie J, Janssens S, Zazulak C, Kotze P, Shekar K. Successful provision of inter-hospital extracorporeal cardiopulmonary resuscitation for acute post-partum pulmonary embolism. *Int J Obstet Anesth.* 2017;30:65–8.

85. Callaway CW et al. Part 8: Post-cardiac arrest care: 2015 American Heart Association Guidelines update for cardiopulmonary resuscitation and emergency cardiovascular care. *Circulation.* 2015;132(suppl 2):S465–82.

86. Banerjea MC, Speer CP. Bilateral thalamic lesions in a newborn with intrauterine asphyxia after maternal cardiac arrest—A case report with literature review. *J Perinatol.* 2001;21:405–9.

87. Rittenberger JC, Kelly E, Jang D, Greer K, Heffner A. Successful outcome utilizing hypothermia after cardiac arrest in pregnancy: A case report. *Crit Care Med.* 2008;36(4):1354–6.

88. Wible EF, Kass JS, Lopez GA. A report of fetal demise during therapeutic hypothermia after cardiac arrest. *Neurocrit Care.* 2010;13(2):239–42.

89. Chauhan A et al. The use of therapeutic hypothermia after cardiac arrest in a pregnant patient. *Ann Emerg Med.* 2012;60:786–9.

90. Oguayo KN, Oyetayo OO, Stewart D, Costa SM, Jones RO. Successful use of therapeutic hypothermia in a pregnant patient. *Tex Hear Inst J.* 2015;42(4):367–71.

91. De Santis V, Negri M. Successful use of targeted temperature management in pregnancy after out-of-hospital cardiac arrest. *Am J Emergency Med.* 2016;34:122.e3–e4.

92. Oami T, Oshima T, Oku R, Nakanishi K. Successful treatment of pulmonary embolism-induced cardiac arrest by thrombolysis and targeted temperature management during pregnancy. *Acute Med Surg.* 2018;25(5):292–5.

93. Nelissen ECM, de Zwaan C, Marcus MAE, Nijhuis JG. Maternal cardiac arrest in early pregnancy. *Int J Obstet Anesth.* 2009;18:60–3.

94. Schuler PK et al. Pregnancy outcome and management of women with an implantable cardioverter defibrillator: A single centre experience. *Europace.* 2012;14:1740–5.

95. Miyoshi T et al. Safety and efficacy of implantable cardioverter-defibrillator during pregnancy and after delivery. *Circulation J.* 2013;77:1166–70.

96. Salman MM, Kemp HI, Cauldwell MR, Dob DP, Sutton R. Anesthetic management of pregnant patients with cardiac implantable electronic devices: Case reports and review. *Int J Obstet Anesthesia.* 2018;33:57–66.

97. Doyle NM, Monga M, Montgomery B, Dougherty AH. Arrhythmogenic right ventricular cardiomyopathy with implantable cardioverter defibrillator placement in pregnancy. *J Matern Fet Neonat Med.* 2005;18:141–4.

98. American College of Obstetricians and Gynecologists (ACOG) Committee on Obstetric Practice. No. 723. *Guidelines for Diagnostic Imaging during Pregnancy and Lactation.* ACOG; Washington, DC; October 2017.

99. Haydon G, van der Riet P, Maguire J. Survivors' quality of life after cardiopulmonary resuscitation: An integrative review of the literature. *Scand J Caring Sci.* 2017;31:6–26.

100. Chan PS et al., for the Get with the Guidelines – Resuscitation Registry Investigators. A validated prediction tool for initial survivors of in-hospital cardiac arrest. *Arch Intern Med.* 2012;172(12):947–53.

101. Lipman SS et al. Deficits in the provision of cardiopulmonary resuscitation during simulated obstetric crises. *Obstet Gynecol.* 2010;203:179.e1–5.

102. Nair M, Nelson-Piercy C, Knight M. Indirect maternal deaths: UK and global perspectives. *Obstet Medicine.* 2017;10(1):10–5.

103. Building U.S. Capacity to Review and Prevent Maternal Deaths. *Report from nine maternal mortality review committees,* 2018. http://reviewtoaction.org/Report_from_Nine_MMRCs. Accessed 1/1/19

104. Andersen LW et al., for the American Heart Association's Get With The Guidelines Resuscitation Investigators. *Resuscitation.* 2016;98:112–7.

105. Mhyre JM et al. The maternal early warning criteria: A proposal from the National Partnership for Maternal Safety. *Obstet Gynecol.* 2014;124:782–6.

106. Lyons PG, Edelson DP, Churpek MM. Rapid response systems. *Resuscitation.* 2018;128:191–7.

107. Gosman GG et al. Introduction of an obstetric-specific medical emergency team for obstetric crises: Implementation and experience. *Am J Obstet Gynecol.* 2008;198:367.e1–e7.

108. Richardson MG, Domaradzki KA, McWeeney DT. Implementing an obstetric emergency team response system: Overcoming barriers and sustaining response dose. *Joint Comm J Quality Pat Safety.* 2015;41:514–21.

109. Talbot L, Maclennan K. Physiology of pregnancy. *Anaesthesia Intens Care Med.* 2016;17:341–5.

110. Ewy GA. The mechanism of blood flow during chest compressions for cardiac arrest is probably influenced by the patient's chest configuration. *Acute Med Surg.* 2018;5:236–40.

111. Farinelli CK, Hameed AB. Cardiopulmonary resuscitation in pregnancy. *Cardiol Clin.* 2012;30:453–61.

112. Marx GF, Murthy PK, Orkin LR. Static compliance before and after vaginal delivery. *Br J Anaesth.* 1970;42:1100–4.

113. Kikuchi J, Deering S. Cardiac arrest in pregnancy. *Semin Perinatol.* 2018;42:33–8.

Index

Note: Page number followed by b, f, and t indicates box, figure and table respectively.